# POWER EATING

## FOURTH EDITION

**Susan M. Kleiner, PhD, RD**

High Performance Nutrition, LLC
Mercer Island, Washington

*with*

**Maggie Greenwood-Robinson, PhD**

Human Kinetics

Library of Congress Cataloging-in-Publication Data

Kleiner, Susan M.
  Power eating / Susan M. Kleiner, PhD, RD, High Performance Nutrition, LLC, Mercer Island, Washington, with Maggie Greenwood-Robinson, PhD. -- Fourth edition.
    pages cm
  Includes bibliographical references and index.
  ISBN-10: 1-4504-3017-1
  ISBN-13: 978-1-4504-3017-3
  1. Athletes--Nutrition. 2. Bodybuilders--Nutrition. I. Greenwood-Robinson, Maggie. II. Title.
  TX361.A8K595 2013
  613.7--dc23
                              2013006261
ISBN-10: 1-4504-3017-1 (print)
ISBN-13: 978-1-4504-3017-3 (print)

This publication is written and published to provide accurate and authoritative information relevant to the subject matter presented. It is published and sold with the understanding that the author and publisher are not engaged in rendering legal, medical, or other professional services by reason of their authorship or publication of this work. If medical or other expert assistance is required, the services of a competent professional person should be sought.

The web addresses cited in this text were current as of April 2013, unless otherwise noted.

**Acquisitions Editor:** Justin Klug; **Developmental Editor:** Anne Hall; **Assistant Editor:** Tyler Wolpert; **Copy-editor:** Patsy Fortney; **Indexer:** Alisha Jeddeloh; **Permissions Manager:** Martha Gullo; **Graphic Designer:** Nancy Rasmus; **Graphic Artist:** Kim McFarland; **Cover Designer:** Keith Blomberg; **Photograph (cover):** © Human Kinetics; **Photographs (interior):** © Human Kinetics unless otherwise noted. Photo on page 74 © Denis Anikin/fotilia.com. Photo on page 169 © sylvaine thomas/fotilia.com. Photo on page 238 © Monteleone/fotolia.com; **Visual Production Assistant:** Joyce Brumfield; **Photo Production Manager:** Jason Allen; **Printer:** Sheridan Books

Human Kinetics books are available at special discounts for bulk purchase. Special editions or book excerpts can also be created to specification. For details, contact the Special Sales Manager at Human Kinetics.

Printed in the United States of America      10 9 8 7 6 5

The paper in this book is certified under a sustainable forestry program.

**Human Kinetics**
Website: www.HumanKinetics.com

*United States:* Human Kinetics
P.O. Box 5076
Champaign, IL 61825-5076
800-747-4457
e-mail: info@hkusa.com

*Canada:* Human Kinetics
475 Devonshire Road, Unit 100
Windsor, ON N8Y 2L5
800-465-7301 (in Canada only)
e-mail: info@hkcanada.com

*Europe:* Human Kinetics
107 Bradford Road
Stanningley
Leeds LS28 6AT, United Kingdom
+44 (0)113 255 5665
e-mail: hk@hkeurope.com

For information about Human Kinetics' coverage in other areas of the world, please visit our website: www.HumanKinetics.com

*In loving memory of Mom and Dad, who showed me
how to gracefully embrace strength and power*

# Contents

Preface   vii

Acknowledgments   ix

## PART I   Foundation

**1**   Eating for Power                                    3

**2**   Manufacturing Muscle                                19

**3**   Fueling Workouts                                    47

**4**   Managing Fat                                        73

**5**   Burning Fat                                         87

**6**   Hydrating
for Heavy-Duty Workouts                                     109

## PART II   Supplements

**7**   Vitamins and Minerals
for Strength Trainers                                       129

**8**   Muscle-Building Products                            163

**9**   Botanicals for Performance                          199

# PART III Plans and Menus

**10** Developing
a Power Eating Plan     219

**11** Planning a Peak     233

**12** Maintaining
Physique Menu Plans     245

**13** Building Muscle Menu Plans     255

**14** Cross-Training Menu Plans     265

**15** Fat-Loss Menu Plans     279

**16** Getting Cut Menu Plans     289

**17** Power Eating Recipes     299

Appendix A   Three-Day Food Record   329
Appendix B   Restaurant Guide and Healthy Fast Food   333
Works Consulted   337
Index   355
About the Authors   363

# Preface

I am so excited to bring you the fourth edition of *Power Eating*. The fields of sport nutrition and exercise physiology are booming as the discovery of the human genome has resulted in an explosion of technology that has deepened our understanding of how the body works. For this edition I have cast a wide net to explain how the chemical properties of food, botanicals, and supplements turn genes on and off to affect our ability to gain muscle, burn fat, and enhance training. I also discuss how you can harness the power of the brain to drive metabolic processes through food, taste, mood, training, environment, and relationships.

As always, input from readers has been invaluable. You asked, and I have answered with a new chapter of menus for cross-trainers. All of the chapters and menus have been updated to stay on the cutting edge of the science for competitive athletes as well as novice and more casual trainers.

*Power Eating* has held its place at the top of the bookshelf because I give you not only the latest published research, but a play-by-play of the research being conducted in laboratories around the world, just as I'm writing the book. Then, I tell you how to put it all together to reach your goals. This edition offers a true insider's view of the latest news on muscle-building supplements and state-of-the-science diet and supplement strategies for gaining energy, getting cut, enhancing mood, and tightening mental focus.

*Power Eating* is the leader in guiding you through all your training periods throughout the year. The Power Eating menus are unsurpassed in their level of detail yet practical to customize and follow in your busy life. Whether you are trying to maintain, build, taper, or cut, the Power Eating diet plans will get your body where you want it to be when you want it to be there, and keep you healthy, safe, and legal. You *can* have it all! Train hard and POWER EAT!

# Acknowledgments

It is humbling that my readers have looked to *Power Eating* as their trusted resource for 16 years, since we published the first edition in 1998. You have inspired me through your stories in person and online, through emails and hand-written notes, encouraging me to write a fresh, fourth edition that once again breaks new ground in the pursuit of strength and power. Thank you once again to my teammate in creating this legacy, Maggie Greenwood-Robinson. You are an all-star writer whose chops only keep getting better. Writing books is like an endurance relay, and your smooth hand-offs make it look easy all the way to the finish line! To Amanda McQuade Crawford, medicine hunter and herbalist extraordinaire, thank you for sharing your elite expertise on botanicals. Thank you to my dear friend, Shar Sault, two-time consecutive winner of the drug-tested World Figure Title of Ms. Natural Olympia, for sharing some of your fast, delicious and nutritious recipes in this fourth edition of *Power Eating*. To our acquisitions editor, Justin Klug, thank you for taking me seriously when I proposed a new edition and for shepherding it through the publication process with understanding and zeal. The entire team at Human Kinetics is fantastic. I always know that the intensive editorial process will produce a final product that is extraordinary. To Anne Hall, Martha Gullo, Tyler Wolpert, Kim McFarland, Sue Outlaw, and others, thank you for your unwavering support of my vision for *Power Eating* and your dedication to excellence. To my entire family, from the bottom of my heart thank you for your support and love. This has been a journey we have all taken together.

# Foundation

Since the publication of the third edition of *Power Eating* several years ago, huge strides have been made in the science of nutrition for strength training, particularly in the "neurobiology" of food. What I mean by that is how food influences the way your brain controls your body and appetite, and how a positive relationship with food helps you focus on building your body up rather than tearing it down. Addressing the neurobiology of food is now a key strategy for championship performance, recovery, and growth. When you put the latest nutritional science into practical application, your body will function at peak levels; your detoxification and cleansing mechanisms will operate optimally; and fat burning, energy metabolism, and muscle growth will move forward at a rapid pace. This is an exciting time in sport nutrition, because we now understand the nutritional needs of muscle, right down to the molecular and genetic level—and with that knowledge athletes like you can perform at higher levels than ever before. Chapters 1 through 6 explore this cutting-edge information and guide you on how to put it to use.

# 1

# Eating for Power

Think about how you'd like to look and feel. Imagine yourself with a body that's fit and firm with just the right amount of muscle. Imagine the joy of high strength and energy that give you the power to perform, day in and day out.

Keep those images in your mind's eye. This book will show you how to achieve them with a few nips and tucks in one of the most important fitness factors of all—nutrition. But we're not talking about just any type of nutrition. This is a book for people who strength train to stay in shape, compete in strength-training sports, or want to improve their athletic ability. In other words, you're a strength trainer if you lift weights a few times a week or train for competition. As a strength trainer, you have specific nutritional needs that depend on your type and level of activity.

So, what kind of strength trainer are you? Are you a bodybuilder, a powerlifter, an Olympic weightlifter, an athlete who strength trains for conditioning and cross-training, or someone who works out with weights to stay in shape? These activities have different physical demands and different nutritional requirements, which is why you will find several individualized strength-training diets in chapters 12 through 16. But the common denominator is that all strength trainers, from competitors to recreational exercisers, are interested in the same thing: building lean muscle.

## What Builds Muscle?

Most certainly, strength training builds muscle. But for this construction to take place, you have to supply the construction material: protein, carbohydrate, and fat. In a process called metabolism, the body breaks down these nutrients and uses the products to generate the energy required for growth and life.

During metabolism, proteins are broken down into amino acids. Cells use amino acids to make new proteins based on instructions supplied by DNA, our genetic management system. The DNA provides information on how amino acids are to be lined up and strung together. Once these instructions have been carried out, the cell has synthesized a new protein.

On the basis of this process, logic would tell you that the more protein you eat, the more muscle your body can construct. But it doesn't work that way. Excess protein is converted to carbohydrate to be used for energy or converted to fat for storage.

The way to make muscles grow is not by gorging on protein but by demanding more from it—that is, by making protein work harder. The muscles will respond by taking up the nutrients they need, including amino acids from protein metabolism, so they can grow. If you work your muscles hard and give them comprehensive nutritional support, your muscle cells will synthesize the protein the muscles need.

# What Fuels Muscle?

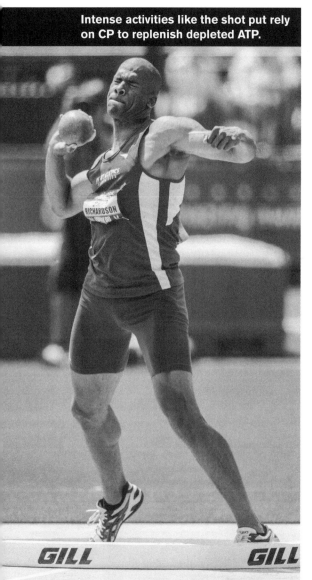

Intense activities like the shot put rely on CP to replenish depleted ATP.

To work your muscles hard, you have to provide the right kind of fuel. Muscle cells, like all cells, run on a high-energy compound known as adenosine triphosphate (ATP). ATP makes muscles contract, conducts nerve impulses, and promotes other cellular energy processes. Muscle cells make ATP by combining oxygen with nutrients from food, mainly carbohydrate. Fat is also used for fuel by muscles, but fat can be broken down only when oxygen is present. Muscle cells prefer to burn carbohydrate, store fat, and use protein for growth and repair.

Your cells generate ATP through any one of three energy systems: the phosphagen system, the glycolytic system, and the oxidative system.

## The Phosphagen System

The phosphagen system rebuilds ATP by supplying a compound called creatine phosphate (CP). Once ATP is used up, it must be replenished from additional food and oxygen. During short, intense bursts of exercise such as weight training and sprinting, the working muscles exhaust the available oxygen. At that point, CP kicks in to supply energy for a few short seconds of work.

CP can help create ATP when ATP is depleted. Any intense exercise lasting for 3 to 15 seconds rapidly depletes ATP and CP in a muscle; these compounds must then be replaced. Replenishing ATP and CP is the job of the other energy systems in the body.

## The Glycolytic System

The glycolytic system makes glucose available to the muscles, either from the breakdown of dietary carbohydrate during digestion or from the breakdown of muscle and liver glycogen, the stored form of carbohydrate. In a process called glycolysis, glycogen is disassembled into glucose in the muscles and, through a series of chemical reactions, ultimately converted into more ATP.

The glycogen reserve in your muscles can supply enough energy for about two to three minutes of short-burst exercise at a time. If sufficient oxygen is available, a lot of ATP will be made from glucose. If oxygen is absent or in short supply, the muscles produce a waste product from glucose called lactic acid. A buildup of lactic acid in a working muscle creates a burning sensation and is part of what causes the muscle to fatigue and stop contracting. Lactic acid exits the muscle when oxygen is available to replenish CP and ATP. A brief rest period gives the body time to deliver oxygen to the muscles, and you can continue exercising.

## The Oxidative System

The third energy system is the oxidative system. This system helps fuel aerobic exercise and other endurance activities. Although the oxidative system can handle the energy needs of endurance exercise, all three energy systems kick in to some degree during endurance exercise. The phosphagen and glycolytic energy systems dominate during strength training.

Oxygen is not a direct source of energy for exercise; it is used as an ingredient to produce large amounts of ATP from other energy sources. The oxidative system works as follows: You breathe in oxygen, which the blood subsequently takes from your lungs. Your heart pumps oxygen-rich blood to tissues, including muscle. Hemoglobin, an iron-containing protein of the blood, carries oxygen to the cells to enable them to produce energy. Myoglobin, another type of iron-containing protein, carries oxygen primarily to muscle cells. Inside muscle cells, carbohydrate and fat are converted into energy through a series of energy-producing reactions.

Your body's ability to produce energy through any one of these three systems can be improved with the right training diet and exercise program. The result is a fat-burning, muscle-building metabolism.

# Nutrition Principles for Strength Trainers

If you are serious about improving your physique and your strength-training performance, you'll do everything you can to achieve success. Unfortunately, advice given to strength trainers today is a hodgepodge of fact and fiction. What I'd like to do is separate one from the other by sharing several principles with you—principles that all strength trainers can follow to get in shape and achieve their personal best in performance. These principles are the same ones I have advocated for world-class athletes, Olympic contenders, and recreational strength trainers for more than 25 years. Let's review them here.

## Eat Enough Calories

A key to feeling energized is to eat the right amount of calories to power your body for hard training. In the United States, the terms *calorie* and *energy* are often used interchangeably. Elsewhere, the joule is used as a measurement of energy. Although this book refers to calories, you can convert to kilojoules by multiplying the number of calories by 4.1868. A lack of calories will definitely make you feel like a wet dishrag by the end of your workout. A diet that provides fewer than 1,600 calories per day, for example, generally does not contain all the vitamins and minerals you need to stay healthy, prevent disease, and perform well. Very low-calorie diets followed for longer than two weeks can be hazardous to your health, and they do not provide the dietary reference intakes (DRIs) of enough of the nutrients needed for basic health.

Historically, the recommended dietary allowances (RDAs) were the national standard for the amount of carbohydrate, protein, fat, vitamins, and minerals we need in our diets to avoid deficiency diseases and to maintain growth and health. The DRIs were established to update the RDAs based on more functional criteria rather than criteria based on deficiency diseases. Rather than focusing on avoiding disease, the DRIs focus on optimal performance both mentally and physically. But under certain conditions—stress, illness, malnutrition, and exercise—we may require a higher intake of certain nutrients. Studies have shown that athletes, in particular, may have to exceed the DRI of many nutrients. Some competitive bodybuilders have estimated their caloric intake to be greater than 6,000 calories a day during the off-season—roughly three times the DRI for the average person (2,000 calories a day for women and 2,700 calories a day for men).

How much you need of each nutrient depends on a number of factors, including your age and sex, how hard you train, and whether you are a competitive or recreational strength trainer. Generally, we find that strength trainers need to eat more protein, more of the right kinds of carbohydrate, and more of the right kinds of fat. What's more, they may be wise to supplement their diet with antioxidants and certain minerals. You'll learn more about these considerations as you read this book. If you are trying to gain muscle and lose body fat, eating enough calories and taking in enough nutrients will make the difference between success and failure.

## Eat the Carbohydrate You Need

It's well known that most athletes, strength trainers included, don't eat enough carbohydrate, the primary fuel for the body. Most athletes follow diets in which less than half of the total daily calories come from carbohydrate, but 5 to 7 grams of carbohydrate per kilogram of body weight should be consumed daily. That's more than half of an athlete's total calories, which is extremely important for a heavyweight competitive bodybuilder or Olympic weight lifter. Lots of bodybuilders practice very low-carbohydrate dieting because they believe it promotes faster weight loss. The problem with these diets is that they deplete glycogen, the body's storage form of carbohydrate. Once glycogen stores are emptied, the body starts burning protein from tissues, including muscle tissue, to meet its energy demands. You lose hard-earned muscle as a result.

Many fitness-minded people shy away from foods high in carbohydrate. They think these foods will make them fat—a myth that is partially responsible for the unbalanced proportion of carbohydrate, fat, and protein in strength-training diets, which are typically too high in protein.

The real story on carbohydrate for weight control and muscle building is that you should select whole-food carbohydrate—natural, complex carbohydrate as close to its natural state as possible—instead of refined, processed carbohydrate. What's the difference? A blueberry is a whole-food carbohydrate; a blueberry toaster muffin is a processed carbohydrate.

One important reason whole foods are better than processed foods has to do with their high fiber content. Fiber is the remnant of plant foods that remains undigested by the body. It's what keeps your bowel movements regular. Fiber is also a proven fat fighter. Research shows that people who eat healthy high-fiber diets have smaller waistlines, for example, and are able to better control their weight. The bottom line is that the right types of carbohydrate can help you manage your weight. The only types of carbohydrate you should shy away from are sugars and highly processed foods. Even so, when used in a targeted way, sugars can be an athlete's best friend by providing the right fuel at the right time. But without a plan, they can be fattening.

You will learn more about carbohydrate in chapter 3, especially how to select the right types of carbohydrate in the right amounts at the right times so that you take in enough to fuel your muscles without gaining fat.

## Sport Nutrition Fact Versus Fiction: Is Carbohydrate Fattening?

Much misinformation exists about whether carbohydrate is fattening. Here's the real deal: Eating too much food is fattening. Further, eating sugary foods and highly processed foods, plus consuming carbohydrate alone (without protein and fat) is what triggers fat gain. By contrast, the right kinds of carbohydrate, meaning natural, unprocessed carbohydrate, will help you build muscle and get lean. What's more, these foods are low in calories, and the healthiest diet for weight loss, disease prevention, and physical performance is one that combines carbohydrate, protein, and fat. So the problem does not lie in high-carbohydrate foods; the problem is poor selection of carbohydrate, in particular, and food, in general.

## Vary Your Diet

You have probably admired the physiques of bodybuilders in magazines, and for good reason. They are muscular, well defined, and in near-perfect proportion—they look like the picture of health. But in many cases, bodybuilders follow incredibly unhealthy diets. The first study I ever conducted investigated the training diets of male competitive bodybuilders. What I found was that they ate a lot of calories, roughly 6,000 a day or more. The worrisome finding from this study was that they ate, on average, more than 200 grams of fat a day. That's almost as much fat as you'd find in two sticks of butter! In the short term, that's enough to make most people sick. Eaten habitually over time, such an enormous amount of unhealthy fat may lead to heart disease.

Bodybuilding diets, especially precontest diets, tend to be monotonous, with the same foods showing up on the plate day after day. The worst example I've ever seen was a bodybuilder who ate chicken, pepper, vinegar, and rice for three days straight while preparing for competition. The problem with such a diet is that it lacks variety, and without a variety of foods, you miss out on nutrients essential for peak health. By contest day you certainly are not the picture of health, either.

Most bodybuilders don't eat much fruit, dairy products, and red meat. Fruit, of course, is packed with disease-fighting, health-building antioxidants and phytochemicals. Dairy products supply important nutrients such as bone-building calcium and bioactive proteins that promote lean muscle growth. And red meat is an important source of vital minerals such as iron and zinc.

When people limit or eliminate such foods from their diet, potentially serious deficiencies begin to show up. In studies conducted by myself and others, the most common deficiencies observed are those of calcium and zinc, particularly during the precompetition season. Many female bodybuilders have dangerous shortages of these minerals year round. A chronic short supply of calcium increases the risk of osteoporosis, a crippling bone-thinning disease. Although a woman's need for zinc is small (8 mg a day), adequate zinc is an impenetrable line of defense when it comes to protecting against disease and infection. In short, deficits of these minerals can harm health and performance. But the good news is that skim milk, red meat, and dark-meat poultry will help alleviate some of these problems. A 3-ounce (90 g) portion of lean sirloin beef has about 6 milligrams of zinc; nonfat, 1 percent, or 2 percent milk has about 1 milligram of zinc in one 8-ounce (240 ml) glass; and 3 ounces (90 g) of dark-meat turkey have about 4 milligrams of zinc.

Another nutritional problem among bodybuilders is fluid restriction. Just before a contest, bodybuilders don't drink much water, fearing it will inflate their physique to the point of blurring their muscular definition. Compounding the problem, many bodybuilders take diuretics and laxatives, a practice that flushes more water, as well as precious minerals called electrolytes, from the body. Generally, bodybuilders compete in a dehydrated state. At one contest, I saw two people pass out on stage—one because of severe dehydration, the other because of an electrolyte imbalance.

After a competition, bodybuilders tend to go hog wild with food. There's nothing wrong with this, as long as it's a temporary splurge for a few days or a week. But such dietary indulgence over a long time can lead to extra body fat.

Most bodybuilders, however, do a lot of things right, especially during the training season. For one thing, they eat several meals throughout the day—a practice that nutritionists recommend to the general public.

## Time and Combine Your Food and Nutrients

To achieve superb shape and maximum performance, forgo the usual approach of three meals a day. Active people must fuel themselves throughout the day, eating small meals and snacks every two to three hours, preferably timed around their workout schedules. As we'll see, these meals don't include just any type of food.

When eating multiple meals, you always want to combine protein with carbohydrate and fat. Examples would be a turkey sandwich, a sprouted grain bread with peanut butter, or an apple with nuts. Eating multiple meals also promotes variety in your diet and keeps your blood sugar levels even so that you avoid peaks and valleys throughout the day (a cycle that happens to promote fat storage).

By including small amounts of protein in meals and snacks, you can control your appetite, feed your muscles more efficiently, and maintain muscle when you're trying to lose fat. You also burn fat better because protein, as well as eating multiple small meals, has been shown to increase thermogenesis, the process by which your body converts ingested calories and stored fat into heat. Another advantage of multiple meals is mental performance. Eating regular, timed meals helps you think and process information more effectively, increases your attention span, and boosts your mood.

The bottom line is that eating small, frequent meals throughout the day is the best fat-burning, muscle-building strategy you can integrate into your lifestyle. Table 1.1 provides a look at how to time your meals properly and the benefits of doing so. The supplements listed in the table are discussed in detail elsewhere in this book.

## Use a Food Plan

Any nutritional program aimed at losing body fat and building muscle should be based on a food plan that emphasizes lean protein, natural carbohydrate, and good fat. It should also include sample menus and recipes as well as information on how to make healthy selections that are personalized to your lifestyle. It should be neither so restrictive that it invites failure nor so unstructured as to be confusing. These are precisely the guidelines for food planning that you will find here.

More specifically, if your goals are to develop lean muscle while reducing body fat, then your plan should take into consideration several factors, including balancing protein, carbohydrate, and fat; increasing your water intake; organizing your food into multiple meals; timing your intake; and incorporating certain dietary supplements into the mix.

## TABLE 1.1  Timing Meals

| **Throughout the day** |
|---|
| Fluids: 8-12 cups (2-3 L) a day; at least 5 cups (1 L) should be water. |
| Breakfast: Never skip this meal! It improves physical and mental performance and helps regulate weight. |
| Meals: Small, frequent protein–carbohydrate meals and snacks every 2-3 h. |
| **Before exercise** |
| Fluids: At least 8 oz (240 ml) before exercise. |
| Preexercise meal: At least 4 h before exercise so that the body properly assimilates carbohydrate for use by muscles. |
| Preexercise snack: 30-90 min before exercise. Snack should consist of 200-400 calories, including 30-50 g carbohydrate, 10-20 g protein, and no more than 5-7 g fat. Snack can be food or meal-replacement supplement. This snack will provide additional energy for prolonged stamina and help decrease exercise-induced breakdown of muscle protein. |
| **During exercise** |
| Fluids: 7-10 oz (210-300 ml) every 10-20 min |
| Glucose–electrolyte sport drinks: Sipping these during a workout has been shown to extend endurance. Use them during phases when you're trying to build muscle but not when you're trying to lose fat. |
| **After exercise** |
| Fluids: Replace each pound (0.5 kg) of fluid lost with 16-24 oz (480-720 ml) of water or sport drink. |
| Carbohydrate: Consume 0.5 to 1 g/kg depending on what phase you're in. |
| Protein: Consume 0.5 g/kg protein with carbohydrate to encourage muscle growth. Postexercise snacks can be in the form of meal-replacement beverages with 0.5 to 1 g/kg of a high glycemic–index and high glycemic–load carbohydrate and 0.5 g/kg protein. Follow this within 2 h of exercise with a meal containing lots of unprocessed carbohydrate and high-quality protein sources (e.g., fish, lean meats, low-fat dairy products, eggs). |
| Recovery supplements: Consume these with your meal replacement: creatine (2-5 g); glutamine (4-10 g); vitamin C (up to 500 mg); zinc (up to 25 mg); beta-alanine (amount depends on daily dosing); probiotic. |

You have to be exact about what you eat, and you need to make the right choices. Each calorie that you put into your mouth has to be results oriented. To drive your fat-burning machinery and lose weight, for example, you need to eat specific foods, such as dairy foods, whey protein, fish, soy, nuts, olives and olive oil, and green tea, to name a few. With the information you'll learn here, you can create a healthy diet that promotes fat loss and muscle gain.

# Protein, Strength, and Muscle Building

For generations, athletes have believed that a high-protein diet will increase strength. This belief can be traced to a famous Greek athlete, Milo of Crotona, in the sixth century BCE. One of the strongest men in Greece, Milo was the wrestling victor in five Olympic Games and many other festivals. As the legend goes, he applied progressive resistance training by lifting a growing calf daily. When the calf was four years old, he carried it the length of the Olympian stadium, killed it, roasted it, and ate it. It is written that his normal daily intake of meat was about 20 pounds (9 kg).

In the 1960s and 1970s, many people thought protein was a miracle food because muscle magazines hyped it so much. Bodybuilders and other athletes would follow diets made up mostly of meat, milk, and eggs. The raw-egg milkshake was particularly popular, thanks to Rocky Balboa. Why would anyone swill such a concoction? The answer is simple: misinformation. Articles and advertising from those days falsely communicated the notion that protein from raw foods, particularly eggs, is more available to the body for building muscle than protein from cooked foods is.

Not only is this notion absolutely untrue, it is dangerous. Eating raw eggs is a hazardous practice because eggs may be contaminated with the microorganisms that cause salmonella poisoning. Cooking eggs destroys bacteria, eliminating the risk of contracting this serious illness. Raw eggs should be avoided completely. If you want to add eggs to a supplemental drink, try pasteurized egg-white products instead of raw eggs, which is a safer practice. This form of egg whites can be cooked as well.

Cooking also makes protein more readily available to your body. A protein molecule is a string of amino acids connected like a strand of pearls. If two strands of pearls were wound together and then twisted to double up on each other, they would resemble a protein molecule. Heating or cooking the protein molecule unwinds the string of amino acids, straightens it out, and separates it into smaller pieces. This is the process of heat denaturing, which is similar to the process of chemical denaturing, otherwise known as digestion. Cooking foods with protein can begin the digestive process and can actually decrease the net energy that the body must expend during digestion.

Protein is extremely vital in your diet, but by itself, it is not the magic bullet for muscle gain. Instead, protein and carbohydrate together are the magic bullet, especially in combination with the right kinds of fat. In other words, you must place equal emphasis on the right types of protein, carbohydrate, and fat in your diet. These nutrients work in concert to give you the edge on building body-firming muscle.

To build lean, quality muscle, strength train to trigger muscle growth and follow my recommended diet, which includes lean protein to repair damaged tissue and carbohydrate to fuel the rebuilding process. Beyond those critical factors, your ultimate success or failure boils down to your ability to recover—that is, how fast and effectively you can bounce back from your training efforts.

Training promotes inflammation in the body. The two main types of inflammation are classic and systemic. Classic inflammation, which accompanies physical injuries, results in swelling and pain; this is part of the protection and repair process and is considered relatively benign. Systemic inflammation, which can't be seen by the naked eye, can increase the risk for a number of diseases, including allergies, cancer, joint pain, heart disease, Alzheimer's disease, periodontal disease, and irritable bowel syndrome. Recent research suggests that systemic inflammation of systems or tissues may be the root of the fastest-growing preventable diseases: type 2 diabetes and obesity. These are generally considered lifestyle diseases because of their linked risk factors and the habits that have been proven to help prevent and reverse them (diet and exercise).

Both types of inflammation exist throughout your body in various degrees and are influenced by external factors such as the food you eat, your workouts, and even the air you breathe. Researchers in South Korea found that eating large quantities of sugar and fats, even from just a few meals, causes an increased concentration of free radicals in the bloodstream, which creates inflammation in the body.

## POWER PROFILES: Calorie Sources

Calories are certainly important in building muscle mass; however, the source of those calories is crucial if you want to maximize muscle and minimize body fat. A case in point is a professional rookie football player who wanted to lose weight to improve his speed on the field. Unless he trimmed down, his chance to be on the team was in jeopardy, so he needed a dramatic nutritional rescue.

This football player was eating slightly more than 7,000 calories a day. Broken down, those calories figured out to about 17 percent protein, 32 percent fat, and 49 percent carbohydrate. In daily fat grams, he was consuming a whopping 250 grams a day. The composition of his calories was an impediment to losing fat. I reconfigured his diet to 5,680 calories a day; 15 percent of those calories came from protein, 25 percent from fat, and 60 percent from carbohydrate. That mix slashed his fat grams to a healthier 142 grams a day.

He was eating a lot of unhealthy fat in foods such as fried chicken, whole milk, and fast foods. For the high-fat foods, we substituted skinless chicken breasts, 1 percent milk, and fast-food choices such as salads and frozen yogurt that were lower in fat. In addition, we modified some of his favorite dishes such as sweet potato pie into healthier versions. He also began to load up on foods containing complex carbohydrate, such as brown rice, whole-wheat bread, fruits, and vegetables. Plus, he was using leaner protein sources with a wider variety of choices.

The upshot of these dietary changes was that he lost the weight, made the team, and had a great season. He is still a professional football player today.

# The Scoop on Supplements and Functional Foods

So many people ask me why we need to supplement if our diets are so complete. The answer goes back to the science of nutritional anthropology. According to investigators of early human life and lifestyles, our ancestors consumed and expended approximately 3,500 calories per day, at least on average. These calories were not necessarily consumed daily, but the foods they ate were very dense in nutrients and low in calories. Overall, a high amount of nutrient-dense foods made up the daily diet. When early humans exercised, it was in short bursts such as when spearing a predator, in very long-duration, low-intensity activity such as when tracking prey, or in long, moderate-intensity activity such as when seeking new hunting grounds or foraging for roots and berries. At the same time, they also had long periods of recovery.

Today, most people can't consume 3,500 calories a day without gaining a lot of body fat. And anyone exercising to burn off 3,500 calories a day probably doesn't get enough recovery time. By consuming that many calories each day, our ancestors were taking in enough nutrients, fiber and phytochemicals for good health. They had virtually the same bodies we have today, yet because we eat fewer than 3,500 calories daily, we definitely don't get in the nutrition we need. And if we do consume 3,500 calories to replace our daily energy needs, we don't get the density of nutrients or the recovery time we need. The answer to this conundrum lies in supplementation. We need to supplement to achieve optimum performance and to continually enhance our performance and our health.

Today, the supplement industry has recognized that consumers are looking for better-quality supplements. Some companies have pulled the supplement industry up by its bootstraps, conducting third-party laboratory testing for purity and potency and raising the bar of consumer expectations and quality guarantees. These companies have even conducted scientific studies on their products to ensure that they are pure, and that they work. These are very promising developments in the supplement industry.

Another promising development is occurring in a category of foods called functional foods. These are foods or food ingredients that can prevent disease or improve health. Some well-known examples are calcium-fortified orange juice and fiber-enhanced cereal. But practically everything from milk to protein shakes to chocolate is being upgraded to functional food status through the addition of nutrient all-stars such as calcium, antioxidants, omega-3 essential fat, and probiotics. Other foods, such as Greek yogurt, green tea, berries, and most vegetables, are naturally functional. Functional foods provide extra nutrients, vitamins, minerals, protein, phytochemicals, enzymes, and other elements that give you energy, help fight disease and aging, and, for strength trainers, build muscle. So along with eating clean and pure food, taking targeted, high-quality supplements and enhancing your diet with functional foods most definitely will give you an edge.

# How to Be a Power Eater
# if You're a Vegetarian

As I travel around the United States, one of the most common questions I'm asked is how to follow my Power Eating plan as a vegetarian. If you still eat fish, dairy, and eggs, the plan is really easy to follow. There is no need to eat meat or poultry. Whenever you see lean or very lean protein servings in the menu plan, just substitute fish or plant protein from such sources as beans or legumes. One-half cup of beans is equivalent to one very lean protein serving, plus one starch serving.

If you've eliminated fish, dairy, and eggs from your diet, you will have to put in a bit of extra effort to follow the Power Eating plan, but you probably already have noticed that about your diet. Substitute soy foods for eggs in the menu. They both contain the important phospholipids (i.e., types of fat) that are critical for brain health. Just make sure to eat soy foods that contain all the natural fat, such as soybeans, edamame, tofu, tempeh, and whole soy milk or yogurt with the fat still in it.

Substituting for dairy is just as easy as substituting for protein. Use soy milk or other plant-based milks such as rice milk, almond milk, or coconut milk. Make sure they are fortified with calcium and vitamins A and D, all of which are very important for brain and body health. Milks other than soy milk are not really great substitutes for cow's milk because they are lower in protein and higher in fat and sugar. However, if you account for that otherwise in your diet, you will benefit from the fortification of calcium and vitamins that these milks provide.

Unfortunately, there is no good substitute for fish. Only 5 percent of the type of omega-3 fat from flaxseed and other vegetable sources (alpha-linolenic acid, ALA) is converted into the two omega-3 fats found in fish (docosahexaenoic acid, DHA, and eicosapentanoic acid, EPA). These are the two critical fats needed by the heart, brain, and central nervous system, and for all-around general health. Although the protein from fish is excellent, you can substitute other protein for a similar benefit. However, nothing that we currently know of substitutes for marine oils.

If you don't eat fish because of taste preferences, then use a fish oil supplement. If you are allergic to fish, then you must consult your physician before using a supplement. Some of my vegan clients (those who eat no animal products of any kind) have decided to use fish oil supplements because it is such an important health issue, and they feel the difference. But this is certainly a personal choice.

Alternatively, there is a supplemental algae source of docosahexaenoic acid (DHA). The algae has been modified to produce the marine oil, DHA. It is available only in supplement form, not from the algae itself. Currently, this supplement can be quite expensive, and because of the amount of DHA in each pill, you may need to take 5-10 or so daily to consume what you need. But the product is available if all other options are not viable. As a result of increasing consumer demand, these products are quickly improving in cost and dosage.

If you have eliminated all animal products from your diet, you must add some important nutrients back in. To add vitamins $B_{12}$ and D to your diet, you can purchase foods fortified with them, or you can take a multivitamin–mineral supplement. Active women especially may have difficulty taking in enough iron and zinc. These nutrients can be in your supplement, too. Eat plenty of dark green leafy veggies, which contain calcium and iron. Also, choose calcium-fortified soy milk and orange juice. A supplement can also cover your calcium needs.

Adopting a plant-based vegetarian diet can be a great weight-loss strategy. One of the hardest things about losing weight is keeping it off. Several studies have identified many diet plans that can help you lose weight, but the problem is finding one you can stick with for longer than a few months. Some studies have shown that people on vegetarian weight-loss plans were able to stick with them longer than people who undertook some of the well-known diet fads. A study conducted at the University of North Carolina at Chapel Hill investigated the difference in weight-loss outcomes after one and two years between a group of postmenopausal women who followed a vegan diet and a group who followed a more moderate low-fat diet. The study also compared women who were offered support group follow-up and those who were on their own. Vegans lost more weight and maintained a greater weight loss after one and two years. Those participants who received follow-up support maintained an even greater weight loss.

A study published in the *International Journal of Obesity* (2008) showed no greater weight loss or maintenance over 18 months in participants following a lacto-ovo vegetarian diet pattern than in those following a standard calorie- and fat-reduced diet. The authors noted, however, that those following the vegetarian diet pattern "had a significantly greater reduction in animal protein and greater increases in vegetable protein and in dietary fiber, all beneficial changes."

You're doing your health a huge favor by emphasizing more fruits, vegetables, and whole grains in your diet. Plant-based diets appear to be protective against several types of cancer, including cancers of the breast, ovaries, lung, colon, esophagus, and stomach. Vegetarian-style eating may protect you from cardiovascular disease, diabetes, age-related macular degeneration, and overall mortality.

These studies raise a number of questions. Should athletes or people trying to increase muscle size, strength, and power restrict their intake of animal protein foods? Can they achieve their goals by adopting vegetarian diets or vegan diets? Or should they adopt a more varied diet following a more omnivorous pattern, including both animal protein and plant protein?

There has been quite a bit of research in this area, but the questions remain largely unanswered.

Studies do show that you can build muscle on both types of diets. What I have found in my own practice, however, is that it is very difficult to create a high-performance nutrition program if you are a vegan (i.e., you eat no animal products of any type). The time required to shop, plan, and prepare a vegan diet is excessive if you are an athlete living on your own and responsible for your own meals. Vegan diets are high in fiber, which promotes health; however, that much fiber is filling, making it difficult to exercise at peak capacity. The vegan concept may sound good philosophically and in theory, but in practice, it is virtually impossible to carry out. Of course someone always points to a famous vegan athlete as their reason for wanting to follow a vegan diet, but it's no surprise that you can count the number of successful vegan athletes on one hand. There just aren't very many, and the reason is that it's simply too difficult to stay healthy and competitive on such a restrictive diet.

## Sport Nutrition Fact Versus Fiction: Are Organic Foods Better for You?

With the amount of food strength trainers eat, many are opting to go organic to avoid the chemical fertilizers, pesticides, and additives used in many foods. Do you get an advantage in buying organic foods?

In general, organically grown foods are grown in soil enriched with organic fertilizers rather than synthetic fertilizers and treated only with nonsynthetic pesticides. Organic farms use a soil-building program that promotes vibrant soil and healthy plants, usually including crop rotations and biological pest control.

We tend to think of the term *organic* as pertaining to fruits and vegetables only. However, organic meat, poultry, and egg products also exist. These foods come from farms that have been inspected to verify that they meet rigorous standards mandating the use of organic feed, prohibiting the use of antibiotics, and giving animals access to the outdoors, fresh air, and sunlight.

You can tell the difference between organically produced food and conventionally produced food by looking at package labels. The United States Department of Agriculture (USDA) has developed strict labeling rules to help consumers know the exact organic content of the food they buy. Look for the USDA Organic seal; it tells you that a product is at least 95 percent organic.

Organic foods may have some advantages over conventionally produced foods. Here is what some of the latest research shows:

- Organic foods may be highly nutritious. Organic food may be somewhat higher in vitamin C and perhaps other minerals, antioxidants, and phytochemicals.

- Consuming organic food appears to lower concerns over the health hazards associated with pesticide contamination. In one study, children who ate organic produce and juice had only one-sixth the level of pesticide by-products in their urine, compared to children who ate conventionally produced food. There are thus some important safety justifications for eating organic food.

- Organic foods have little pesticide residue, and may be potentially safer than nonorganic foods. One study found that farmworkers who apply pesticides as part of conventional farming have higher concentrations of pesticides in their bodies. Conceivably, a continuation of the trend toward organic farming may help protect farmworkers from unhealthy exposures.

- Organic foods are not only good for you—they are also good for the planet. Organic farming methods are less harmful to the environment than conventional methods. The use of natural products helps to improve the soil. Organic pest control generally relies on preventive measures such as crop rotation and biological controls. These methods place little to no stress on the earth or its wildlife inhabitants. With organic agriculture now being embraced as environmentally sound and more sustainable than mainstream agriculture, consumers believe they are contributing to a better future and an improved environment, according to one survey.

Also, organic produce often tastes better than nonorganic produce. Here in Seattle, where I live, lots of organic food is grown locally. Consequently, the produce is very fresh, because it doesn't have to be transported vast distances.

Whether you decide to go organic, the most important move you can make health-wise is to eat more fruits and vegetables, organic or not. Much research shows that people can improve their health and the quality of their lives by consuming more plant foods. Despite the use of pesticides, populations that eat large amounts of fruits and vegetables have lower rates of cancer and other life-threatening illnesses than populations that eat few fruits and vegetables.

In the end, the choice is yours. Purchasing organic foods is not just a nutritional issue but a political, social, and personal issue as well. If you want to treat the earth well and potentially protect workers from pesticide exposure, speak with your pocketbook: Buy organic.

You'll pay more for organic produce, so if your pocketbook is light, buy fresh conventional produce and follow these guidelines for reducing pesticide residues in foods:

- Wash fresh produce in water. Use a scrub brush, and rinse the produce thoroughly under running water.
- Use a knife to peel an orange or grapefruit; do not bite into the peel.
- Discard the outer leaves of leafy vegetables such as cabbage and lettuce.
- Peel waxed fruit and vegetables; waxes don't wash off and can seal in pesticide residues.
- Peel vegetables such as carrots and fruits such as apples when appropriate. (Peeling removes pesticides that remain in or on the peel but also removes fibers, vitamins, and minerals.)

---

Those vegan athletes who are successful typically are already genetically gifted in their sport, and they often have a support team to help them plan, shop, and cook. Whenever possible, I encourage my clients to follow a mixed-protein diet that is plant centered but not exclusively plant based.

## Where Do You Stand Now?

Analyze your present diet now to see exactly what you're eating, particularly in terms of the three energy nutrients. You should also analyze how much water you're drinking, because water is a critical nutrient. This analysis will make the following chapters more relevant and interesting. For example, when you're reading about protein, you may wonder how much protein you're eating now. With this analysis handy, you can find out quickly.

Using the form provided in appendix A, record everything you eat over the course of three days. Choose days that best represent your typical diet. Be as accurate as you can in terms of the amount of food you eat. Use the information in chapters 10 and 11 to help you figure out nutrients and calories.

# 2

# Manufacturing Muscle

Inside your body, a marvelous process of self-repair takes place day in and day out, and it all has to do with protein, the nutrient responsible for building and maintaining body tissues.

Protein is present everywhere in the body—in muscles, bones, connective tissue, blood vessels, blood cells, skin, hair, and fingernails. This protein is constantly being lost or broken down as a result of normal physiological wear and tear and must be replaced. For example, about half of the total amount of protein in muscle tissue is broken down and replaced every 150 days.

The mechanism by which this repair occurs is really quite amazing. During digestion, protein in food is dismantled by other proteins (enzymes) into subunits called amino acids. Amino acids then enter cells, and other enzymes, acting on instructions from DNA, put them back together as the new proteins needed to build and repair tissue. Virtually no other system in the world repairs itself so wonderfully. Every day, this process goes on and life continues.

Under any condition of growth—childhood, pregnancy, muscle building—the body manufactures more cells than are lost. From an energy source such as carbohydrate or fat, the body can manufacture many of the materials needed to make new cells. But to replace and build new protein, it must have protein from food. Unlike carbohydrate and fat, protein contains nitrogen, and nitrogen is required to synthesize new protein.

Protein, therefore, is absolutely necessary for the maintenance, replacement, and growth of body tissue. But protein has other uses, too. The body uses protein to regulate hormone secretion, maintain the body's water balance, protect against disease, transport nutrients in and out of cells, carry oxygen, and regulate blood clotting.

# Protein and Muscle Building

Protein is a key player in the repair and construction of muscle tissue, and we now know more about how to use protein to drive anabolic (tissue building or growth)machinery right down to the molecular level. Keep in mind that a balance is needed between protein synthesis and protein degradation; to build lean muscle, synthesis must be greater than degradation.

A messaging system in your brain directly affects protein synthesis in your muscles. When you stress your muscles through resistance training, your brain tells your muscle cells to start making new proteins, which ultimately leads to larger muscle tissue. However, enough amino acids must be available to jump-start this process. By supplying your body with protein, particularly right after exercise and for the next 48 hours, you can keep yourself in an anabolic state.

A 2009 review article published in the journal *Applied Physiology and Nutrition Metabolism* pointed out that you can maximize this process by doing high-intensity interval training (HIIT). This involves resistance-type exercise performed at a very high intensity for a short duration with brief periods of rest between bouts. HIIT induces rapid changes that initiate genetic responses and messages to ultimately alter muscle cell proteins and generate new proteins. The net effect is increases in muscle size, strength, and power. HITT should not replace your heavy lifting.

There's more: when muscle cells are stressed through exercise, they increase their capacity to shore up their antioxidant systems as a protective reaction. Thus, it is vital to supply the body with antioxidant-rich foods, along with protein, after exercise. With this knowledge, you can target the protein and antioxidant needs of your muscles during and after training.

# Protein and Fat Burning

Studies have suggested that, compared with diets high in carbohydrate and low in fat, diets high in protein and low in fat promote greater weight loss. One reason is that lean protein helps stoke your fat-burning fires. Its thermogenic (heat-producing) effect may be as high as 22 percent, compared with as low as 0.8 percent for carbohydrate. In other words, you burn more calories by doing nothing more than eating slightly more protein and less carbohydrate.

A research article published in 2002 by Dr. Carol Johnston and colleagues from Arizona State University East in Mesa, Arizona, helps to explain the mechanism. Ten women aged 19 to 22 consumed either a high-protein or high-carbohydrate diet, and then their energy production was measured two and a half hours after the meal. The study found that energy production was 100 percent higher on the high-protein diet than on the high-carbohydrate diet. Over the course of the day, postmeal energy production on the high-protein diet totaled 30 more calories at each test time. Johnston speculated that if this energy differential actually lasted for two to three hours after each meal (because each test point was two and a half hours after each meal), the added thermogenic effect of the high-protein diet may have been as high as 90 calories. What that means is that you can potentially burn more calories with extra protein in your diet. The high-protein diet contained 2 grams of protein per kilogram of body weight per day.

An increased sense of satiety is associated with the thermogenic effect of protein. Women on high-protein, moderate-carbohydrate meals have a greater sensation of fullness during meals that lasts for longer periods compared with women on low-protein meals. The difference is associated with the thermogenic effect of the meal. By following a high-protein, moderate-carbohydrate diet, you will feel more satisfied and have greater control over what and how much you eat.

To capitalize on the thermogenic effect of high-protein meals, you should consume protein in frequent meals and snacks throughout the day. This allows for the most efficient absorption and use of protein, and it helps to maintain higher levels of energy production to promote weight loss.

## Protein and Strength-Training Performance

It would seem that the more construction material (protein) you supply your body, the more muscle you'll build. At least that's the train of thought strength athletes have followed for ages. But it doesn't quite work that way. Eating twice as much protein won't make your muscles twice as big. Furthermore, one problem with eating too much protein is that the excess can be stored as body fat.

To build muscle, you must maintain a positive nitrogen balance. Nitrogen leaves the body primarily in the urine and must be replaced by nitrogen taken in from food. Protein contains a fairly large concentration of nitrogen. Generally, healthy adults are in a state of nitrogen equilibrium, or zero balance—that is, their protein intake meets their protein requirement. A positive nitrogen balance means that the body is retaining dietary protein and using it to synthesize new tissue. If more nitrogen is excreted than consumed, the nitrogen balance is negative. The body has lost nitrogen—and therefore protein. A negative nitrogen balance over time is dangerous, leading to muscle wasting and disease.

Achieving a positive nitrogen balance doesn't necessarily mean that you have to eat more protein. Muscle cells take up the exact amount of nutrients (including amino acids from dietary protein) they need for growth, and strength training helps them make better use of the protein that's available.

This fact was clearly demonstrated in 1995 by a group of Tufts University researchers led by Wayne W. Campbell. The researchers took a group of older men and women (aged 56 to 80) who had never lifted weights before, placed them on either a low-protein diet or a high-protein diet, and measured their nitrogen balance before and after participation in a 12-week strength-training program. The low-protein diet was actually based on the RDA for protein (0.8 g per kg of body weight daily). The high-protein diet was twice the RDA (1.6 g per kg of body weight daily). The researchers wanted to see what effects each diet had on nitrogen balance during strength training.

What they discovered was interesting. Strength training enhanced nitrogen retention in both groups—protein was being retained and used to synthesize new tissue.

However, in the low-protein group, there was even better use of protein. Strength training caused the body to adapt and meet the demand for protein—even when the bare minimum requirement for protein was met each day. Although this low level of protein intake may not be optimal for building muscle, this study shows how marvelously the body adjusts to what is available and how strength training makes muscle cells more efficient at using available protein to synthesize new tissue.

So, exactly how much protein should you eat for maximum performance and results? That question has been hotly debated in science for more than 100 years and by athletes since the time of the ancient Greeks. Nutrition scientists have had difficulty reaching a consensus on protein intake for several reasons. One has to do with the type and frequency of exercise. In endurance exercise, for example, protein can act as kind of a spare fuel tank, kicking in amino acids to supply fuel. If protein is in short supply, endurance athletes can peter out easily. In strength sports, additional dietary protein is needed to provide enough amino acids to synthesize protein in the muscles.

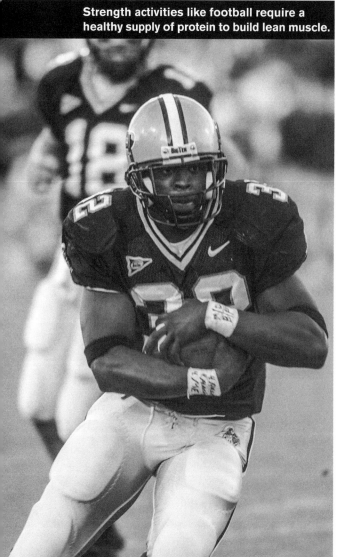

Strength activities like football require a healthy supply of protein to build lean muscle.

For generations, strength trainers have looked to protein as the nutritional panacea for muscle building. Is there any scientific basis to this belief? New research shows that as a strength trainer, you may benefit from eating some extra protein.

## Age and Protein Intake

It's no secret that as you age, you can lose muscle mass, strength, and function, partly because of inactivity. One way to reverse the downhill slide is to strength train. Study after study has shown that you can make significant muscle gains well into your 90s if you strength train.

Scientific research indicates that senior strength trainers can get a real boost from additional protein. At Tufts University, researchers gave supplemental protein to a group of elderly strength trainers, while a control group took no supplements. Based on CAT scans of muscle, the supplement group gained much more muscle mass than the control group did.

But what if you're not yet in your golden years? Can you get the same benefits from extra protein? Many studies say yes. Two groups of young bodybuilders following a four-week strength-training program followed the same diet, but with one exception. One group ate 2.3 grams of protein per kilogram of body weight (much more than the DRI), and the other group ate 1.3 grams of protein per kilogram of body weight. By the end of the study, both groups had gained muscle, but those eating the higher amount of protein had gained five times more!

## Protein Requirements for Endurance: Sexual Inequality

Requirements for carbohydrate and protein differ among men and women involved in endurance exercise. Women don't use as much carbohydrate during exercise as men do, and they don't use as much carbohydrate after exercise for recovery growth and repair as men do. Contrary to popular belief, women are great fat burners; that's why they don't need as much carbohydrate for exercise as men do.

A study of female cyclists looked into how much protein women actually need. Interestingly, researchers discovered that women don't use as much protein as men do, either. Men get a huge muscle protein synthesis boost from consuming protein after exercise; women do not. These female cyclists had a total protein requirement of 1.28 grams, or approximately 1.3 grams per kilogram of body weight per day to maintain nitrogen balance. Men have a requirement much closer to 1.8 to 2.0 grams per kilogram of body weight per day to maintain positive nitrogen balance during endurance exercise. Using the data, we can extrapolate for men and lower the amount of protein for women to 1.4 to 1.6 grams per kilogram of body weight per day for endurance exercise. I like to give a little extra leeway in order to stay in a positive nitrogen balance in case, as happens frequently, endurance athletes do not consume their full need for calories. With a calorie deficit, protein needs are always higher.

## Proper Protein Levels

At Kent State University, researchers divided strength trainers into three groups: (1) a low-protein group on a diet of 0.9 gram of protein per kilogram of body weight, which approximates the recommendation of 0.8 gram per kilogram for sedentary people; (2) a group on a diet of 1.4 grams of protein per kilogram of body weight; and (3) a group on a diet of 2.4 grams of protein per kilogram of body weight. Control groups with both sedentary participants and strength-training participants were also included.

Two exciting findings emerged. First, increasing protein intake to 1.4 grams triggered protein synthesis (an indicator of muscle growth) in strength trainers. There were no such changes in the low-protein group. Second, upping protein intake from 1.4 grams to 2.4 grams produced no further protein synthesis. This latter finding suggests that a plateau was reached, meaning that the participants got more protein than they could use from 2.4 grams.

The research appears to indicate that if you strength train and eat more protein, you are going to enhance muscle development and preservation. But this doesn't necessarily mean that you should start piling protein on your plate. Studies should always be interpreted with caution. Let's talk about how much protein you really need based on your activity level.

**Functions of Protein in Exercise**

- Promotes growth and repair of tissue
- Provides bodily structure (muscle, connective tissue, bone, and organs)
- Supports metabolic and hormonal activities
- Enhances immunity
- Maintains bodily protein to prevent muscle tissue breakdown
- Minimizes fatigue by providing branched-chain amino acids as fuel

## Your Individual Protein Requirements

As a strength trainer or bodybuilder, you need more protein than a less active person does. Your requirement is higher than the current DRI of 0.8 gram of protein per kilogram of body weight a day, which is based on the needs of nonexercisers, but it's only slightly higher. (Don't forget, your body can work with a protein intake that meets the DRI.) Plus, individual protein requirements vary, depending on whether you're building muscle, doing aerobic exercise on a regular basis, or dieting for competition. Here's a closer look.

### Muscle Building

With increases in training intensity, you need additional protein to support muscle growth and increases in certain blood compounds. On the basis of the latest research with strength trainers, I recommend that you eat 2.0 grams of protein per kilogram of body weight a day. Here's how you would figure that requirement if you weigh 150 pounds, or 68 kilograms (a kilogram equals 2.2 pounds):

$$2 \text{ g of protein} \times 68 \text{ kg} = 136 \text{ g of protein a day}$$

Strength trainers living in high altitudes need even more protein: 2.2 grams per kilogram of body weight daily. If you're a vegan, your protein needs are also 10 percent higher to make sure your diet is providing all the necessary amino acids:

$$2.2 \text{ g of protein} \times 68 \text{ kg} = 150 \text{ g of protein a day}$$

If you are new to strength training, you may need to eat more than a veteran strength trainer typically consumes—as much as 40 percent more.

### Aerobic Exercise

On average, most strength trainers and bodybuilders perform an hour or two of intense weight training daily, plus five or more hours a week of aerobic exercise. If you are in this category, your protein needs are further elevated. Here's why.

During aerobic exercise lasting 60 minutes or more, certain amino acids—the branched-chain amino acids (BCAAs)—are used for energy in small amounts, particularly when the body is running low on carbohydrate, its preferred fuel source. One of the BCAAs, leucine, is broken down to make alanine, another amino acid, which is converted by the liver into blood sugar (glucose) for energy. This glucose is transported to the working muscles to be used for energy. The harder you work aerobically, the more leucine your body breaks down for extra fuel. In addition, studies show that obtaining amino acids such as leucine stimulates muscle repair, as well as muscular development, in the period following exercise.

Given this special use of amino acids as an energy and recovery source, you should increase your protein intake if your training program includes more than five hours a week of an endurance program. You may require as much as 2.2 grams of protein per kilogram of body weight. With the preceding example, you would calculate your requirements as follows:

$$2.2 \text{ g of protein} \times 68 \text{ kg} = 150 \text{ g of protein a day}$$

## Cross-Training

If you're a marathoner, a triathlete, or even an ultramarathoner, you engage in cross-training, which consists of taking part in a variety of activities geared for your sport, including running, cycling, and long-distance swimming. And you may be lifting weights as a part of it all.

Although years ago cross-training athletes were encouraged to load up on carbohydrate, in more recent years experts have contended that protein is equally essential for reaching new performance heights. However, protein is slightly lower in order to leave room in the diet for increased carbohydrate, which is critical in the diet of an endurance athlete who is cross-training. Cross-training athletes thus need 1.6 to 1.8 grams of protein per kilogram of body weight a day, depending on the frequency and intensity of exercise. For example:

1.6 to 1.8 g of protein per kg of body weight × 68 kg = 109 to 122 g of protein a day

Cross-trainers, like endurance athletes, use more carbohydrate during training and competition than pure strength athletes do. Like endurance athletes, they need higher intakes of dietary carbohydrate than strength athletes do, and they can benefit from some carbohydrate loading before competition. Cross-trainers should use the updated, shorter version of carbohydrate loading, which entails long duration training one week prior to the event to deplete muscle glycogen stores. They should then begin tapering their exercise and increase carbohydrate consumption three or four days prior to the event, reaching a pre-event rest day during which they take in about 600 grams of dietary carbohydrate.

## Competition Dieting or Trimming Fat

When cutting calories to get lean for looks or for competition, you risk losing body-firming muscle. Because muscle is the body's most metabolically active tissue, losing it compromises the ability of your body to burn fat. What's more, no bodybuilder wants to lose muscle before competition. One way to prevent diet-related muscle loss is to consume adequate protein while you're preparing for competition. Dieting bodybuilders need 2.2 to 2.5 grams of protein per kilogram of body weight a day; I recommend 2.3 grams per day. Here is an example:

$$2.3 \text{ g of protein} \times 68 \text{ kg} = 156 \text{ g of protein a day}$$

Incidentally, the distribution of calories in this kind of plan will be 30 percent protein, 40 percent carbohydrate, and 30 percent fat (30–40–30). For more information on getting cut for competition, see chapter 16.

## Benefits of Properly Timing Your Protein Intake

Let's say you've just finished an intense strength-training workout. If you could zoom in to the microscopic level of your muscles, you'd be astounded by the sight. There are tears in the tiny structures of your muscle fibers and leaks in your muscle cells. Over the next 24 to 48 hours, muscle protein will break down, and additional muscle glycogen will be used.

These are some of the chief metabolic events that occur in the aftermath of a hard workout. And although these events might look like havoc, they are actually a necessary part of recovery—the repair and growth of muscle tissue that take place after every workout. During recovery, the body replenishes muscle glycogen and synthesizes new muscle protein. In the process, muscle fibers are made bigger and stronger to protect themselves against future trauma.

You can do much to enhance the recovery process—including consuming protein before and after your workout. Having a small meal that includes protein and carbohydrate before your strength-training workout is very beneficial. In a review study (a study that looks at a bundle of research) of the role of protein in the athlete's diet, Dr. Peter W. Lemon, who has done cutting-edge research on protein, noted that protein meals consumed before exercise can result in greater gains in both muscle mass and strength than with training alone. The evidence here is too compelling to ignore, which is why I recommend small preexercise meals that include protein.

The next step is to eat a small meal immediately after exercise. Your body has already digested your preexercise protein, and it is working for you at the muscular level. Two or three hours later, as that effect wears off, your body begins to demand protein for the repair and recovery phase following a workout. According to research, you can jump-start the glycogen-making process by eating 0.5 gram of protein per kilogram of body weight, along with a high-glycemic carbohydrate, such as dextrose, maltodextrin, sucrose, or even honey, within 30 minutes of exercise. For example, if you weigh 150 pounds (68 kg), you should eat 34 grams of protein.

When protein is consumed along with carbohydrate, there's a surge in insulin. Insulin is like an acceleration pedal. It races the body's glycogen-making motor in two ways. First, it speeds up the movement of glucose and amino acids into cells, and second, it activates a special enzyme crucial to glycogen synthesis. Additional research shows that a carbohydrate and protein supplement ingested after exercise triggers the release of growth hormone in addition to insulin. Both are conducive to muscle growth and recovery.

Also, the availability of essential amino acids (see table 2.1) after exercise boosts the rate of muscle protein resynthesis in the body. On the basis of these findings, I recommend that you consume 0.5 to 1 gram per kilogram of body weight of a high-glycemic carbohydrate with 0.5 gram per kilogram of a protein food or a quality protein supplement—preferably one that contains all the essential amino acids. (See table 3.2 for a glycemic index of foods.)

**TABLE 2.1   Essential, Conditionally Essential, and Nonessential Amino Acids**

| Essential | Conditionally essential | Nonessential |
|---|---|---|
| Isoleucine* | Arginine | Alanine |
| Leucine* | Cysteine (cystine) | Asparagine |
| Lysine | Glutamine | Aspartic acid |
| Methionine | Histidine | Citruline |
| Phenylalanine | Proline | Glutamic acid |
| Threonine | Taurine | Glycine |
| Tryptophan | Tyrosine | Serine |
| Valine* | | |

*Branched-chain amino acid.

Adapted from M.G. Di Pasquale, 2000, Proteins and amino acids in exercise and sport. In *Energy-yielding macronutrients and energy metabolism in sports nutrition*, edited by J.A. Driskell and I. Wolinsky (Philadelphia: CRC Press), 119-162.

## Staying Anabolic All Day

Imagine walking around in an anabolic (growth) stage all day long, with your body in a tissue-building and fat-burning mode, continually. Is this possible? Yes—and I'll let you in on a few scientifically proven secrets.

The first secret to staying anabolic is planning regular meals with the right carbohydrate-protein combination. Your next secret weapon, though, is supplementing with leucine. Along with valine and isoleucine, leucine is one of the branched-chain amino acids (BCAAs). BCAAs are unique among amino acids in that they are used predominantly by muscle (most amino acids are processed and dismantled in the liver). Scientists have established that BCAAs produce energy during exercise, as well as promote protein synthesis. Recent research further underscores the importance of leucine for both muscle growth and muscle maintenance while dieting.

A recent review of the role of leucine points out that leucine and insulin appear to work together to promote protein synthesis in skeletal muscle. In addition, this same review noted that leucine taken alone after a workout is sufficient to "switch on" protein synthesis. Yet, although leucine alone is a potent activator of muscle growth, you still need the other essential amino acids to make those muscle proteins.

Other research has pointed out the importance of leucine during dieting. To make a long story short, when calories are reduced, leucine in muscle is used to produce the amino acid alanine, which is used to produce glucose in the liver. It seems logical to hypothesize that high leucine intakes while dieting help spare protein and improve blood glucose control. The research has shown that 2.5 grams of leucine stimulates the metabolic pathways that catalyze muscle proteins synthesis, thereby enhancing muscle growth and maintaining lean body mass.

This function of leucine, in addition to its anticatabolic function, may be critical in preventing overtraining. Although total energy intake is paramount, protein intake should not be ignored or limited during reduced training. If you have slowed training in an effort to prevent overtraining, don't drop your protein intake. Overtraining can be a result of and a state of catabolism. Optimal protein levels may decrease the risk of and enhance recovery from overtraining. In fact, it may even be more important at this time.

Of the commonly available dietary proteins, whey isolate has the highest leucine content (14 percent of its total protein content). Animal proteins contain 10 percent leucine, whereas other proteins contain around 8 percent. Therefore, approximately 25 grams of animal or whey protein typically contains 2.5 grams of leucine. Strive to take in 10 grams of leucine per day from food and supplementation. If you are consuming soy protein or other plant proteins, you would need slightly more. Consuming proteins at every meal and snacks throughout the day, approximately every three to four hours, allows for adequate energy and protein consumption to remain anabolic. This includes around exercise, both before and after.

## Protein, Mood, and Sleep

Protein foods contain an amino acid called tryptophan. It is a building block for the calming, feel-good brain chemical, serotonin. Typically, unless you are on a protein-restricted diet, you have enough tryptophan circulating to raise serotonin levels. A lack of carbohydrate in the diet, which initiates the cascade of biochemical events that allow tryptophan to cross the blood–brain barrier and enter the brain, is the most common dietary reason for low levels of serotonin. But it's important to know that protein plays a role in elevated mood. Serotonin is also responsible for helping the body prepare for rest and sleep. During the day serotonin receptors stimulate a sense of alertness and elevated mood. In the evening those receptors power down, and the receptors responsible for preparing the body for rest and sleep power up. So it is a combination of protein and carbohydrate that enhances both of these effects.

# Beware of High-Protein, Low-Carbohydrate Diets

The high-protein, low-carbohydrate approach to weight control is a defeatist strategy if you are a strength trainer or bodybuilder. Not eating enough carbohydrate can lower your calorie intake, and when calories are restricted, your body will use protein from the diet to meet its energy demands. This reduces the amount of protein available for the physiological functions that only protein can perform. Without enough protein, more muscle is lost during weight loss, resulting in the undesirable effect of reduced metabolic rate. The bottom line is that you need carbohydrate along with protein to maintain muscle mass. Following a fat-loss diet that is 30 percent protein, which I recommended earlier in this chapter, is a win–win strategy. In this diet, you're lowering carbohydrate intake only slightly to make room for the extra protein, which will help drive fat burning.

The high-protein diets I object to are those that omit or drastically cut carbohydrate. Such diets promising quick weight loss continue to be the rage. These diets let you fill up on beef, chicken, fish, and eggs, with little emphasis on other foods such as vegetables and grains.

What's wrong with such diets? To begin with, they're high in fat. The protein in animal foods is often coupled with large amounts of saturated fat and cholesterol. Excess dietary fat can make you gain body fat and can damage your heart. Most extreme protein diets are low in fiber, too. Without enough bulk to move things along, your whole digestive system slows to a crawl, which can lead to constipation, diverticulosis, and other intestinal disorders.

In addition, most protein diets are dehydrating. During the first week on a high-protein diet, you can lose a lot of weight, depending on your initial weight and body-fat percentage. You get on the scale, see an exhilarating weight loss, and feel wonderful, but most of this loss is water. You could be very dehydrated as a result, which spells trouble. If you weigh 150 pounds (68 kg), a mere 3-pound (1 kg) loss of water weight can make you feel draggy and hurt your exercise performance. The minute you go off this diet and eat some carbohydrate, water surges back into your tissues and you regain the lost water weight.

Clearly, your focus should not be on protein, but on a balance of nutrients. For an athlete, weight loss is an outcome of getting your diet and training dialed in; it is not a goal. Your goal is enhanced performance. Don't let the diet world fool you into believing that popular diet fads will put you on the podium. In fact, it's just the opposite. In chapters 12 through 16, you'll learn how to design your own personal eating plan, one that contains the right amount of protein, carbohydrate, and fat to help you build muscle and stay lean.

# Fish Protein

Unless you've been stranded on a desert island, you know about the importance of fish oils and the omega-3 fat that comes from fish. But there is something else special about fish protein—it helps keep you lean.

The effect is partially from the omega-3 fat in fish, but scientists have learned that it may be the fish protein that is making the difference. In a Canadian study titled "Prevention of Skeletal Muscle Insulin Resistance by Dietary Cod Protein," researchers found that when cod protein was fed to rats on a high-fat diet that led to muscle insulin resistance, the cod protein protected against the insulin resistance.

The same researchers went back and looked into whether all fish had the same effects that cod had on insulin resistance. The goal of this new study was to determine whether other fish protein presents similar beneficial effects. So rats were put on a high-fat and high-sugar diet containing protein from casein or fish protein from bonito, herring, mackerel, or salmon. After 28 days, oral glucose tolerance tests were performed on the rats, and the tissues were biochemically analyzed. All the rats were fed diets of equal energy, but the salmon protein group had significantly less weight gain, which was associated with less fat gain. Whole-body insulin sensitivity for glucose improved also. In addition, the fish protein–fed group experienced a very powerful anticancer effect compared with the casein-fed control group. The anticancer effects were attributed to the anti-inflammatory properties that fish protein carries; the same protein may also protect against obesity-linked metabolic complications. Lastly, the salmon-fed group exhibited a rise in the circulating hormone calcitonin. This hormone plays a role in helping to control weight gain and may be the reason for the reduced weight gain in the salmon-fed rats. Although done in rats, this study sheds significant light on the role of fish protein might play in human metabolism.

Researchers in Norway conducted a study to determine whether the amino acid content of various proteins may account for the ability of fish protein to enhance fat loss. It is understood that the amino acids taurine and glycine increase liver bile acid secretion and modulate bile acid metabolism, enhancing fecal bile acid excretion in rats. In this study, rats fed a diet containing fish protein hydrolysate from the saithe fish (pollock), which is high in taurine and glycine, experienced enhanced fat burning. This research enhances our understanding of the mechanisms behind the effect of fish protein on body composition.

I have watched the influence of fish in my clients' diets for decades. It is clear to me that when you eat fish five times a week, you get lean quickly. Of course, you have to do everything else right as well, but eating fish really helps spur the rate at which you can accomplish weight-loss goals.

Eating fish five times a week does not have to mean five fish dinners a week. You can have fish for breakfast in the form of smoked fish or a tuna melt on toast. It's easy to have canned salmon or canned tuna, or even fish tacos, for lunch. There are plenty of ways to vary the fish meals you eat during the week.

I am always asked about the safety of fish. How can we eat fish when there are so many problems with contamination? There are two primary concerns with fish safety: mercury and pesticide contamination. The mercury problem is a matter of contaminated waters and food chain hierarchy. Mercury is a by-product of heavy industry and manufacturing. It is released as pollution into the air, where it is trapped in the clouds and released in rainwater into the oceans, becoming methylmercury. Methylmercury is toxic to humans, and poisoning results in neurological disorders in adults. High levels of mercury will harm an unborn baby's or young child's developing nervous system. Because fish feed in these waters, the mercury builds up in them. The larger and longer lived the fish is, the greater the amount of smaller fish it consumes. Over years, methylmercury builds up in large predatory fish and can reach relatively unsafe levels.

Nearly all fish contain trace amounts of mercury, as do all living things. However, large predatory fish such as swordfish, shark, tuna, king mackerel, and tilefish pose the greatest risks. Some shellfish can also be high in methylmercury based on their very small size in proportion to the contaminants they contain, the waters they feed in, and their key food sources.

Here is the advice from the U.S. Food and Drug Administration and the Environmental Protection Agency:

- Do not eat shark, swordfish, king mackerel, or tilefish because they contain high levels of mercury.
- Eat up to 12 ounces (two average meals) a week of a variety of fish and shellfish that are lower in mercury.
- Five of the most commonly eaten fish that are low in mercury are shrimp, canned light tuna, salmon, pollock, and catfish.
- Another commonly eaten fish, albacore ("white") tuna has more mercury than canned light tuna. So, when choosing your two meals of fish and shellfish, you may eat up to 6 ounces (180 g, or one average meal) of albacore tuna per week.
- Check local advisories about the safety of fish caught by family and friends in your local lakes, rivers, and coastal areas. If no advice is available, eat up to 6 ounces (180 g, or one average meal) per week of fish you catch from local waters, but don't consume any other fish during that week.
- Follow these same recommendations when feeding fish and shellfish to young children, but serve smaller portions.

What the advisory doesn't tell you is that noncontaminated tuna is available from independently owned fishing vessels that sail out of the Pacific Northwest. These fishermen catch small tuna, 7- to 12-pound (3 to 5.4 kg) fish versus the 40- to 70-pound (18 to 32 kg) fish caught by the longlining large commercial canneries. Rather than processing the tuna out in the ocean and boiling off the wonderful omega-3 fat to throw them overboard into the ocean, these small tuna are flash frozen and canned with all their healthy fat intact. (The large canneries really do boil off omega-3 fat. One major cannery now has its own omega-3 fat supplement; it takes it out of the fish and bottles it.) The fish caught by these independent fishermen are virtually mercury free because of their size and the waters in which they are caught. These fisherman are also very environmentally responsible, catching only tuna (not sea turtles or other by-catch) and sticking to sustainable catch sizes. You get a delicious tuna with all the healthy fat and none of the mercury. The large nationwide canneries can't say that about their products. (See the sidebar for resources.)

# Tuna Safety Q&A

**Q.** What is the best and safest method for catching tuna?

**A.** The safest and most sustainable tuna is caught by hand polling or trolling

**Q.** What about tuna steaks and sushi? Are those safe?

**A.** The most common method of catching these fish is longline fishing. All types of longline-caught albacore tuna, bigeye tuna (also known as ahi), and yellowfin tuna are considered high sources of mercury, regardless of whether they are canned or served as steaks or sushi. If you eat just a piece or two of tuna sushi every once in a while, this shouldn't be a problem. But if you make tuna sushi your meal twice a week, your mercury levels may be high.

Bluefin and skipjack tunas are considered safe for health, but the longline fishing technique is considered unsafe for the environment. Longline fishing leads to overfishing of the waters and high levels of by-catch (sea turtles, sea birds, sharks, and occasionally marine mammals). Hand poling and trolling are considered the most environmentally safe fishing methods.

"Light" canned tuna typically contains skipjack tuna, which is why it has been considered safer to eat than other tuna. However, a *Chicago Tribune* investigation discovered that "light" tuna sometimes contains yellowfin tuna without labeling it as such, and yellowfin is significantly higher in mercury than skipjack.

**Q.** Can sushi bars hide the fact that they serve fish of inferior quality?

**A.** One easy way to disguise less-than-top-quality tuna is to mix it with other ingredients. The spicy tuna roll is notorious in the sushi industry for using this method. There are also methods to make fish look fresher than it really is. "Gassing" or "smoking" tuna can make it look rosier than it is. Fish that is not processed using very high-quality methods can naturally lose its redness after death, even with freezing. After the tuna is butchered into loins or fillets and before it is frozen, it is exposed to carbon monoxide. The gas binds with hemoglobin to prevent any change in the flesh from red to brown or even to gray. This misrepresents the product to the consumer, making it difficult to evaluate the age of the fish based on the color of the flesh.

Although we hope that you get what you pay for, price is not always an indicator of the quality of the fish in a sushi restaurant. Here are a few tips to guide you:

- Fresh fish is rarely delivered on the weekend. Rule out Sundays and Mondays when considering a meal at a sushi restaurant.

- Fresh never means fishy. You should never know by walking in the door with your eyes closed that the restaurant serves fish. If there's a fishy smell, walk out.

Fresh fish should be translucent and shiny. If the tuna looks as though it was painted red, it may have been gassed. Ask the chef if it has been smoked. If so, don't eat it.

Busy is better. A busy restaurant will have higher customer turnover and fresher fish.

The other major concern about fish is pesticide contamination. This is particularly a problem in the farmed salmon industry. Wild salmon are born in the cold rivers that run from Alaska to California. After hatching, they struggle their way to the ocean, where they grow into mature fish, returning to their natal rivers to spawn. Most wild salmon is caught in a short period in the late spring through the summer when the fish migrate back from the oceans to the rivers. This natural life process produces a lean, high-quality fish that is high in vitamins D and E and omega-3 fatty acids.

Contrary to wild salmon, farm-raised salmon are raised in an industrialized and contained habitat that allows for mass production. They are fed an artificial diet of small fish that are ground up into fishmeal. An artificial dye is added to the fishmeal to give the fish the pinkish hue that wild salmon develop naturally from their diet in the wild.

Pollutants get into farmed salmon through the small fish used in the fishmeal they are fed. Pollutants, such as factory runoff, enter the habitat of the small fish, which absorb them. These pollutants are then highly concentrated in the fishmeal, which is fed to the farmed salmon; the pollutants are stored in the salmon's fat.

In a recent study, 700 salmon from around the world were analyzed for more than 50 contaminants. The greatest difference between farmed and wild salmon was in the presence of organochlorine compounds, and particularly the cancer-causing polychlorinated biphenyls (PCBs), dieldrin and toxaphene. Farmed salmon in Europe had the highest levels, followed by those from North America. Farm-raised Chilean salmon were the cleanest. And what about eating smoked salmon? Although smoked salmon probably has lower omega-3 fat levels and may contain some carcinogens as part of the smoking process (cold smoking may alleviate this), it is still a good choice if it is wild salmon.

The authors stated that eating more than one meal of farmed salmon per month may increase the risk of cancer. Then they got down to specifics. Table 2.2 lists the safe limits for salmon consumption.

These recommendations are for the average person. Recommendations for pregnant women are still under debate. These pollutants can damage the developing endocrine system, immune system, and brain. The compounds build up in body fat

## TABLE 2.2   Safe Levels for Salmon Consumption

| Source of salmon | Serving and frequency |
| --- | --- |
| Scotland and Faroe Islands farm raised | 2 oz (60 g) per month |
| Canada and Maine farm raised | 4 oz (120 g) per month |
| Chile and Washington State farm raised | 8 oz (240 g) per month |
| Wild salmon | 64 oz (1,920 g) per month (1 lb or 480 g per week) |

Adapted from R.A. Hites, J.A. Foran, D.O. Carpenter, et al., 2004, "Global assessment of organic contaminants in farmed salmon," *Science* 303: 226-229.

and linger there for decades—where they can be passed to a woman's fetus during pregnancy or fed to the baby through breast milk. Farmed salmon in the diets of women of childbearing age is a definite concern.

Isn't wild salmon expensive? Can you buy organic salmon instead? Wild salmon is definitely more expensive than farm-raised salmon, but it's well worth the price when you consider the risks involved and the benefits of eating salmon. But you do have some choices. During the salmon fishing season, you should be able to find half-fish fillets of wild salmon at large warehouse stores such as Costco. I buy 5 pounds (2.3 kg) at a time, cut it into portions, and freeze it. Salmon will stay fresh in a frost-free freezer for at least six weeks as long as it is well sealed.

There is still no definitive word on the organic labeling of fish. Any fish that you see that is labeled organic is not controlled by the U.S. government labeling standards the way other organic foods are. There is considerable speculation of fraud on the issue of organic fish labeling.

Finally, remember that many fish besides tuna and salmon contain omega-3 fat. Sardines, mackerel, herring, black cod, catfish, and shrimp are all excellent sources of omega-3 fat. And any fish has more omega-3 fat than a hot dog!

# Red Meat

You may have shied away from red meat in the past because it tends to be high in fat and dietary cholesterol. Red meat, however, is a good source of protein, as well as iron, zinc, and other nutrients. Incidentally, so are dark-meat turkey and chicken.

Iron is necessary for manufacturing hemoglobin, which carries oxygen from the lungs to the tissues, and myoglobin, another transporter of oxygen found only in muscle tissue. The iron in red meat and other animal proteins is known as heme iron. The body absorbs heme iron better than it absorbs iron from plant foods, known as nonheme iron.

Zinc is a busy mineral. As one of the most widely distributed minerals in the body, zinc helps the body absorb vitamins, especially the B-complex vitamins. It is also involved in digestion and metabolism and is essential for growth. Like iron, zinc from animal protein is absorbed better than zinc from plant foods.

It may surprise you to learn that red meat can be very lean. In fact, 20 of the 29 lean beef cuts have, on average, only 1 more gram of saturated fat than a skinless chicken breast per 3-ounce (90 g) serving (see table 2.3).

Red meat clearly has some nutritional pluses. The key is to control the amount of fat you get from meat. Here's how.

## Serving Size

Keep the serving size moderate, because about 3 ounces (90 g) of lean beef contains just 8.4 grams of total fat and 21 grams of total protein and is about the size of a deck of cards or the palm of a woman's hand. To get 3 ounces (90 g) of cooked meat, start with 4 ounces (120 g) of uncooked, boneless meat.

### TABLE 2.3   The 20 Leanest Cuts of Beef*

| Cut | Saturated fat (g) | Total fat (g) |
| --- | --- | --- |
| Eye of round roast and steak | 1.4 | 4.0 |
| Sirloin tip side steak | 1.6 | 4.1 |
| Top round roast and steak | 1.6 | 4.6 |
| Bottom round roast and steak | 1.7 | 4.9 |
| Top sirloin steak | 1.9 | 4.9 |
| Brisket, flat half | 1.9 | 5.1 |
| 95% lean ground beef | 2.4 | 5.1 |
| Round tip roast and steak | 1.9 | 5.3 |
| Round steak | 1.9 | 5.3 |
| Shank cross cuts | 1.9 | 5.4 |
| Chuck shoulder pot roast | 1.8 | 5.7 |
| Sirloin tip center roast and steak | 2.1 | 5.8 |
| Chuck shoulder steak | 1.9 | 6.0 |
| Bottom round steak | 2.2 | 6.0 |
| Top loin (strip) steak | 2.3 | 6.0 |
| Shoulder petite tender and medallions | 2.4 | 6.1 |
| Flank steak | 2.6 | 6.3 |
| Shoulder center (ranch) steak | 2.4 | 6.5 |
| Tri-tip roast and steak | 2.6 | 7.1 |
| Tenderloin roast and steak | 2.7 | 7.1 |
| T-bone steak | 3.0 | 8.2 |

*Per 3 oz. (85 g) cooked portion trimmed of visible fat

Data from U.S. Department of Agriculture, Agricultural Research Service. 2008. USDA National Nutrient Database for Standard Reference, Release 21.

## Grade

Beef is graded according to fat marbling: prime, choice, and select. Select is the leanest grade. When choosing beef, look for lean cuts closely trimmed of fat, or trim them yourself at home before cooking them. Pork is also a leaner meat than it used to be. The leanest cuts of pork come from the loin and leg areas, and a 3-ounce (90 g) cooked and trimmed portion of any of these cuts contains fewer than 9 grams of fat and 180 calories. Lamb and veal are also lower in fat than beef. Follow the same guidelines for selecting lean cuts.

## Preparation

To keep a lean cut tasty after cooking, you must handle and prepare it properly. Because leaner cuts have less fat to keep them moist and juicy, the method of preparation is important. More tender cuts, such as loin cuts, can be broiled or grilled and served immediately. Avoid overcooking. Beef can also be marinated to tenderize it. Because it is the acid in the marinade (vinegar, citrus juice, or wine) that tenderizes the meat, oil can be replaced with water without diminishing the tenderizing effect. To improve the tenderness of roasts, carve them into thin slices on the diagonal and across the grain when possible.

## Beef Safety Tips

Consumer confidence in beef is fairly high despite concerns around the globe regarding mad cow disease. Even so, you should take precautions to protect yourself against any meat-related disease, including food-borne illnesses. Here's what you can do to take charge of beef safety:

- Choose beef cuts that are likely to be free of bone tissue and nervous system tissue (the brain, spinal cord, and nerve endings). These tissues are the most infectious part of a cow with mad cow disease. Safer beef cuts include boneless cuts such as boneless steaks, chops, and roasts, as well as beef products from grass-fed and organic cattle. T-bone steaks, porterhouse steaks, prime ribs with bone, beef tips, and bone-in roasts carry miniscule risk.

- Avoid ground beef as much as possible; it may contain bone and nervous system tissue. If you do eat ground beef, use a food thermometer to make sure it is cooked to 160 degrees Fahrenheit (71 degrees Celsius), eliminating any food-borne bacteria in the meat. Wash the thermometer immediately after using it. If you order ground beef in a restaurant, ask your server if it has been cooked to at least 155 degrees Fahrenheit (68 degrees Celsius) for 15 seconds (a safe option for restaurants).

- Be wary of products that contain beef extracted by advanced meat recovery (AMR) machines that squeeze out as much meat as possible from cow carcasses. AMR meat may be used in hot dogs, taco fillings, pizza toppings, sausages, and beef jerky made from ground or chopped meat. Unfortunately, manufacturers are not yet required to identify AMR beef on food labels.

## Going Meatless, Staying Muscular

Can you be a vegetarian and still build muscle? Absolutely—as long as you plan your diet properly. The key is to mix and match foods so that you get the right balance of amino acids.

You can think of amino acids as a construction crew building a house. Each crew member has a specific function, from framing to wiring. If just one crew member calls off, then the construction job doesn't get finished. It's the same with amino acids. There are 22 amino acids, all of which combine to construct the proteins required for growth and tissue repair. For your body to build protein, all of these amino acids must be on the job. If just one amino acid is missing or even if the concentration of an amino acid is low, protein construction comes to a halt.

Of the 22 amino acids, 8 cannot be made by the body; they must be supplied by the food you eat. These 8 amino acids are called the essential amino acids. Seven of the 22 amino acids are termed conditionally essential amino acids. This means that they are made by the body but, under certain conditions, are required in greater amounts. The remaining 7, which can be manufactured by the body, are known as the nonessential amino acids. Your body makes nonessential amino acids from carbohydrate and nitrogen and by chemically re-sorting essential and nonessential amino acids. (The essential, conditionally essential, and nonessential amino acids are listed in table 2.1.)

Foods that contain all the essential amino acids in the amounts required for health and growth are called complete proteins. Proteins found in dairy products, eggs, meat, poultry, fish, and other animal sources are complete proteins. Various plant foods typically provide incomplete proteins that either completely lack or are low in a particular essential amino acid. The essential amino acid that is missing or in short supply is called the limiting amino acid.

To get enough essential amino acids from a vegetarian diet, select foods that complement one another's limiting amino acids. In other words, mix and match foods during the day so that foods low in one essential amino acid are balanced by those that are higher in the same amino acid. It's not necessary to combine these proteins at one meal; you can simply eat a variety of protein sources throughout the day. For example, grains contain a limited amount of lysine but a higher amount of methionine. Legumes such as navy beans, kidney beans, and black beans are high in lysine but low in methionine. Thus, by combining grains and legumes, you create a complete protein meal. Soybeans are an exception and are considered a complete protein. Other fully nutritious protein combinations are as follows:

- Rice and beans
- Corn and beans
- Corn and lima beans
- Corn tortillas and refried beans
- Pasta and bean soup

If you are a vegetarian who chooses to eat milk and eggs, you needn't worry about combining foods. The protein in milk, eggs, cheeses, and other dairy products contains all the essential amino acids you need for tissue growth, repair, and maintenance. A word of caution, though: Dairy products can be high in fat, so be sure to choose low-fat or nonfat dairy foods such as milk, cheese, and yogurt. As for eggs, limit yourself to one egg yolk a day. Most of the protein is found in the egg white anyway.

Whether you choose to include or exclude meat in your diet is a matter of personal choice. If you decide to go meatless, plan your diet carefully to avoid certain nutritional danger zones—namely, iron, zinc, and vitamin $B_{12}$ deficiencies. These deficiencies can hurt exercise performance. It is important to consider the following nutrients to help you avoid deficiencies if you're a vegetarian strength trainer.

- **Protein.** A challenge for vegetarian strength trainers is to obtain the 2 grams of high-quality protein per kilogram of body weight required daily to support muscle growth. You can do this by including plenty of low-fat dairy products and protein-rich plant sources in your diet. If you are a pure vegan (you eat no animal foods at all), increase your daily protein intake to 2.2 grams of protein per kilogram of body weight.

- **Heme iron.** Include some sources of heme iron in your diet. As noted, all types of animal protein contain the more easily absorbed form of iron, heme iron. If you're a semivegetarian—that is, still eating fish or chicken but no red meat—you're in luck, because chicken and fish contain heme iron. If you avoid animal protein, you won't be consuming heme iron. That means you have to work harder to get all the iron you need. No easy absorption tactics will be available to you.

- **MFP factor.** Meat, fish, and poultry (MFP) contain a special quality called the MFP factor that helps your body absorb more nonheme iron. When meat and vegetables are eaten together at the same meal, more nonheme iron is absorbed from the vegetables than if the vegetables had been eaten alone. If you're a semivegetarian, your slightly lower iron intake will signal your body to absorb extra iron from vegetables.

- **Vitamin C.** Fruits, vegetables, and other foods that contain vitamin C help the body absorb nonheme iron. For example, if you eat citrus fruits with an iron-fortified cereal, your body will absorb more iron from the cereal than if it had been eaten alone.

- **Vitamin $B_{12}$.** Guard against a vitamin $B_{12}$ deficiency. Vitamin $B_{12}$ is one of the most significant nutrients typically missing from the diets of vegans. That's because it is available only from animal products. Fortunately, the body needs only tiny daily amounts of this vitamin (the DRI is 2.4 mcg for adults), which is used in the manufacture of red blood cells and nerves. Even so, a deficiency is serious, potentially causing irreversible nerve damage.

  Fermented foods, such as the soybean products miso and tempeh, supply some vitamin $B_{12}$ from the bacterial culture that causes fermentation, but generally not enough. Vegans should eat foods fortified with $B_{12}$ or take supplements to ensure a healthy diet.

- **Iron and Zinc.** Some foods contain phytates, oxalates, or other substances that block the absorption of iron and zinc in the intestine. Coffee and tea (regular and decaffeinated), whole grains, bran, legumes, and spinach are a few examples of foods containing blockers. These foods are best eaten with sources of heme iron or vitamin C to help your body absorb more iron and zinc. In addition, consider iron and zinc supplements. Our bodies don't absorb the iron that comes from vegetables as easily as the iron that comes from animal foods. Non-meat eaters, especially active people or menstruating women, must pay attention to their dietary iron needs. Animal flesh is the major source of zinc in most diets, so all vegetarians may be at greater risk of having low intakes of this mineral.

Although dietary supplements are not replacements for food, it may be a good idea to supplement if iron and zinc are in short supply in your diet. Daily supplementation of iron and zinc at 100 percent of the DRI is insurance against harmful deficiencies.

## POWER PROFILES: Vegetarianism

I once worked with a professional basketball player who, for philosophical reasons, was a lacto-ovo vegetarian (i.e., he ate no animal foods except dairy and egg products). He was determined to stick to his vegetarian game plan both on the road and at home.

Unexpectedly, this player's biggest problem was not protein. He was getting plenty of protein from dairy products. But he wasn't getting enough iron, selenium, and zinc—minerals that are plentiful in meat. In addition, his diet was high in fat because he was eating a lot of cheese-laden vegetable lasagna.

To solve the mineral problem, he began taking a mineral supplement containing the RDA of the minerals he was lacking. After basketball practice, he started drinking one or two meal-replacement beverages, which contain extra nutrients and fit perfectly into a lacto-ovo vegetarian diet.

With my help, he discovered several new low-fat recipes, such as vegetarian chili, that he could pack for road trips as long as he had a microwave oven in his hotel room. He took dried fruit on the road, too, which can be eaten anywhere and is loaded with minerals and energy-packed calories.

At home, he began to vary his diet using vegetarian staples such as beans, tofu, rice, and peanut butter. By varying his diet, he was also getting plenty of quality calories to fuel both training and competition. Equally important, he learned that he didn't have to sacrifice his beliefs for athletic performance.

## Protein Quality and Types

As an exerciser or athlete, you should be concerned about the quality as well as the type of protein you eat. The bottom line is that you need either high-quality protein or a variety of protein sources to ensure adequate intake of all eight essential amino acids—particularly after exercise.

# How Do You Rate Protein Quality?

Protein is rated on its quality, or the content of essential amino acids. To rate the quality of the protein in foods, scientists have developed a number of measurement methods. Here's a rundown of the three most common methods.

### Protein Digestibility Corrected Amino Acid Score (PDCAAS)

The protein values you read on food labels are calculated using the PDCAAS. It describes the proportion of amino acids in a protein source, as well as its digestibility, or how well a protein is used by the body. In calculating the PDCAAS, the food is first assigned a score based on its amino acid composition. The score is then adjusted to reflect its digestibility.

Digestibility, which varies from food to food, is important. Generally, more than 90 percent of the protein in animal foods is digested and absorbed, whereas about 80 percent of the protein in legumes is used. Between 60 and 90 percent of the protein in fruits, vegetables, and grains is digested and absorbed. With the PDCAAS, the highest possible score is 100. For reference, egg whites, ground beef, milk powder, and tuna have scores of 100; soy protein has a score of 94.

### Protein Efficiency Rating (PER)

The PER reflects a particular protein's ability to support weight gain in test animals and gives researchers a good indication of which foods best promote growth. The yardstick for comparison is the growth produced by the complete protein found in egg whites or milk. Egg protein, in particular, is considered the perfect protein, because it contains all eight essential amino acids in the ideal proportions and is the reservoir of nutrients to grow a bird.

### Biological Value (BV)

The BV represents the percentage of protein absorbed from a particular food that your body can use for growth and repair rather than for energy production. As with the PER, the BV of egg whites serves as the yardstick by which other protein sources are compared. Complete proteins tend to have high biological values, whereas incomplete proteins have lower values. Lower BV foods are used mainly for fuel rather than for growth and repair.

# What Kind of Protein?

To bump up the protein in your diet, consider some additional sources of protein (besides lean choices such as fish, poultry, or meat) such as low-fat dairy and soy proteins. I am a major proponent of milk in the diets of athletes—for two important reasons. First, when taken after strength training, milk proteins have been shown in research to affect the development of muscle. Specifically, these proteins work by stimulating the uptake of amino acids by the muscle—a process that leads to the building of muscle. The two proteins found in milk are whey and casein; both have beneficial actions in producing muscle gains (see the following discussion).

Also, research with animals hints that lactose, a sugar found in milk, may also be instrumental in stimulating muscle development. This is probably because lactose slightly elevates insulin, and insulin is necessary for pushing protein into muscle cells for energy, growth, and development.

The second reason I advocate that athletes drink milk is that milk is naturally high in the amino acid tryptophan. This amino acid elevates brain levels of serotonin, a natural chemical that makes you feel good mentally and emotionally. And milk has a small amount of natural carbohydrate, lactose. The protein-carbohydrate partnership supports the manufacture of serotonin in the brain. When you're in a good mood, you just feel more motivated to work out and achieve your fitness goals.

That said, what follows is a rundown on the benefits of various types of protein to consider as additions to your diet.

### Whey

Whey is a natural, complete protein derived from cow's milk and available in protein supplements, and it provides numerous benefits if you strength train. Whey is considered a "fast protein" because it is digested and absorbed quickly, making amino acids readily available for muscle repair. Whey is thus ideal to consume immediately after exercise because of its rapid uptake. As noted earlier, whey is high in leucine—a branched-chain amino acid that can help you maintain an anabolic state. In recent years there has been a tremendous amount of research on whey protein and its influence on muscle protein synthesis and degradation. To briefly summarize this research, whey protein does the following:

- Enhances protein synthesis, outperforming most other sources of protein in this regard
- Limits the degradation or the damage that occurs from exercise
- Enhances recovery repair and growth
- Promotes cellular growth and immunity
- Is vital for a healthy nervous system and brain
- Is an abundant source of the amino acid leucine, which is directly involved in muscle growth
- Boasts an ideal proportion of essential amino acids to stimulate synthesis and enhance the training response
- Stimulates fat-burning mechanisms in the liver and muscle, as well as making more fat available for fuel during exercise

Of course, for anyone who is a vegan, whey protein is not an option. If you are lactose intolerant, however, whey protein isolate or soy protein is a very good option (discussed later).

### Casein

Casein is another milk-derived protein that is also available in protein supplements. It is considered to be a "slow protein" because it generally forms into a solid in the stomach and is delivered to the muscles more slowly—in a timed-release fashion. Consuming casein prior to working out is a good move because of this sustained action in feeding your muscles. Both milk proteins are high in glutamine, an amino acid that assists in muscle building and in fortifying your body's immune system.

### Soy Protein

Soy protein is a complete protein extracted from soybeans that provides the essential amino acids to meet basic protein needs. However, a diet that is 100 percent dependent on soy protein may not be adequate to meet the needs of a person trying to gain muscle and strength. Soy, however, is a good substitute if you are a vegetarian or have a sensitivity to milk proteins. Soy protein also contains isoflavones, which have a number of potential health benefits.

Recent research with strength trainers has investigated a blend of dairy and soy protein supplementation. Only one animal study showed any benefit to the blend of whey, casein, and soy in extending muscle protein synthesis posttraining. It is much too early to make any evidence-based recommendations regarding blended protein supplements that include soy.

Several recent studies of the influence of soy protein in weight-loss diets appear to conclude that soy protein doesn't confer an advantage. The biggest advantage of soy protein is that it is an alternative protein supplement when whey protein can't be used, isn't available, or is unpalatable to an athlete. This doesn't mean that soy protein should not be used. As a food source, it offers important nutrients and phytochemicals and is an excellent source of plant protein, giving variety to the diet as well as these important compounds. As a supplement, soy protein also offers variety. It is still a good protein source, nurturing the body and providing the essential amino acids required for muscle repair, recovery, and growth.

Finally, a discussion of soy protein cannot exclude the questions regarding genetically modified organisms (GMOs) and soy foods. It would take a treatise to give this topic the discussion that it deserves, but in a nutshell, we still don't really know for sure whether genetic modification helps or harms us, society, or the environment. In fact, the process may do a little bit of both depending on who you are, where you live, and where the crops are grown. Because I want to be an informed consumer, I believe that products containing GMO ingredients should be labeled as such so that I can make an informed choice.

### Egg Protein

Egg (ovalbumen) protein was once considered the best source of protein, especially in supplements. But because egg protein is fairly expensive compared with other forms of quality protein, its popularity has decreased.

## The Bottom Line on Protein

Protein is definitely a key to manufacturing muscle, and the latest research shows that strength trainers who are building muscle, are vegetarians, or do cross-training require slightly elevated amounts of protein. You don't have to go overboard, though, because your body will extract exactly what it needs. By following the recommendations here, you'll get the optimal amount of protein to build muscle and maintain strength.

## Sport Nutrition Fact Versus Fiction: Supplemental Amino Acids Build Muscle

For a long time, a debate has raged as to whether exercisers and athletes should take amino acid supplements as a natural way to enhance the muscle-building process. Today, the talk focuses more on the importance of the timing and type of protein and amino acid intake relative to muscle growth and performance. A mound of research validates the need to take protein prior to and after exercise to activate the repair and growth of lean muscle mass.

As for amino acids, in particular, researchers at the University of Texas tested the hypothesis that taking 6 grams of essential amino acids orally one to two hours after strength training stimulates the manufacture of lean muscle. The two amino acids used in the study were leucine and phenylalanine. When volunteers took a drink containing these amino acids following strength training, there was a positive increase in net muscle protein in their muscles—an indication that new muscle was being manufactured.

Another amino acid, arginine, has been shown in research to initiate recovery following exercise. In one study, exercisers consumed either a carbohydrate supplement or a carbohydrate–arginine supplement one, two, and three hours after exercise. The supplements were formulated with either 1 gram of carbohydrate per kilogram of body weight or 1 gram of carbohydrate plus 0.08 gram of arginine per kilogram of body weight. During the four-hour recovery period, the increase in muscle glycogen was more rapid in those who had consumed the carbohydrate–arginine formula.

The researchers attributed this response to arginine's ability to increase the availability of glucose for muscle glycogen storage during recovery. There were some untoward side effects associated with the carbohydrate–arginine supplement, however. These included bitter taste and diarrhea.

As for the BCAAs—leucine, isoleucine, and valine—they make up about one third of your muscle protein. They work together to rebuild muscle protein, which is dismantled by exercise, and act as fuel for exercise. The harder you work out, the more leucine your body will use. After aerobic exercise, plasma leucine levels drop 11 to 33 percent; after strength-training exercise, they drop 30 percent. Furthermore, high-intensity aerobic exercise drains skeletal muscle stores of leucine.

For strength trainers, supplementing with leucine (50 mg per kg of body weight a day), along with a daily protein intake of 1.26 kilograms of protein per kilogram of body weight, can prevent a decrease in leucine during five weeks of speed and strength training, according to one study.

> *continued*

> *continued*

Other research indicates that consuming BCAAs (30 to 35 percent leucine) before or during endurance training may decrease, or even prevent, the rate of protein degradation in the muscle, plus spare muscle glycogen.

So should you supplement with BCAAs? Consider these facts: Your body starts drawing on BCAAs for fuel during exercise only if you're not eating enough or taking in sufficient carbohydrate (carbohydrate keeps the body from burning up too much of its BCAA supply). In other words, you should be able to get all the BCAAs you need from food. That's easy to do. Each of the following foods contains all the BCAAs you need daily to prevent protein breakdown during aerobic exercise:

- 3 ounces (90 g) of water-packed tuna
- 3 ounces (90 g) of chicken
- 1 cup (230 g) of nonfat yogurt
- 1 cup of cooked legumes

In addition, a great way to replace BCAAs lost during exercise is to consume dairy products or whey protein after your workout.

Although the research into individual amino acid supplements is very compelling, I am still not an absolute proponent of using these supplements. I would rather see you get your amino acids naturally—from food, or at least whole protein supplement sources. And just as important, time your protein intake by having a small mixed meal of protein, carbohydrate, and some fat prior to and after your strength-training session.

Food remains the best protein source for your body. One of the main reasons has to do with absorption. All nutrients are absorbed better when they come from real food. There are substances in foods, which scientists have coined "food factors," that help the body absorb and use nutrients. We don't even know what many of these food factors are, but we do know that they aren't found in food supplements.

As for protein, it is one of the best-absorbed foods, particularly animal protein. Scientific research has found that 95 to 99 percent of animal protein is absorbed and used by the body. Even protein from plant sources is well absorbed: more than 90 percent of the protein from high-protein plants is taken up and put to use by the body.

If you eat a variety of protein sources (see table 2.4), you don't need to take protein or amino acid supplements. However, protein supplements are an important convenience in the diets of most active people. Just 1 ounce (30 g) of chicken contains 7,000 milligrams of amino acids. To get that much, you might pay $20 for an entire bottle of amino acid supplements!

## TABLE 2.4 Good Sources of Protein

| Food | Amount | Protein (g) | Calories |
|------|--------|-------------|----------|
| **Animal foods** | | | |
| Beef, lean, sirloin, broiled | 3 oz (90 g) | 26 | 172 |
| Roasted chicken breast (boneless, no skin) | 3 oz (90 g) | 26 | 140 |
| Sole or flounder, baked or broiled | 3 oz (90 g) | 21 | 100 |
| Turkey | 3 oz (90 g) | 25 | 145 |
| **Dairy products** | | | |
| Cheese | 1 oz (30 g) | 8 | 107 |
| Cottage cheese, 2% | 1/2 cup (105 g) | 16 | 101 |
| Egg, boiled | 1 large | 6 | 78 |
| Egg white, cooked | 1 large | 4 | 78 |
| Milk, dried nonfat, instant | 1/2 cup (34 g) | 12 | 122 |
| Milk, low-fat, 1% | 1 cup (240 ml) | 8 | 102 |
| Milk, nonfat | 1 cup (240 ml) | 8 | 86 |
| Yogurt, low-fat, plain | 8 oz (230 g) | 13 | 155 |
| Yogurt, low-fat, fruit | 8 oz (230 g) | 11 | 250 |
| **Nuts, seeds, and nut products** | | | |
| Peanuts, dry roasted | 1 oz (30 g) | 7 | 166 |
| Peanut butter | 2 tbsp | 8 | 190 |
| Pumpkin seeds, dry roasted | 1/2 cup (114 g) | 6 | 143 |
| Sunflower seeds, dry roasted, hulled | 2 tbsp | 3 | 93 |
| **Soy products** | | | |
| Soybeans, cooked | 1/2 cup (90 g) | 15 | 149 |
| Soy milk | 1 cup (240 ml) | 8 | 79 |
| Tofu | 1/2 cup (126 g) | 10 | 94 |
| **Vegetables, high protein** | | | |
| Black beans, boiled | 1/2 cup (86 g) | 8 | 114 |
| Chickpeas (garbanzos), boiled | 1/2 cup (82 g) | 7 | 135 |
| Lentils, boiled | 1/2 cup (99 g) | 9 | 115 |
| Pinto beans | 1/2 cup (86 g) | 7 | 117 |

# 3

# Fueling Workouts

From the oatmeal you eat for breakfast to the baked potato you eat for dinner, carbohydrate is the leading nutrient fuel for your body. During digestion, carbohydrate is broken down into glucose. Glucose circulates in the blood, where it is known as blood sugar, to be used by the brain and nervous system for energy. If your brain cells are deprived of glucose, your mental power will suffer, and because your brain controls your muscles, you might even feel weak and shaky.

Glucose from the breakdown of carbohydrate is also converted to glycogen for storage in either liver or muscle. Two thirds of your body's glycogen is stored in the muscles, and about one third is stored in the liver. When muscles use glycogen, they break it back down into glucose through a series of energy-producing steps.

It is no surprise that vegetables, fruit, cereal, pasta, grains, sport drinks, energy bars, and other forms of carbohydrate are the foods of choice for endurance athletes, who load up on carbohydrate to improve their performance in competition. But carbohydrate is just as necessary for strength trainers as it is for endurance athletes—in the right amounts, and combined with protein and fat. The glycogen provided by carbohydrate is the major source of fuel for working muscles. When carbohydrate is in short supply, your muscles get tired and heavy. Carbohydrate, particularly in combination with protein and fat, is thus a vital nutrient that keeps your mind and muscles powered up for hard training and muscle building.

The amount of carbohydrate you need in your diet each day varies, depending on your training goals, how frequently and intensively you train, your gender, and your own individual needs. After decades of working with athletes at all levels and in all kinds of sports, I have noted that carbohydrate is needed in highly variable amounts from one individual to another even doing the same level of exercise. In general, to fuel performance, athletes need from 4.5 to 10 grams of carbohydrate per kilogram of body weight every day. This very large range depends on the factors noted earlier, including the type of exercise; exercise goals; the frequency, intensity, and duration of exercise; gender; and the weight requirements of the sport. Carbohydrate needs are different still when the goal of the diet and training program is to lose fat. That discussion can be found in chapters 4 and 5 of this book.

# The Force Behind Muscle Building and Fat Burning

Among the nutrients, carbohydrate is the most powerful in affecting your energy levels. But it also affects your muscle-building and fat-burning power. It takes about 2,500 calories to build just 1 pound (0.5 kg) of muscle. That's a lot of energy! The best source of that energy is carbohydrate. It provides the cleanest, most immediate source of energy for body cells. In fact, your body prefers to burn carbohydrate over fat or protein. As your body's favored fuel source, carbohydrate spares protein from being used as energy. Protein is thus free to do its main job—building and repairing body tissue, including muscle.

Carbohydrate is a must for efficient fat burning, too. Your body burns fat for energy in a series of complex chemical reactions that take place inside cells. Think of fat as a log on a hearth waiting to be ignited. Carbohydrate is the match that ignites fat at the cellular level. Unless enough carbohydrate is available in key stages of the energy-producing process, fat will just smolder—in other words, not burn as cleanly or completely.

Carbohydrate also raises carnitine levels in muscle cells. Carnitine is an amino acid–like nutrient that carries fat into the mitochondria of cells (the machinery that burns fat for fuel). Researchers at the University of Nottingham gave healthy young men carnitine, as well as insulin and glucose, intravenously at the same time. The researchers supplied just enough glucose to keep the blood sugar levels of their subjects constant. The treatment lasted for five hours.

The more insulin is circulating in the body, the higher the level of carnitine in the muscles following carnitine supplementation. This suggests that carnitine probably works best when taken with a well-balanced meal that includes carbohydrate.

The implication here is that endurance athletes who load up on carbohydrate before a race might be further helped by carnitine supplements. The same may be true for high-power athletes such as downhill mountain bike racers, who operate in the anaerobic zone almost exclusively. These athletes may even be helped more by carnitine supplementation. Strength trainers who want to give their muscles a glycogen boost before training may also find a benefit. Keep in mind that the research in this area is very young, and we don't know whether the results from dietary consumption are specific to the type of carnitine and carbohydrate used in the study, or that it's a generalized effect. Clearly, the insulin spike is a key component to getting carnitine into muscle cells.

# Increase Carbohydrate Calories

The most important nutritional factor affecting muscle gain is calories—specifically, calories from carbohydrate. Building muscle requires a rigorous strength-training program. A tremendous amount of energy is required to fuel this type of exercise—energy that is best supplied by carbohydrate. A carbohydrate-dense diet allows for the greatest recovery of muscle glycogen stores on a daily basis. This ongoing replenishment lets your muscles work equally hard on successive days. Studies continue to show that carbohydrate-dense diets give strength-training athletes an edge in their workouts; and the bottom line is, the harder you train, the more muscle you can build.

To build 1 pound (0.5 kg) of muscle, add 2,500 calories a week. This means introducing extra calories into your diet. Ideally, women must increase their calorie intake by 300 a day; and men, by 400. Research has shown this to be the optimal increase to begin building muscle and minimize fat gain.

You should increase your calorie consumption gradually so that you don't gain too much fat. What I suggest to strength trainers in a building phase is to start by introducing only 300 to 350 more calories per day. Then after a week or two, add another 300 to 400 calories a day. As long as you're not gaining fat, start introducing extra calories into your diet weekly, again at the same rate of 300 to 400 calories. (Incidentally, for losing fat, you can drop calories by the same amount—300 calories a day for women and 400 calories a day for men.)

But back to increasing calories: Most of these additional calories should come from carbohydrate in the form of food and liquid carbohydrate supplements. An example of 300 to 400 calories worth of carbohydrate from food is 1/2 cup (70 g) of whole-grain pasta, 1/2 cup of yams (68 g) and one banana. It just doesn't take that much additional food to increase your carbohydrate intake. Later in the book, I'll show you how to time your carbohydrate intake properly and how to combine the additional carbohydrate with the right foods to enhance muscle building.

When I'm working with athletes, I make sure their protein and fat needs are taken care of; then I look at their carbohydrate intake. I adjust calories by increasing or decreasing carbohydrate calories. Carbohydrate calories are the fuel, so if someone wants to gain weight, carbohydrate calories go up; to lose fat, carbohydrate calories go down. Remember, you should always eat carbohydrate in combination with the right amounts of protein and fat; it should not be consumed alone except perhaps in a sport drink when you just can't eat any additional solid food. (Sport drinks, however, should only be consumed during training, not as a beverage during the day.)

To be really exact, you can match your carbohydrate intake to your weight. If you are a strength trainer and want to build muscle, you should take in about 4.5 to 7 grams of carbohydrate per kilogram of body weight a day, depending on whether you are female or male and the stage of your training. An athlete who cross-trains with strength training, wants to build, and does any type of endurance activity needs anywhere from 5 to more than 10 grams per kilogram of body weight a day based on the same factors.

Supplementing with liquid carbohydrate, including smoothies, is an excellent way to increase those calories, boost carbohydrate and protein consumption, and take in nutrients conveniently. It's also a great way to consume nutrients when you don't feel like eating, particularly after a heavy weight-training session. In addition, liquid nutrition is absorbed faster than nutrition from solid foods is. Liquid supplementation also appears to support muscle growth.

In a landmark experiment, competitive weightlifters took a liquid high-calorie supplement for 15 weeks. The goal of the study was to see how the supplement affected the athletes' weight gain, body composition, and strength. The weightlifters were divided into three groups: those using the supplement and no anabolic steroids, those using the supplement plus anabolic steroids, and a control group taking no supplements or steroids but participating in exercise. (This study was conducted many years ago and obviously could not be repeated today because of the drug use.) The supplement contained 540 calories and 70.5 grams of carbohydrate, plus other nutrients.

All of the participants followed their usual diets. The steroid group and the control group ate most of their calories in the form of fat rather than carbohydrate (45 percent fat, 37 percent carbohydrate). The supplement group ate more carbohydrate and less fat (34 percent fat, 47 percent carbohydrate). What's more, the supplement group ate about 830 more calories a day than the control group and 1,300 more calories a day than the steroid group.

Here's what happened: The weight gain in both supplemented groups was significantly greater than in the control group. Those in the supplement-only group gained an average of 7 pounds (3 kg); those in the supplement and steroid group, 10 pounds (4.5 kg); and those in the control group, 3.5 pounds (1.6 kg). Lean mass in both the supplement and steroid groups more than doubled compared with the control group. The supplement group lost 0.91 percent body fat, whereas the steroid group gained 0.5 percent body fat. Both the supplement and steroid groups gained strength—equally.

These results are amazing. They prove that ample calories and carbohydrate are essential for a successful strength-training and muscle-building program. Even more astounding is the fact that you can potentially attain the same results with diet alone as you can with drugs. That's powerful news for drug-free strength trainers everywhere. In chapter 13, you'll learn how to plan your own carbohydrate-dense diet to support muscle growth.

## Choose the Right Carbohydrate

Not just any type of carbohydrate is appropriate for building lean mass and developing a fit, streamlined physique. The right types of carbohydrate come from unrefined, whole foods such as fruits, vegetables, legumes, and whole grains. There is also some carbohydrate in milk from lactose, the milk sugar. By contrast, the wrong types of carbohydrate come from processed foods, including sugar, high-fructose corn syrup, white flour, white rice, commercial baked goods, many packaged foods, and alcohol. Processed foods have been stripped of their important nutritional factors, including fiber. Because they lack fiber, it is easy to eat huge quantities of calories without feeling full. Foods with processed carbohydrate are the ones you should mostly avoid.

Not surprisingly, people who eat the right types of carbohydrate tend to have lower body weights and better control of blood lipids and carbohydrate metabolism when compared with those who eat predominantly simple sugars. Increased whole-grain intake in particular is associated with decreased risks of obesity, coronary heart disease, type 2 diabetes, insulin resistance, and many causes of illness. Thus, by replacing bad types of carbohydrate with good ones, you gain better control over most of the physiological and metabolic risk factors associated with the development of obesity and chronic disease.

## Sport Nutrition Fact Versus Fiction: Does Carbohydrate Make You Fat?

The media is currently beating the drum about the contention that carbohydrate-dense diets make people fat and are therefore bad. This is based on the fact that overweight and obesity are risk factors for the development of insulin resistance, a condition in which the pancreas oversecretes insulin to maintain normal blood levels of glucose after a carbohydrate-dense meal. This oversecretion causes carbohydrate to be converted to stored body fat, leading to more overweight and obesity, and ultimately landing people on the pathway to the development of type 2 diabetes.

Although this may be true for a sedentary population, it's just not the same case with athletes and other active people. In fact, for bodybuilders, insulin is an anabolic hormone that helps build muscle mass by fueling the muscles.

As someone who's active, you're already keeping your insulin levels in line. Although the exact mechanism isn't clear, exercise makes muscle cells more sensitive to insulin. For glucose to enter muscle cells, it has to have help from insulin. Once insulin gets to the outer surface of the cell, it acts like a key and unlocks tiny receptors surrounding the cell. The cell opens and lets glucose in for use as fuel. Maintaining muscle tissue through strength training helps normalize the flow of glucose from the blood into muscle cells, where it can be properly used for energy.

Should you be worried about eating pasta and bread? No! But you should concentrate on a variety of whole-carbohydrate foods such as beans, whole grains, fruits, and vegetables in addition to whole-grain bread and pasta. Even in the unlikely event that you are insulin resistant, the variety minimizes the effects, as does mixing carbohydrate with protein and fat. Also, staying active helps control body weight and builds muscle tissue, which helps regulate the body's use of glucose.

Insulin and carbohydrate are not the bad guys when it comes to fat—calories, poor diet planning, and a sedentary lifestyle are. You gain body fat when you remain inactive, make poor choices, and eat more calories than you burn. It's just that simple.

## High in Fiber

The right carbohydrate is high in fiber, which is found only in plant foods, primarily whole foods and largely unprocessed foods. It is a structural and storage form of carbohydrate and is not digested as it passes through the human digestive system. Fiber is classified by its ability to dissolve in water, and there are two types: water soluble and water insoluble. Soluble fibers, which come primarily from beans, fruits, and whole grains, can be dissolved in water and include plant material such as gums, mucilages, pectin, and some hemicelluloses. Insoluble fibers, which come primarily from vegetables, beans, whole wheat, and fruit skins, do not dissolve in water and include lignins, cellulose, and some hemicelluloses. Both types of fiber improve the work of the intestines, although in different ways. Water-soluble fiber is generally sticky and viscous and slows down the movement of food through the digestive tract. Water-insoluble fiber acts like a stool softener and bulk former and keeps things moving through the system.

Want to know an easy way to stay lean and healthy? Add 5 more grams of fiber to your diet every day. Just 5 more grams a day will reduce your chances of experiencing an expanding waistline and becoming overweight. The latest research out of France has shown that a 5-gram increase in total dietary fiber can reduce the risk of becoming overweight by almost 11 percent and reduce the risk of an expanding waistline by almost 15 percent. This relationship was particularly strong with insoluble fiber from fruit, dried fruit, nuts, and seeds.

Another study published by a research group from Harvard showed that women who increased fiber intake by about 8 grams per day ate 150 fewer calories per day than those who decreased their fiber intake by 3 grams per day during the study. During the 12 years of the study, the women with the highest fiber consumption lost about 8 pounds (3.6 kg), compared with a nearly 20-pound (9 kg) weight gain for those who cut their fiber intake during those years.

How does fiber work its weight-controlling wonders? First, high-fiber foods take longer to eat, resulting in a full, satisfied feeling. Second, they lower levels of insulin, a hormone that stimulates appetite. Third, more energy (calories) is used up during the digestion and absorption of high-fiber foods. Fourth, high-fiber diets are lower in calories and help you naturally manage your weight. In addition, studies have substantiated that one of the primary reasons people succeed at keeping weight off is that they stick to a high-fiber diet over time. One more important point: By avoiding obesity through a high-fiber diet, you lower your risks for the development and progression of cardiovascular disease, cancer, hypertension, and diabetes. Table 3.1 provides a list of the best high-fiber foods for strength trainers, bodybuilders, exercisers, and other athletes.

Here's a question a lot of my clients ask me when I advise upping their fiber intake: How do you get a lot of fiber in your diet without feeling bloated or being in the bathroom all the time? The answer is to stick to your regimen of smaller multiple meals that include carbohydrate, protein, and fat. These small, frequent meals give you timed-release energy while lowering the total volume of fiber you take in at any one time.

## TABLE 3.1 Food Sources of Dietary Fiber Ranked

| Food, standard amount | Dietary fiber (g) | Calories |
|---|---|---|
| Navy beans, cooked, 1/2 cup (91 g) | 9.5 | 128 |
| Bran ready-to-eat cereal (100%), 1/2 cup (30 g) | 8.8 | 78 |
| Kidney beans, canned, 1/2 cup (89 g) | 8.2 | 109 |
| Split peas, cooked, 1/2 cup (98 g) | 8.1 | 116 |
| Lentils, cooked, 1/2 cup (99 g) | 7.8 | 115 |
| Black beans, cooked, 1/2 cup (86 g) | 7.5 | 114 |
| Pinto beans, cooked, 1/2 cup (86 g) | 7.7 | 122 |
| Lima beans, cooked, 1/2 cup (85 g) | 6.6 | 108 |
| Artichoke, globe, cooked, 1 each | 6.5 | 60 |
| White beans, canned, 1/2 cup (90 g) | 6.3 | 154 |
| Chickpeas, cooked, 1/2 cup (82 g) | 6.2 | 135 |
| Great northern beans, cooked, 1/2 cup (89 g) | 6.2 | 105 |
| Cowpeas, cooked, 1/2 cup (83 g) | 5.6 | 100 |
| Soybeans, mature, cooked, 1/2 cup (90 g) | 5.2 | 149 |
| Bran ready-to-eat cereals, various, ~1 oz (~30 g) | 2.6-5.0 | 90-108 |
| Crackers, rye wafers, plain, 2 wafers | 5.0 | 74 |
| Sweet potato, baked, with peel, 1 medium | 4.8 | 131 |
| Asian pear, raw, 1 small | 4.4 | 51 |
| Green peas, cooked, 1/2 cup (80 g) | 4.4 | 67 |
| Whole-wheat English muffin | 4.4 | 134 |
| Pear, raw, 1 small | 4.3 | 81 |
| Bulgur, cooked, 1/2 cup (91 g) | 4.1 | 76 |
| Mixed vegetables, cooked, 1/2 cup (82 g) | 4.0 | 59 |
| Raspberries, raw, 1/2 cup (62 g) | 4.0 | 32 |
| Sweet potato, boiled, no peel, 1 medium | 3.9 | 119 |
| Blackberries, raw, 1/2 cup (72 g) | 3.8 | 31 |
| Potato, baked, with skin, 1 medium | 3.8 | 161 |
| Soybeans, green, cooked, 1/2 cup (90 g) | 3.8 | 127 |
| Stewed prunes, 1/2 cup (124 g) | 3.8 | 133 |
| Figs, dried, 1/4 cup (37 g) | 3.7 | 93 |

> continued

TABLE 3.1  > *continued*

| Food, standard amount | Dietary fiber (g) | Calories |
|---|---|---|
| Dates, 1/4 cup (45 g) | 3.6 | 126 |
| Oat bran, raw, 1/4 cup (18 g) | 3.6 | 58 |
| Pumpkin, canned, 1/2 cup (123 g) | 3.6 | 42 |
| Spinach, frozen, cooked, 1/2 cup (95 g) | 3.5 | 30 |
| Shredded wheat ready-to-eat cereals, various, ~1 oz (~30 g) | 2.8-3.4 | 96 |
| Almonds, 1 oz (30 g) | 3.3 | 164 |
| Apple with skin, raw, 1 medium | 3.3 | 72 |
| Brussels sprouts, frozen, cooked, 1/2 cup (78 g) | 3.2 | 33 |
| Whole-wheat spaghetti, cooked, 1/2 cup (70 g) | 3.1 | 87 |
| Banana, 1 medium | 3.1 | 105 |
| Orange, raw, 1 medium | 3.1 | 62 |
| Oat bran muffin, 1 small | 3.0 | 178 |
| Guava, 1 medium | 3.0 | 37 |
| Pearled barley, cooked, 1/2 cup (79 g) | 3.0 | 97 |
| Sauerkraut, canned, solids and liquids, 1/2 cup (71 g) | 3.0 | 23 |
| Tomato paste, 1/4 cup (131 g) | 2.9 | 54 |
| Winter squash, cooked, 1/2 cup (103 g) | 2.9 | 38 |
| Broccoli, cooked, 1/2 cup (78 g) | 2.8 | 26 |
| Parsnips, cooked, chopped, 1/2 cup (78 g) | 2.8 | 55 |
| Turnip greens, cooked, 1/2 cup (72 g) | 2.5 | 15 |
| Collards, cooked, 1/2 cup (95 g) | 2.7 | 25 |
| Okra, frozen, cooked, 1/2 cup (92 g) | 2.6 | 26 |
| Peas, edible pod, cooked, 1/2 cup (80 g) | 2.5 | 42 |

Source: ARS Nutrient Database for Standard Reference, Release 17. From the U.S. Department of Health and Human Services and the U.S. Department of Agriculture, 2005, *Dietary guidelines for Americans 2005*. Available: http://www.health.gov/dietaryguidelines/dga2005/document/html/appendixB.htm.

You'll also experience less gas with smaller, more frequent meals. That's because the friendly bacteria in your gut feeds off fiber. A by-product of bacterial digestion can be gas, but if you take in fiber in smaller amounts, less gas is produced. If you have trouble with bloating, the following list includes the high-fiber foods that form the least gas:

- Fresh fruits with skin, dried fruits, and fruit juices with pulp
- Potatoes, sweet potatoes, and yams with skin
- Peas
- Carrots
- Winter squash
- Tomatoes
- Romaine, leaf, Boston, and Bibb lettuces
- Whole grains and cereals

## Low Glycemic Ratings

In addition to being high in fiber, the right types of carbohydrate are also low on the glycemic index, and when portion sizes are controlled, they have low glycemic loads. The glycemic index is a measure of how quickly sugar is released into the bloodstream after eating a food containing 50 grams of digestible carbohydrate. Foods high on the index raise blood sugar levels rapidly; foods lower on the index cause a slower response. Highly refined foods are generally digested more quickly compared with whole foods and raise blood sugar levels more rapidly. However, this is not always the case. The volume of carbohydrate consumed is also a big factor. Although the creators of the glycemic index understood that and kept the volume constant to 50 grams, many of the normal portion sizes contain less than 50 grams of carbohydrate.

The concept of glycemic load was created to more specifically understand the metabolic response to carbohydrate. The glycemic index uses a constant 50-gram portion of digestible carbohydrate, but all foods do not contain equal volumes of digestible and indigestible (fiber) carbohydrate. The volume of food that a subject eats to get the right amount of digestible carbohydrate varies from food to food, making portion sizes and the index measure inconsistent with what the average person might actually eat. Glycemic load combines the glycemic index with the amount of food typically eaten, or the load, and it has been shown to be physiologically related to increases in blood sugar and insulin levels. Table 3.2 provides the glycemic index and load for common foods.

Nibbling, or eating smaller meals more frequently, allows you to eat smaller portions and reduces the amount of carbohydrate you eat at one time, or the load. Choosing foods lower on the glycemic index and load that are less processed, such as whole fruit instead of fruit juice or beans instead of bread, will give you that timed-release response to digestion that keeps your blood sugar levels more even. Because carbohydrate is digested more rapidly than protein or fat, when you eat combinations of foods such as an apple with peanut butter or bread with cheese, you mimic the whole-food response and slow digestion down, while still getting that slow release of sugar into the bloodstream and preventing weight gain. Rather than having to follow a diet devoid of carbohydrate, you can still enjoy carbohydrate and get the same weight-loss benefit.

## TABLE 3.2   Glycemic Index by Glycemic Load

| Foods | Glycemic load | Glycemic index |
|---|:---:|:---:|
| **Low glycemic–load breads, cereals, and grains** | | |
| All-Bran cereal | 8 | 42 |
| Whole-meal rye bread | 8 | 58 |
| Hamburger bun | 9 | 61 |
| Cinnamon, raisin, pecan bread | 9 | 63 |
| Barley flour bread | 9 | 67 |
| Gluten-free bread | 9 | 69 |
| White bread | 10 | 70 |
| Whole-wheat bread | 9 | 71 |
| Popcorn | 8 | 72 |
| Waffles | 10 | 76 |
| **Low glycemic–load fruits** | | |
| Apples | 6 | 38 |
| Pears | 4 | 38 |
| Strawberries | 1 | 40 |
| Oranges | 5 | 42 |
| Peaches | 5 | 42 |
| Grapes | 8 | 46 |
| Raw apricots | 5 | 57 |
| Pineapple | 7 | 59 |
| Cantaloupe | 4 | 65 |
| Watermelon | 4 | 72 |
| **Low glycemic–load vegetables** | | |
| Peanuts | 1 | 14 |
| Chickpeas | 8 | 28 |
| Pinto beans | 10 | 39 |
| Carrots | 3 | 47 |
| Sweet corn | 9 | 54 |
| Beets | 5 | 64 |
| Pumpkin | 3 | 75 |
| **Low glycemic–load miscellaneous foods** | | |
| Fat-free milk | 4 | 32 |
| Reduced-fat chocolate milk | 9 | 34 |
| Honey | 10 | 55 |
| Sucrose (table sugar) | 7 | 68 |
| Popcorn, plain | 8 | 72 |

| Foods | Glycemic load | Glycemic index |
|---|---|---|
| **Medium glycemic–load breads, cereals, and grains** | | |
| Fettuccine | 18 | 40 |
| Sourdough wheat bread | 15 | 54 |
| Buckwheat | 16 | 54 |
| Wild rice | 18 | 57 |
| Raisin Bran cereal | 12 | 61 |
| Rye Crisp crackers | 11 | 63 |
| Puffed wheat cereal | 13 | 67 |
| Cheerios | 15 | 74 |
| Shredded Wheat | 15 | 75 |
| **Medium glycemic–load fruits** | | |
| Apple juice | 12 | 40 |
| Orange juice | 12 | 50 |
| Bananas | 12 | 52 |
| Apricots, canned in light syrup | 12 | 64 |
| Lychee, canned in syrup | 16 | 79 |
| **Medium glycemic–load vegetables** | | |
| New potatoes | 12 | 57 |
| Sweet potatoes | 17 | 61 |
| Parsnips | 12 | 97 |
| **Medium glycemic–load miscellaneous foods** | | |
| Vegetarian pizza, thin crust | 12 | 49 |
| Cheese pizza | 16 | 60 |
| Gatorade | 12 | 78 |
| **High glycemic–load breads, cereals, and grains** | | |
| Spaghetti | 20 | 42 |
| Macaroni | 23 | 47 |
| Linguine | 23 | 52 |
| White rice | 23 | 64 |
| Couscous | 23 | 65 |
| Oatmeal, quick-cooking | 24 | 69 |
| Plain white bagel | 25 | 72 |
| White rice, instant | 31 | 74 |
| Cornflakes | 21 | 81 |
| **High glycemic–load vegetables** | | |
| Baked russet potatoes | 26 | 85 |

Because you may never memorize the list of foods with the lowest glycemic load, here are a few pointers to give you a general sense of which foods are lower on the scale:

- Whole, unprocessed foods in their natural state are lower on the glycemic-load scale than processed foods.
- Raw, uncooked foods are lower than cooked foods.
- Solid foods are lower than liquid foods.
- Foods higher in fiber, fat, and protein are lower on the glycemic-load scale than those lower in these elements.
- A smaller portion provides a lower load than a larger portion.

Exact glycemic index and load numbers are available at www.glycemicindex.com.

## Sugar and Your Health

So what's the scoop on sugar? To eat it or not eat it? If you're active, there is certainly a place for sugar in your diet—a small place. Anyone who is consuming at least 2,000 calories a day can tolerate some added sugar, as long as exercise is part of the program.

What do I mean by "added sugar"? It's the sugar not found naturally in foods that is added either by you (such as the table sugar you add to your coffee or tea) or the food manufacturer (to sweeten foods).

Although it's fine to eat a tiny bit of sugar, your goal should always be to eat as much whole food as possible to support your training and your health. Downplay processed foods, which tend to be loaded with added sugar.

You can, however, put sugar to work for you. Eat it before, during, or after your workouts. That's when it is best used as fuel, and you will burn it off quickly. But too much added sugar takes away calories from your diet that could otherwise be spent on whole foods.

If eaten too frequently, not burned off, or not used to replenish muscle glycogen, sugar becomes an empty food that makes you feel poorly. It increases the stress response in your body, for example, which ultimately diminishes both physical and mental performance.

How much sugar should, or can, you eat and still achieve your goals? If you look at the building diet in chapter 13, you'll see that on a 2,000-calorie diet, you can have 3 teaspoons (1 tbsp) of added sugar. You should put it to work for you immediately after exercise to begin recovery. You need the rest of those calories for robust, nutrient-dense carbohydrate, protein, and high-performance fats. As the amount of calories increases, the amount of added sugar increases to allow for greater refueling of a more active and larger, more muscular body. The added sugars are almost completely for recovery nutrition: before, during, and after exercise. That's when they work for you.

Besides the fact that sugar provides almost no nutrients but plenty of calories, too much of it in your diet can harm your health in various ways. What follows is a list of detrimental effects, culled from the scientific literature on sugar consumption. Sugar does the following:

- Decreases levels of the helpful, protective cholesterol, HDL
- Increases triglycerides (elevated triglycerides increase your risk of coronary artery disease)
- Causes fluctuations in blood glucose levels—a situation that can be problematic in people with diabetes
- Contributes to the formation of advanced glycation end products (AGEs) in a process in which sugar links to protein. AGEs are implicated in aging, diabetic nerve damage, vascular problems, and impaired cellular function
- Increases the risk of obesity
- Is directly related to the formation of dental cavities
- Displaces the intake of whole foods in the diet

Source: B.V. Howard and J. Wylie-Rosett, 2002, "Sugar and cardiovascular disease: A statement for healthcare professionals from the Committee on Nutrition of the Council on Nutrition, Physical Activity, and Metabolism of the American Heart Association," *Circulation* 106(4): 523-527.

# Carbohydrate: How Much, How Often?

Clearly, there are plenty of reasons to fill up on carbohydrate, particularly the whole, unrefined kind. First, though, you have to understand that there is a ceiling on how much carbohydrate your body will stock. Think of a gas tank; it can hold only so many gallons. If you fill it with more than it can hold, it will only overflow. Once your carbohydrate stores fill up in the form of glycogen, the liver turns the overflow into fat, which is then stored under the skin and in other areas of the body.

The amount of muscle glycogen you can store depends on your degree of muscle mass. Just as some gas tanks are larger, so are some people's muscles. The more muscular you are, the more glycogen you can store.

To make sure you get the right amount of carbohydrate and not too much, figure your daily carbohydrate intake as follows: To build muscle, consume 4.5 to 7 grams of carbohydrate per kilogram of body weight daily. Divide your body weight in pounds by 2.2 to get your body weight in kilograms; then multiply by 4.5 to 7. If you want to maintain your weight, lose fat, or cut, you can find your customized carbohydrate needs in chapters 12, 15, and 16.

Once you increase your carbohydrate to the right level, you should start making additional strength gains. Ample amounts of carbohydrate will give you the energy to push harder and longer for better results in your workout.

## Bread, Cereal, Rice, and Pasta

Along with many fruits and vegetables, the grain food group contains complex carbohydrate, which you know best as starch. Starch is to the plant what glycogen is to your body, a storage form of glucose that supplies energy to help the plant grow. At the molecular level, starch is actually a chain of dozens of glucose units. The links holding the starch chain together are broken apart by enzymes during digestion into single glucose units that are circulated to the body's cells.

Although primitive humans probably gnawed on whole kernels, today we grind or mill grains to ease their preparation and improve their palatability—hence the term *refined grains.* Milling subdivides the grain into smaller particles. For example, the wheat kernel can be milled to form cracked wheat, fine granular wheat, or even finer whole-wheat flour. Refining processes also remove the germ or seed, as well as the bran, a covering that protects the germ and other inner parts of the grain.

When the endosperm, a starch layer that protects the germ, is separated from a corn kernel, you get such products as grits and cornmeal. Another processing technique is abrasion, in which the bran of rice or barley is removed and the remaining portion is polished. The result is white rice or pearled barley.

As parts of the kernel such as the germ or bran are removed, so are the nutrients they contain—fiber, unsaturated fat, protein, iron, and several B-complex vitamins. These are replaced in cereal products in a process known as enrichment. However, enriched cereals are not nearly as nutritious as the original grains, so you should minimize your consumption of them. Furthermore, they lack the fiber found in whole grains.

I recommend that most of the starchy foods in your diet be whole grains. First, they are higher in fiber. Second, unlike refined foods, whole grains are less likely to cause insulin resistance, when elevated blood sugar circulates in the blood because body cells respond abnormally to the action of insulin. High intakes of refined foods can lead to insulin resistance, even in active people.

As a strength trainer, you're probably used to eating a lot of oatmeal, rice, and other common grains. For variety, you might experiment with grains that are less well known but are now widely available in supermarkets. For instance, tabbouleh, a Middle Eastern dish, is a delicious cold salad made from bulgur wheat. The Russians traditionally use kasha, or roasted buckwheat groats, to make both warm and cold dishes and stuffings. Barley makes a hearty soup. Quinoa, more of a seed than a grain, is cooked like a grain but is higher in protein, calcium, magnesium, iron, and phosphorus than typical grains. Its nutty flavor adds variety and nutrition to warm and cold dishes.

## Fruits and Vegetables

You've heard it since grade school: Eat your fruits and vegetables and you'll be healthy. Somewhere between then and now, you may have become skeptical of that advice. It seems too simplistic. After all, human health and nutrition science must be more complicated than that! But science has put grade school advice to the test and turned up some provocative findings. In a nutshell, the advice you heard as a kid is not only sound, it may also be lifesaving.

Thanks to continuing research, there are now more reasons than ever to eat lots of fruits and vegetables. In addition to their high vitamin, mineral, and fiber content, fruits and vegetables are full of other nutritional treasures such as the following:

- **Antioxidants.** Vitamins and minerals such as vitamin A, beta-carotene, vitamins C and E, and selenium fight disease-causing substances in the body called free radicals. Antioxidants have some real benefits for strength trainers; see chapter 7 for more details.

- **Phytochemicals.** These plant chemicals protect against cancer, heart disease, and other illnesses. Table 3.3 lists some of the important phytochemicals found in various types of carbohydrate.

- **Phytoestrogens.** These are special phytochemicals found in tofu and other soy foods that in moderation may protect against some cancers, lower dangerous levels of cholesterol, and promote bone building. Phytoestrogens are also listed in table 3.3.

There are lots of reasons for piling more fruits and vegetables on our plates. First, plant foods provide significant protection against many types of cancer. People who eat greater amounts of fruits and vegetables have about half the risk of getting cancer and less risk of dying of cancer than those who eat lesser amounts.

**TABLE 3.3 Phytochemicals for Fitness**

| Phytochemical | Food source | Protective action |
| --- | --- | --- |
| Allyl sulfides | Garlic, onions, shallots, leeks, chives | Lower risk of stomach and colon cancers |
| Sulforaphanes, indoles, isothiocyanates | Broccoli, cabbage, brussels sprouts, cauliflower, kohlrabi, watercress, turnips, Chinese cabbage | Lower risk of breast, stomach, and lung cancers |
| Carotenes | Carrots, dried apricots and peaches, cantaloupe (rock melon), green leafy vegetables, sweet potatoes, yams | Lower risk of lung and other cancers |
| Lycopene, p-coumaric acid, chlorogenic acid | Tomatoes | Lower risk of prostate and stomach cancers |
| Alpha-linolenic acid, vitamin E | Vegetable oils | Lower risk of inflammation and heart disease |
| Monoterpenes | Cherries, orange-peel oil, citrus-peel oil, caraway, dill, spearmint, lemongrass | Lower risk of breast, skin, liver, lung, stomach, and pancreatic cancers |
| Polyphenols | Green tea | Lower risk of skin, lung, and stomach cancers |
| Phytoestrogens | Soy foods, including tofu, miso, tempeh, soybeans, soy milk, isolated soy protein | Lower risk of breast and prostate cancers; decrease in symptoms of menopause |

For example, tomatoes may protect against prostate cancer. In a study sponsored by the National Cancer Institute, researchers identified lycopene as the only carotenoid associated with a lower risk of prostate cancer. Cooked tomato products are concentrated sources of lycopene. Thus, tomato sauce, stewed tomatoes, tomato paste, tomato juice, pizza sauce, and spaghetti sauce are rich in lycopene. People who consumed more than 10 servings of these combined foods per week had a significantly decreased risk of developing prostate cancer compared with those who ate fewer than one and a half servings per week.

Here's more proof of the cancer-fighting power of fruits and vegetables: A study of 2,400 Greek women showed that women with the highest intake of fruit (six servings a day) had a 35 percent lower risk of breast cancer compared with women who had the lowest fruit intake (fewer than two servings a day).

The number of fruits and vegetables in your daily diet makes a difference in cardiovascular health, too. Researchers tracked 832 men aged 45 to 65 as part of the famous Framingham Heart Study, which has followed the health of residents of a Boston suburb since 1948. For every increase of three servings of fruits and vegetables that the men ate per day, there was approximately a 20 percent decrease in their risk of stroke. A previous study reported a similar finding among women. Those who ate lots of spinach, carrots, and other vegetables and fruits rich in antioxidants had a 54 percent lower risk of stroke than other women.

There's more: In the United States, men with low vitamin C intakes have a significantly higher risk of cardiovascular disease and death compared with men who eat the highest levels of vitamin C. Risk of heart disease appears to be the lowest in people who eat an average of at least 11 pounds (5 kg) of citrus fruit per year.

Want to better control your blood pressure? Eat more fruit. It's loaded with potassium and magnesium—two minerals that have been credited with possibly lowering blood pressure. Research shows that people who follow the dietary patterns of various ethnic backgrounds tend to have lower blood pressure than those who follow the typical American diet. The reason is that people who maintain their traditional diet patterns eat twice as many servings of fruits and vegetables as people who transition to the average American diet. Other research indicates that high blood pressure can be lowered—without medication—if you eat a diet packed with fruits and vegetables.

Can you get the same health benefits from popping supplements as you can from food? Not exactly. New research has discovered that factors such as antioxidants and phytochemicals work best to fight disease when you get them from food rather than when they are isolated as supplements. In other words, a vitamin and mineral supplement, or any other kind of nutritional supplement, can't match the power of food.

To get the disease-fighting benefits of fruits and vegetables, you should eat a minimum of three servings of vegetables and two servings of fruit every day. One serving of a vegetable is equal to 1/2 cup (91 g) of cooked or chopped raw vegetables; 1 cup (38 g) of raw, leafy vegetables; 1/2 cup (90 g) of cooked legumes; or 3/4 cup (178 ml) of vegetable juice. One serving of a fruit is equal to one medium piece of raw fruit, half of a grapefruit, one melon wedge, 1/2 cup (62 g) of berries, 1/4 cup (37 g) of dried fruit, or 3/4 cup (180 ml) of fruit juice.

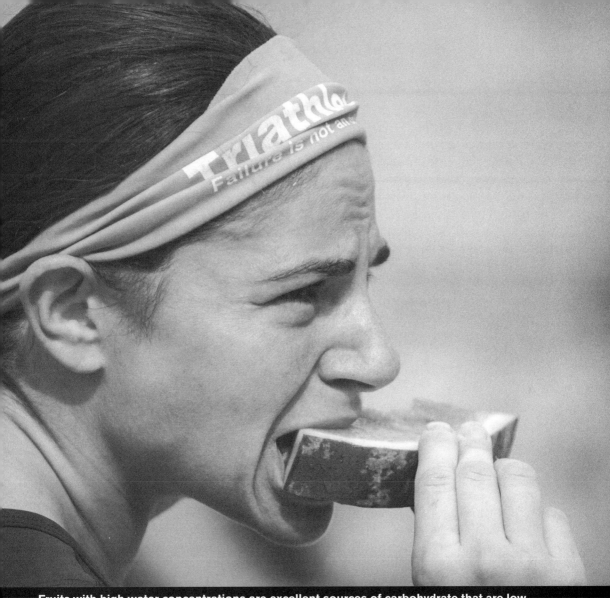

Fruits with high water concentrations are excellent sources of carbohydrate that are low in calories.

## Energy Bars

Energy bars, which are a convenient, ready-to-eat source of carbohydrate, have come a long way since I first ate a PowerBar close to 30 years ago. There was no question then that food was a better choice, but it was hard to eat a cheese sandwich and an apple while cycling along the rugged coast of Maine. A PowerBar was desirable because I could wrap it around my handlebars, peel it off, and eat it as I rode. Although still not my favorite source of nutrition, bars have now become specialized to boost energy for activity, add protein for dieting or building muscle, or generally replace a small meal or snack. Most important, they are convenient to have with you when you need them.

For the most part, energy bars come in three varieties: those containing lots of carbohydrate and little fat; those formulated with a more equal combination of carbohydrate, protein, and fat; and those that emphasize protein.

For strength trainers, eating energy bars is a fast way to replace glycogen stores (which are depleted during heavy exercise) to help your body recover. If you need to add fiber to your diet, look for bars that contain fiber-rich whole foods such as oats, nuts, and fruit, whose carbohydrate content provides a steady release of energy. Some of these often have as much as 5 grams of fiber in them. You'd be wise to check the calorie counts of these products, however. They can contain anywhere from 200 to 400 calories or more per bar. So if you're trying to shed body fat, you could unwittingly sabotage your diet by eating bars as snacks instead of whole foods such as fruits and vegetables.

With some planning you might be able to avoid bars most of the time by having a convenient food source of carbohydrate that you take with you in the morning. Pair it with a rich protein source and you'll be eating whole, natural food rather than an engineered bar. Table 3.4 lists good food sources of carbohydrates.

## Carbohydrate Before and During Your Workout

Preworkout carbohydrate: Is it a good idea? It depends. If you're in a mass-building phase and want to push to the max, fuel yourself with carbohydrate before and during your workout. The best timing recommendations for eating before exercise is to eat a small meal of carbohydrate and protein one and a half to two hours before working out (for building). This meal should contain about 50 grams of carbohydrate (200 calories) and 20 grams of protein (80 calories).

If you are trying to taper or cut, you want to minimize the amount of carbohydrate you take in prior to your workout, because you are training to burn fat. I suggest cutting your carbohydrate–protein meal in half. Thus, your meal would contain about 25 grams of carbohydrate and 20 grams of protein.

And, of course, you should make sure you are always well hydrated. Drink 2 cups (480 ml) of fluid within two hours of working out and another cup (240 ml) 15 minutes before exercise. Following this pattern will ensure that you gain the greatest energy advantage from your preexercise meal without feeling full while you exercise.

If you want a little extra boost, try drinking a liquid carbohydrate beverage just before your workout. In a study of strength trainers, one group consumed a carbohydrate drink just before training and between exercise sets. Another group was given a placebo. For exercise, both groups did leg extensions at about 80 percent of their strength capacity, performing repeated sets of 10 repetitions with rests between sets. The researchers found that the carbohydrate-fed group outlasted the placebo group, performing many more sets and repetitions.

Another study turned up a similar finding. Exercisers drank either a placebo or a 10 percent carbohydrate beverage immediately before and between the 5th, 10th, and 15th sets of a strength-training workout. They performed repeated sets of 10 repetitions, with three minutes of rest between sets. When fueled by the carbohydrate drink (1 g per kg of body weight), they could do more total repetitions (149 vs. 129) and more total sets (17.1 vs. 14.4) than when they drank the placebo.

## TABLE 3.4 Good Food Sources of Carbohydrate

| Food | Amount | Carbohydrate (g) | Calories |
|------|--------|------------------|----------|
| **Fruits** | | | |
| Apple | 1 medium | 21 | 81 |
| Orange | 1 medium | 15 | 62 |
| Banana | 1 medium | 28 | 109 |
| Raisins | 1/4 cup (36 g) | 29 | 109 |
| Apricots, dried | 1/4 cup (33 g) | 25 | 107 |
| **Vegetables** | | | |
| Corn, canned | 1/2 cup (82 g) | 15 | 66 |
| Winter squash | 1/2 cup (103 g) | 10 | 47 |
| Peas | 1/2 cup (80 g) | 13 | 67 |
| Carrot | 1 medium | 7 | 31 |
| **Breads** | | | |
| Whole wheat | 2 slices | 26 | 138 |
| Bagel, plain | 1 whole (3.5 in. or 9 cm diameter) | 38 | 195 |
| Whole-wheat English muffin | 1 whole | 27 | 134 |
| Pita pocket, whole wheat | 1 whole (6.5 in. or 16 cm diameter) | 35 | 170 |
| Bran muffin, homemade | 1 small | 24 | 164 |
| Matzo | 1 sheet | 24 | 112 |
| Granola bar, hard | 1 bar | 16 | 115 |
| Granola bar, soft | 1 bar | 19 | 126 |
| Low-fat granola bar, Kellogg's | 1 bar | 29 | 144 |
| PowerBar Original | 1 bar | 45 | 240 |
| PowerBar Pria | 1 bar | 16 | 110 |
| **Grains and cereals** | | | |
| Grape Nuts | 1/4 cup (29 g) | 22 | 97 |
| Raisin Bran | 1/2 cup (31 g) | 21 | 86 |
| Granola, low-fat | 1/4 cup (26 g) | 19 | 91 |
| Oatmeal, plain, instant | 1 packet | 18 | 104 |
| Oatmeal, cinnamon spice, instant | 1 packet | 35 | 177 |
| Shredded Wheat (spoon sized) | 1/2 cup (25 g) | 20 | 83 |
| Kashi puffed cereal | 1 cup | 20 | 99 |

> continued

TABLE 3.4   > *continued*

| Food | Amount | Carbohydrate (g) | Calories |
|---|---|---|---|
| **Sport drinks** | | | |
| 6% glucose–electrolyte solution | 8 oz (240 ml) | 14 | 50 |
| High-carbohydrate replacer | 12 oz (360 ml) | 70 | 280 |
| Meal replacer | 11 oz (325 ml) | 59 | 360 |
| **Pasta and starches** | | | |
| Baked potato, with skin | 1 large | 46 | 201 |
| Baked sweet potato | 1 cup (200 g) | 49 | 206 |
| Whole-wheat spaghetti, cooked | 1 cup (140 g) | 37 | 174 |
| Brown rice, cooked | 1 cup (195 g) | 46 | 218 |
| **Legumes** | | | |
| Baked beans, vegetarian, canned | 1 cup (254 g) | 52 | 236 |
| Navy beans, canned | 1 cup (182 g) | 54 | 296 |
| Black beans | 1 cup (172 g) | 34 | 200 |
| Baby lima beans, frozen, cooked | 1 cup (182 g) | 35 | 189 |
| Lentils, cooked | 1 cup (198 g) | 40 | 230 |

All this goes to show that carbohydrate clearly give you an energy edge when consumed before and during a hard workout lasting longer than one hour. The harder you can work out, the more you can stimulate your muscles to grow.

If you sip a carbohydrate drink over the course of a long workout, be aware that you can take in too many calories. When counseling clients, I recommend that they alternate between drinking a carbohydrate beverage and drinking water during training, especially if their workouts last more than an hour. That way, they don't consume too many calories from the carbohydrate drink.

The real key is to figure out how many grams of carbohydrate you need daily. If you supplement with a sport drink, be sure to count the carbohydrate in that drink as well. Consider your goals—mass building or fat burning—and listen to your body for signs of fatigue. Adjust your carbohydrate intake accordingly, depending on your goals and energy level.

## Recovery Nutrition

After working out, you want your muscles to recover. Recovery is essentially the process of replenishing muscle glycogen. The better your recovery, the harder you'll be able to train during your next workout. There are three critical periods in which to "feed" your muscles with carbohydrate. These three periods are explained in the following discussion.

## Go for Carbohydrate

As you plan to include carbohydrate in your diet, keep in mind these important principles:

- Choose the right source of carbohydrate (unrefined, whole foods) to get the best elevations of insulin for muscle building.
- Combine carbohydrate with protein and fat, and eat multiple meals featuring this combination throughout the day.
- Use sugars such as honey, sport drinks, and other high-glycemic foods in a targeted way, usually just after a workout to accelerate the recovery process. The most important dietary factor that will influence your strength-training performance is the amount of carbohydrate in your daily diet.

Giving careful thought to what you eat—and making sure you get plenty of carbohydrate—will provide a solid foundation for optimizing both your performance and your health.

What type of carbohydrate should you consume during cross-training exercise? The answer is a carbohydrate that digests quickly, absorbs into your bloodstream rapidly, and reaches your muscle cells fast. This translates into high-glycemic carbohydrate sources such as a sport drinks, or even bagels or white potatoes while you are on your bike. High-glycemic carbohydrate sources cause an insulin surge that reverses the catabolic state associated with training. This type of carbohydrate also helps the body quickly enter an anabolic state by carrying amino acids into muscle cells.

Plenty of research has been conducted into the effect of consuming high-glycemic carbohydrate sources around exercise, but the research often conflicts. Case in point: When eight untrained healthy men underwent three experimental conditions (consuming low-glycemic carbohydrate sources, high-glycemic carbohydrate sources, or a placebo), it didn't matter what type of carbohydrate sources were ingested. This indicates that what matters is that you consume carbohydrate to fuel your workout, and not the glycemic rating.

Other research does indicate that consuming high-glycemic carbohydrate foods increases the resynthesis of glycogen in the muscle cells, however. Based on current findings, I recommend that you use your own personal experience and examine your own practical issues to decide which type of carbohydrate works best for you.

## Immediately After Your Workout

Your muscles are most receptive to producing new glycogen within the first few hours after your workout. That's when blood flow to muscles is much greater, a condition that makes muscle cells practically sop up glucose like a sponge. Muscle cells are also more sensitive to the effects of insulin during this time, and insulin promotes glycogen synthesis. You should therefore take in some carbohydrate, along with protein, immediately after your workout. (Remember that protein helps jump-start the manufacture of glycogen.) The question is this: What's the best type of carbohydrate for refueling? Answer: Carbohydrate with a high glycemic index because it will be rapidly absorbed.

If you are in a building phase, I suggest that you consume 1.0 to 1.5 grams of carbohydrate per kilogram of body weight as soon as possible after exercise. If you are in a tapering phase, consume 0.5 to 1 gram of carbohydrate per kilogram of body weight as soon as possible after exercise if you are a man; consume less if you are a woman or have a smaller body size.

Think of it this way: Have a 3:1 ratio of carbohydrate to protein as soon as possible after exercise. Protein is the big key to building muscle after exercise; carbohydrate is more about refueling. The more you are trying to enhance performance, the more you'll depend on carbohydrate. If weight and fat loss are the goals of your current training, then the goal is to depend less on carbohydrate.

The following recipe is for a smoothie that contains the proper ratios of carbohydrate, protein, and fat for refueling.

## Kleiner's Muscle Formula PLUS

21 g isolated whey protein

1 cup frozen unsweetened strawberries

1 medium banana

1 cup (240 ml) nonfat vanilla soy milk fortified with calcium and vitamins A and D

1 cup (240 ml) orange juice fortified with calcium and vitamin C

Blend for 60 seconds until smooth.

*One serving contains:*

| Nutrients | Food Group Servings |
|---|---|
| 436 calories | 4 fruit servings |
| 86 g carbohydrate | 3 very lean protein servings |
| 27 g protein | 1 nonfat milk serving |
| 0 g fat | 3 tsp added sugar (from soy milk) |
| 8 g dietary fiber | |

Honey, particularly in the form of a carbohydrate gel, is also a good postworkout choice because it is a high-glycemic carbohydrate. A research study published in the *Journal of the International Society of Sports Nutrition* in 2007 found that combining honey with a whey protein supplement may boost postworkout recovery and help prevent drops in blood sugar after exercise. In this particular study, honey powder performed as well as maltodextrin—a starch that has been the standard among recovery carbohydrates.

Among the newer supplemental carbohydrate sources on the block is a patented amylopectin (starch) fraction called Vitargo, a unique complex carbohydrate ingredient included in some new bodybuilding products. It's derived and fractionated from any source of food starch, such as barley or potatoes, and contains no sugar. Fractionation separates a naturally-occurring unique starch molecule from the other common starch molecules. Unlike other types of carbohydrate added to drinks and powders, such as maltodextrin, this fractionated starch is emptied from the stomach, enters the small intestine, and arrives in the bloodstream twice as fast as any other carbohydrate. Glycogen is replenished in muscle cells within two hours—twice as fast as any other carbohydrate, and performance studies have shown up to a 23 percent higher work output two hours postexercise. Therefore, recovery is very rapid.

## Every Two Hours After Your Workout

Continue to take in carbohydrate every two hours after your workout until you have consumed at least 100 grams within four hours after exercise and a total of 600 grams within 24 hours after your workout. That equates to roughly 40 to 60 grams of carbohydrate an hour during the 24-hour recovery period. (Many women and smaller athletes may not need this much. Follow the menu plans for customized postworkout meals.)

A word of caution: There is a drawback to high-glycemic foods consumed at times other than exercise. They may produce a fast, undesirable surge of blood sugar. When this happens, the pancreas responds by oversecreting insulin to remove sugar from the blood. Blood sugar then drops too low, and you can feel weak or dizzy.

Low-glycemic foods, on the other hand, provide a more constant release of energy and are unlikely to lead to these reactions. By mixing and matching low- and high-glycemic foods in your diet, you can keep your blood sugar levels stable from meal to meal. The watchword here is *moderation*. Don't overdose on high-glycemic foods or beverages.

## Throughout the Week

So what kind of carbohydrate should you eat all day long and through the week? Because the goal of Power Eating is to help you increase muscle and reduce body fat, the type of carbohydrate you eat, the timing of your eating, and the carbohydrate combination are all very important. All forms of whole-food carbohydrate are important: fruits, vegetables, beans and legumes, and starchy vegetables such as potatoes, yams, and winter squash. But one type of carbohydrate shines: whole grains.

Whole grains, first of all, are best known for their fiber content, as discussed earlier. Fiber increases fullness, reduces transit time through the gut, and helps in blood sugar management. But there's more to whole grains than fiber, according to recent scientific research. Whole grains

- have strong antioxidant an anticancer properties;
- are excellent sources of minerals, trace elements, vitamins, and phytochemicals;
- are high in B vitamins and thus help enhance the nervous system;

- supply "prebiotics," food factors that feed probiotics (healthy bacteria) in the gut and thus are integral to the health of the gastrointestinal system;
- help reduce abdominal fat, body weight, and body fat; and
- decrease the risk of developing metabolic syndrome, especially in the teen years.

Clearly, whole grains are a super-carbohydrate!

## Should You Practice Carbohydrate Loading?

Endurance athletes practice a type of nutritional jump start known as carbohydrate loading. Basically, it involves increasing the amount of glycogen stored in the muscle just before an endurance competition. With more glycogen available, the athlete can run, cycle, or swim longer before fatigue sets in and thus gain a competitive edge. When done properly, carbohydrate loading works wonders for endurance athletes.

Among strength athletes, bodybuilders have experimented the most with carbohydrate loading. Their goal is not endurance, but bigger muscles. In general, about seven days before the contest, the bodybuilder cuts back on carbohydrate. This is the depletion stage. Then, a few days before the contest, the bodybuilder starts increasing carbohydrate intake. This is the loading stage. The depletion stage theoretically prepares the muscles to hold more glycogen once more carbohydrate is eaten just before competition. With more glycogen, the muscles supposedly look fuller.

But does this actually happen? Not really, says one study. Researchers put nine men, all bodybuilders, on a carbohydrate-loading diet. The diet involved three days of heavy weight training (designed to deplete muscle glycogen) and a low-carbohydrate diet (10 percent of the calories were from carbohydrate, 57 percent from fat, and 33 percent from protein). This was followed by three days of lighter weight training (to minimize glycogen loss) and a diet of 80 percent carbohydrate, 5 percent fat, and 15 percent protein. A control group followed the same strength-training program but followed a standard diet. At the end of the study, the researchers measured the muscle girth of all the participants. The results? Carbohydrate loading did not increase muscle girth in any of the bodybuilders.

Data in the sport nutrition literature allow us to conclude that strength athletes derive no real benefit from carbohydrate loading. Your diet should contain ample carbohydrate on a daily basis, but this is not carbohydrate loading. Keep in mind, too, that carbohydrate depletion can actually result in the loss of hard-earned muscle.

# The Gluten Issue

Today, no discussion of whole wheat and whole grains in the diet can sidestep the topic of gluten, a protein component of wheat, rye, and barley. Some people are sensitive to gluten and may have either a gluten intolerance or celiac disease, which is inherited. For those who have an inherited tendency to develop celiac disease, eating foods that contain gluten damages the lining of the small intestine, which leads to nutritional deficiencies and possibly other diseases. Celiac disease, which may affect 1 percent of the population, is an immune system response to gluten that causes severe abdominal pain, bloating, and appetite loss. A lifelong illness, it begins at birth, although the symptoms may not appear for years. If you have celiac disease, which is diagnosed through an endoscopic biopsy and a special blood test, you must avoid all gluten-containing foods.

People with an intolerance to gluten make up approximately 10 percent of the population. Whereas people with celiac disease can take months to recover from exposure to gluten, those with an intolerance can recover quickly, within a few days. Symptoms of a gluten intolerance include upset stomach, rash, heartburn, and nausea.

If you think you have an intolerance to gluten, include some gluten-containing foods in your diet for several months; then follow that with a gluten-free diet. Carefully record your responses. Then add gluten-containing foods back into your diet and document what happens. You must be very strict to get a clear picture of what your body is actually responding to. If you suspect celiac disease, see your physician.

Be very careful about eliminating such important foods from your diet unnecessarily. Although 10 percent of the population may be gluten sensitive, that means that 90 percent is not; however, we are all being targeted by Madison Avenue to buy gluten-free foods. Highly processed gluten-free foods can still be high in sugar and low in nutrition just like other processed foods. You can still eat whole grains even if you must eliminate gluten. The following list is from the Whole Grains Council (www.wholegrainscouncil.org/whole-grains-101/gluten-free-whole-grains):

## Grains With Gluten

Wheat, including varieties such as spelt, kamut, farro, and durum; and products such as bulgur and semolina

Barley

Rye

Triticale

Oats*

Quinoa

Sorghum

Teff

## Gluten-Free Grains

Amaranth

Buckwheat

Corn

Millet

Montina (Indian rice grass)

rice

Wild rice

*Oats are inherently gluten free, but are frequently contaminated with wheat during growing or processing. Six companies—Bob's Red Mill, Cream Hill Estates, GF Harvest (Gluten-Free Oats), Avena Foods (Only Oats), Legacy Valley (Montana Monster Munchies), and Gifts of Nature—currently offer pure, uncontaminated oats. Ask your physician whether these oats are acceptable for you. Visit GlutenFreeDiet.ca for a discussion of oats in the gluten-free diet.

# Mental Muscle

When I worked for the great coach Pat Riley, he said that 50 percent of athletic performance is the result of mental focus—the ability to concentrate throughout an athletic event all the way to the final moments. This ability is what differentiates an athlete from a champion.

One key way to enhance mental alertness, focus, and mood is through food. Nutrients can affect cognitive processes and emotions, and studies confirm that brain health relies on many factors, including nutrients from our everyday diets.

An important brain chemical affecting mental processes is serotonin. It is made from the amino acid tryptophan, which is found in protein-rich foods (meats, dairy, eggs, and legumes). Ironically, eating a protein-rich meal lowers brain tryptophan and serotonin levels, whereas eating a carbohydrate-rich meal has the opposite effect. Tryptophan competes with other amino acids for entry into the brain after eating a lot of protein, resulting in very little tryptophan getting through the blood–brain barrier, so serotonin levels do not rise appreciably.

A carbohydrate-rich meal triggers insulin release. This causes most amino acids to be absorbed from the blood into the body's (not the brain's) cells, especially muscle cells, where we want those proteins to go. This is true of all amino acids except tryptophan, which now faces little competition to enter into the brain, with a resulting rise in serotonin levels. So carbohydrate and protein, working together, play a very important role in helping you maintain your mental focus.

How much carbohydrate do you need to boost your mental focus? Most studies on the subject agree that at least 40 percent of your total daily calories should come from carbohydrate sources to promote mental alertness and mood. Plus, carbohydrate in the diet helps your body cope with the demands of intense training.

So, while you are spending countless hours training and meticulously monitoring your eating and program to maximize muscle, don't forget that cerebral fitness is within your control, too.

# 4

# Managing Fat

After about an hour of intense exercise, your glycogen supply can dwindle to nothing. But not so with your fat stores—another energy source for muscles. Compared with the limited but ready-to-use glycogen stores, fat stores are practically unlimited. In fact, it's been estimated that the average adult man carries enough fat (about 1 gal, or 4 L) to ride a bike from Chicago to Los Angeles, a distance of roughly 2,000 miles (3,219 km).

If fat stores are nearly inexhaustible, why worry about carbohydrate intake and glycogen replenishment? And why not supplement your diet with fat as an extra source of energy? True, there is a large enough tank of fat on your body to fuel plenty of exercise. (That's one reason there's no need to supplement with extra fat.) But the problem is that fat can be broken down only as long as oxygen is available. Oxygen must be present for your body to burn fat for energy, but not to burn glycogen. In the initial stages of exercise, oxygen is not yet available. It can take 20 to 40 minutes of exercise before fat is maximally available to the muscles as fuel. The glucose in your blood and glycogen in your muscles are pressed into service first.

That's not to say that fat is hard to burn. It isn't. But how efficiently your body burns fat depends on your level of conditioning. One of the advantages of strength training and aerobic exercise is that your body improves its ability to burn fat as fuel in two major ways.

First, exercise (particularly aerobic exercise) enhances the development of capillaries that lead to muscle cells, thus improving blood flow where it's needed. In addition, exercise increases myoglobin, a protein that transports oxygen from the blood into muscle cells. With better blood flow and more oxygen in the muscles, the body becomes more efficient at burning fat, which is why you should not neglect the aerobic portion of your training.

Second, exercise stimulates the activity of hormone-sensitive lipase, an enzyme that promotes the breakdown of fat for energy. The more fat you can break down and burn, the more defined you will look.

Fat is definitely an exercise fuel, but it is a second-string source of energy for strength trainers. During strength training, your body still prefers to burn carbohydrate for energy, either from glucose in the blood or glycogen in the muscles. Fat is certainly one of the more controversial topics in nutrition. It is crucial in your diet, but it also has a bad reputation. Let's try to clear up the confusion once and for all.

## Fat Facts

There are three major types of fatty material in the body: triglycerides, cholesterol, and phospholipids. Triglycerides, true fats, are stored in fat tissue and in muscle. A small percentage of fatty material is found in the blood, circulating as free fatty acids, which have been chemically released from the triglycerides. Of the three types of fatty material, triglycerides are the most involved in energy production. Research with bodybuilders has found that triglycerides, including the fat found in muscle, serve as a significant energy source during intense strength training. Not only will strength training help you build muscle, but it will also help you burn body fat.

Cholesterol is a waxy, light-colored solid that comes in two forms. You might call the first kind "the cholesterol in blood," and the second, "the cholesterol in food." Required for good health, blood cholesterol is a constituent of cell membranes

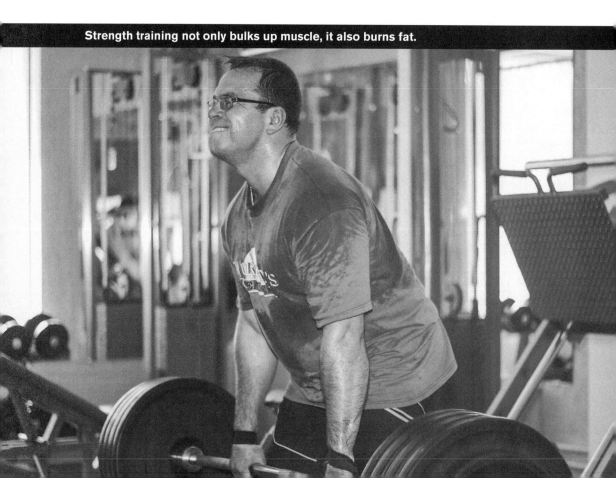

**Strength training not only bulks up muscle, it also burns fat.**

and is involved in the formation of hormones, vitamin D, and bile (a substance necessary for the digestion of fat). Because your body can make cholesterol from fat, carbohydrate, or protein, you don't need to supply any cholesterol from food.

When you eat a food that contains cholesterol, that cholesterol is broken into smaller components that are used to make various fats, proteins, and other substances that your body requires. The cholesterol you eat doesn't become the cholesterol in your blood. Although it is important to reduce your intake of high-cholesterol foods, it is even more important to lower your intake of saturated fat (the kind found mostly in animal foods). That's because the liver manufactures blood cholesterol from saturated fat. The more saturated fat you eat, the more cholesterol your liver makes.

If your liver produces large amounts of cholesterol, the excess circulating in the bloodstream can collect on the inner walls of the arteries. This accumulation is called plaque. Trouble starts when plaque builds up in an artery, narrowing the passageway and choking blood flow. A heart attack can occur when blood flow to the heart muscle is cut off for a long period of time and part of the heart muscle begins to die. High blood cholesterol is therefore a major risk factor for heart disease, but it is one that in many cases can be controlled with exercise and a healthy diet.

Cholesterol may be present in blood as a constituent of low-density lipoprotein (LDL) or of high-density lipoprotein (HDL). LDL and HDL affect your risk of heart disease differently. LDL contains the greater amount of cholesterol and may be responsible for depositing cholesterol on the artery walls. LDL is known as bad cholesterol; the lower your blood value of LDL, the better.

HDL contains less cholesterol than LDL. Its job is to remove cholesterol from the cells in the artery wall and transport it back to the liver for reprocessing or excretion from the body as waste. HDL is the good cholesterol; the higher the amount in your blood, the better.

The science is far more complex and the details about oxidized fractions of LDL may further explain the development of heart disease, but suffice it to say that a total cholesterol reading of greater than 200 milligrams per deciliter of blood may be a danger sign. Generally, your HDL should be greater than 35 and your LDL should be less than 130. High levels of triglycerides in your blood can reflect an excess of alcohol or saturated fat in your diet and can increase your risk of heart disease. It is advisable to have your cholesterol and triglycerides checked annually. In time, scientists and physicians will have even better laboratory tools to predict your risk and protect your health. Table 4.1 shows what your cholesterol numbers mean.

The third type of fatty material, phospholipids, is involved primarily in the regulation of blood clotting. Along with cholesterol, phospholipids form part of the structure of all cell membranes and are critical in the membranes of brain cells and nervous system cells.

## Fat in Foods

As an exerciser, strength trainer, or bodybuilder concerned with your appearance, you may be confused by mixed messages concerning dietary fat. What is the real story? The latest word is that fat is actually good for you and good for weight control,

**TABLE 4.1    Cholesterol Numbers**

| Total cholesterol | |
|---|---|
| <200 mg/dL | Desirable |
| 200-239 mg/dL | Borderline high |
| ≥240 mg/dL | High |
| **LDL cholesterol** | |
| <100 mg/dL | Optimal |
| 100-129 mg/dL | Near optimal/above optimal |
| 130-159 mg/dL | Borderline high |
| 160-189 mg/dL | High |
| ≥190 mg/dL | Very high |
| **HDL cholesterol** | |
| <40 mg/dL | Low |
| ≥60 mg/dL | High |
| **Triglycerides** | |
| <150 mg/dL | Desirable |
| 150-199 mg/dL | Borderline high |
| 200-499 mg/dL | High |
| ≥500 mg/dL | Very high |

Source: National Heart, Lung, and Blood Institute, 2001, *Third report of the National Cholesterol Education Program (NCEP) Expert Panel on Detection, Evaluation, and Treatment of High Blood Cholesterol in Adults (Adult Treatment Panel III) executive summary.* NIH Publication No. 01-3670. [Online]. Available: http://www.nhlbi.nih.gov/guidelines/cholesterol/atp3xsum.pdf [March 5, 2013].

as long as you eat the right kinds. Sure, too much fat, just like too much carbohydrate or protein, can turn into body fat. But the right kinds of fat actually help you lose body fat and keep you healthy in body and mind. You'll need help figuring out how much fat and what kind of fat to eat to stay healthy. Here's a closer look.

Fatty acids from food, the tiny building blocks of fat, are classified into three groups according to their hydrogen content: saturated, polyunsaturated, and monounsaturated. Saturated fatty acids are usually solid at room temperature and, with the exception of tropical oils, come from animal sources. Beef fat and butter fat are high in saturated fatty acids. Butter fat is found in milk, cheese, cream, ice cream, and other products made from milk or cream. Low-fat or skim milk products are much lower in saturated fat. Tropical oils high in saturated fat include coconut oil, palm kernel oil, and palm oil and also the cocoa fat found in chocolate. They are generally found in commercial baked goods and other processed foods.

Polyunsaturated and monounsaturated fats are usually liquid at room temperature and come from nuts, vegetables, and seeds. Polyunsaturated fats such as vegetable shortening and margarines are solid because they have been hydrogenated—a process that changes the chemical makeup of the fat to harden it. The resulting fat is composed of substances known as trans-fatty acids, which recent studies have shown to raise blood cholesterol. Trans-fatty acids are more harmful than saturated fats when it comes to your heart; no levels of trans fat are safe, and they should be avoided altogether. Fortunately, food manufacturers are now required to label the existence of trans fats on their products if their packaged foods enter interstate commerce in the United States. Look at the Nutrition Facts label to see how many grams of trans fats are in your food.

Monounsaturated fatty acids are found in large amounts in olive oil, canola oil, peanut oil, and other nut oils. Monounsaturated fats appear to have a protective effect on blood cholesterol levels. They help lower the bad cholesterol (LDL) and maintain the higher levels of good cholesterol (HDL).

## Essential Fats

Of all dietary fat, certain types of polyunsaturated fat are considered essential. Two of these are linoleic acid and alpha-linolenic acid (ALA). The chemical structure of linoleic acid is referred to as an omega-6 fat, and the chemical structure of linolenic acid is an omega-3 fat. Although these fats are essential, they are not needed in very large amounts. Your body can't make them; you have to get them from food. They are required for normal growth, the maintenance of cell membranes, and healthy arteries and nerves. As well, essential fats keep your skin smooth and lubricated and protect your joints. They also assist in the breakdown and metabolism of cholesterol. Vegetable fats such as corn, soybean, safflower, and walnut oils are all high in essential fats, as are nuts and seeds. The total amount required for good health is 6 to 10 percent of total fat intake, or a total of 5 to 10 grams a day.

In addition to linolenic acid, two other omega-3 fats are considered essential and are found virtually only in fish: eicosapentaenoic acid (EPA) and docosahexaenoic acid (DHA). EPA and DHA are found predominantly in marine oils, whereas ALA is found mostly in plant foods. All three are important and should not be substituted for one another. They are not interchangeable in amounts that will support health and performance.

Unfortunately, most people's intake of omega-3 fat is pitifully low. One reason is that we are eating more omega-6 fat, displacing omega-3 fat and creating an unhealthy imbalance. Sources of omega-6 fat include all the types of oils used in commercial cooking, baking, and food processing, including safflower, sunflower, soybean, corn, and cottonseed oils. Nutrition experts now recommend that we eat omega-6 fat and omega-3 fat in a healthier ratio, increasing our intake of omega-3 oils and decreasing our intake of omega-6 oils. You should substitute olive oil and canola oil, which are lower in omega-6 fat and higher in monounsaturated fat, for the other oils in your diet. Then increase the amount of fish you eat to increase your omega-3 intake. Some have suggested a 1:1 or 2:1 ratio of omega-6 fat to omega-3 fat; others advocate a 4:1 ratio. These ratios have been associated with lower incidences of heart disease and cancer in populations in which the consumption of omega-3 fat is traditionally higher.

Evidence is emerging that when this ratio is out of whack—when there is a high intake of omega-6 fat and a low intake of omega-3 fat—the fatty acid metabolism is altered in the body. The brain releases hormones and neurotransmitters (brain chemicals involved in sending messages) that tell the body to hold on to fat and not to burn it. It appears, then, that by raising levels of omega-3 fat in your diet, you create a better fat-burning effect. You really do need to eat the right kind of fat to feed your brain and burn body fat.

Omega-3 fatty acids, in particular, have far-reaching benefits for health and the management of chronic disease. Current research shows that they lower blood levels of triglycerides and a heart-damaging form of cholesterol called very low-density lipoproteins (VLDL). In addition, omega-3 fat lowers blood pressure in people with high blood pressure and may reduce the risk of sudden cardiac death. Omega-3 fat is also required for the development of the retina. A lack of omega-3 fat in the diets of pregnant women may adversely affect the eyesight of newborns.

## Omega-3 Supplementation

The data are really quite clear about how important the fish oils DHA and EPA are in the treatment of diseases of chronic inflammation. For instance, research has shown that periodontal disease, a chronic inflammatory disease, responds well to DHA treatment. A significant association has been established between periodontal disease and an increased risk for cardiovascular disease, diabetes, hypertension, cancer, low birth weight, and even miscarriage; the connection is chronic systemic inflammation.

It is a good idea to supplement your diet with fish oil. Enough research justifies its use; however, you need to choose wisely. The product you choose should be a good source of EPA and DHA, with at least 500 milligrams of fish oil.

DHA is important for healthy brain function, eyes, and the entire central nervous system. DHA is strongly associated with mood; low levels are associated with depression, loss of mental focus, and loss of memory.

DHA and EPA supplementation is recommended for both the treatment and prevention of virtually all of the chronic diseases. The recommended dose for supplementation or through diet is 1,000 milligrams per day of a combination of DHA and EPA. Under certain circumstances DHA or EPA are recommended alone, but in general the combination works quite well. You should be able to find high-quality supplements that combine DHA and EPA, ideally in a ratio of about 40:60 DHA to EPA.

To consume this much DHA plus EPA daily, you should consume five fish meals per week from predominantly fatty fish. Serving sizes should be 4 to 6 ounces (120 to 180 g). The best fish sources of omega-3 fatty acids are wild salmon, mackerel, black cod, cod, halibut, rainbow trout, shellfish, sardines, herring, and tuna. (See table 4.2 for nutritional information on seafood.)

Omega-3 fat is also found in green leafy vegetables, nuts, canola oil, tofu, and flaxseed. However, it is not the same omega-3 fat as that found in fish oil. It is ALA, the third kind of omega-3 fat besides EPA and DHA. ALA must be converted to EPA and DHA in the body to be useful. On the best of days, when you eat flax or get ALA from any of the other sources, only 5 percent of it is changed into EPA and DHA. Furthermore, you must be well nourished and very healthy to get that 5 percent exchange rate. Most people don't have the capability to fully reach 5 percent. Although flaxseed and other sources of omega-3 fat other than fish have benefits, they are not a good substitute for EPA and DHA.

### TABLE 4.2   Alaska Seafood Nutrition Information[1]

| | Calories | Protein (g) | Fat (g) | Saturated fat (g) | Sodium (mg) | Cholesterol (mg) | Omega-3 (g) |
|---|---|---|---|---|---|---|---|
| **Alaska salmon** | | | | | | | |
| King chinook | 230 | 26 | 13 | 3 | 60 | 85 | 1.7 |
| Sockeye (red) | 220 | 27 | 11 | 2 | 65 | 85 | 1.2 |
| Coho (silver) | 140 | 23 | 4 | 1 | 60 | 55 | 1.1 |
| Keta (chum) | 155 | 26 | 5 | 1 | 65 | 95 | 0.8 |
| Pink | 150 | 25 | 4 | 1 | 85 | 65 | 1.3 |
| **Alaska whitefish** | | | | | | | |
| Halibut | 140 | 27 | 3 | <0.5 | 70 | 40 | 0.5 |
| Cod | 100 | 23 | <1 | <0.5 | 90 | 45 | 0.3 |
| Pollock | 110 | 23 | 1 | <0.5 | 115 | 95 | 0.5 |
| Rockfish | 120 | 24 | 2 | 0.5 | 75 | 45 | 0.4 |
| Flounder | 120 | 24 | 1.5 | <0.5 | 105 | 70 | 0.5 |
| Sablefish | 250 | 17 | 20 | 4 | 70 | 65 | 1.8 |
| **Alaska shellfish** | | | | | | | |
| King crab | 100 | 19 | 1.5 | <0.5 | 1,100 | 55 | 0.4 |
| Snow crab | 115 | 24 | 1.5 | <0.5 | 690 | 70 | 0.5 |
| Dungeness crab | 110 | 22 | 1 | <0.5 | 380 | 75 | 0.4 |
| Pacific oysters | 165 | 19 | 5 | 1.0 | 210 | 100 | 1.4 |
| Shrimp | 100 | 21 | 1 | <0.5 | 220 | 195 | 0.3 |
| **Alaska canned salmon** | | | | | | | |
| Sockeye (red) | 165 | 23 | 7 | 2 | 360 | 45 | 1.4 |
| Pink | 135 | 23 | 5 | 1 | 400 | 80 | 1.1 |

[1] Serving size 3.5 oz/100 g cooked portions.

Adapted, by permission, from Alaska Seafood Marketing Institute, 2011, A guide to nutritional values for Alaska seafood. [Online]. Available: www.alaskaseafood.org/health/experts/pages/chart-nutrition.html [May 20, 2013]. Source: USDA National Nutrient Database for Standard References, Release 22.

## Omega-3 Fatty Acids and Brain Health

Treatment of depression, anxiety, and stress with omega-3 fatty acids is garnering a lot of attention in medical circles. About 60 percent of the brain is composed of fat, and the primary fat in the brain is omega-3 fat. When omega-3 fat is in short supply in the diet, other fat gets involved in brain building, and as a result, the health of brain cells is impaired. The membrane of each brain cell, for example, becomes rigid, and it takes longer for electrical impulses to travel from one cell to another. This means that messages are not being carried rapidly from brain cell to brain cell. Consequently, you don't think clearly, and your memory may become foggy. Depression and anxiety can also set in. Increasing levels of omega-3 fat in the diet has been shown to alleviate these problems.

There is an important ratio of omega-6 to omega-3 fats in the diet that also helps to limit inflammatory processes. In recent years, scientists have discovered that the development of many diseases is influenced by chronic inflammation in the body. Inflammation is an essential part of the body's healing process, brought on when the immune system tries to battle disease-causing germs and repair injured tissue. When that battle is over, the army of inflammation-triggering substances is supposed to withdraw, but in many cases it does not. Chronic inflammation is the result, and it has been implicated in heart disease, diabetes, arthritis, multiple sclerosis, cancer, and even Alzheimer's disease. Omega-3 fat appears to halt chronic inflammation. Omega-6 fat is pro-inflammatory, whereas omega-3 fat is anti-inflammatory. However, omega-6 fat is far more abundant in our food supply. So it takes planning and effort and good choices to create a healthy ratio of omega-6 to omega-3 fat. Although the average American diet reflects a ratio of 20:1, a more ideal ratio is 2:1 to 4:1.

The fat cells in your body create their own inflammatory processes—which is yet another reason to stay lean. In fact, overweight people show symptoms of chronic, low-grade inflammation, perhaps indicating early atherosclerosis, according to research. A study conducted by researchers at the Free University in Amsterdam and scientists at the National Institute on Aging in Bethesda, Maryland, found overweight people to be far more likely than lean ones to have excess concentrations of C-reactive protein (CRP) in their blood—a marker of inflammation. So if you are overweight, losing weight is the first step toward protecting your health.

If you are on the road and can't get fish, I recommend that you supplement your diet with fish oil. For non-fish eaters or vegetarians, other fortified foods contain DHA and EPA, primarily milk and eggs (make sure they are labeled as fortified with these oils). If you cannot consume enough of these foods in your regular diet, I highly recommend supplementation from a fish or algae-based product.

One of the most exciting areas of research with omega-3 fat for physique athletes is the animal research looking at the influence of omega-3 fat on fat burning. Research with mice has shown that omega-3 fat reduces both fat cell numbers and fat cell size. Epidemiological data on humans show that following a Mediterranean-style diet (which includes regular fish meals and plenty of high-performance fat) leads to better total body weight control and better abdominal fat control.

## Enhance Healing Ability

Some interesting laboratory data have shown that fish oil supplementation enhances wound healing. Athletes become injured fairly regularly, so having adequate levels of fish oil is important for healing.

## Olive Oil

Olive oil is one of the "good fats." Please understand, however, that there is a difference between extra-virgin olive oil and olive oil. Extra-virgin olive oil comes from the first pressing and a single variety of olive or fruit, not a blend. That gives it a distinct taste, smell, and color. What is not so well known about extra-virgin olive oil is that it uniquely contains an anti-inflammatory compound called oleocanthal, which is almost identical to the nonsteroidal anti-inflammatory drug ibuprofen. This makes extra-virgin olive oil an excellent anti-inflammatory food. Although olive oil in general is a good anti-inflammatory food, extra-virgin olive oil is significantly better. Use it whenever possible.

## Fat and Your Gut

When you have an upset stomach or uncomfortable intestines, it's tough to train hard day after day, and certainly you will not perform at your best. One solution is to populate your diet with good fat, such as olive oil and omega-3 fat. Remember, these fats exert an anti-inflammatory effect that is healing to your gastrointestinal tract. By contrast, an excess of omega-6 fat promotes inflammation in the gut, which is why you want to steer clear of fried foods, packaged snack foods, foods high in saturated fat, and fast foods. By substituting good fat—or what I like to call high-performance fat—you'll notice a quick improvement in how you feel.

Seeds, another high-performance source of fat, are also helpful in promoting gut health because of their fibrous structure. Lignin, a type of fiber found in plant foods, is present in large amounts in flaxseed. While probiotic bacterial cultures help to promote health in your intestines, lignin keeps the bacterial cultures well fed. For this reason, lignin is called a prebiotic. Including 1 to 2 tablespoons of ground flaxseed in your diet every day is a wonderful way to ingest healthy fibers as well as the strong anti-inflammatory omega-3 fat, ALA. Flaxseed must be ground; our teeth cannot grind the seeds well enough for digestion. If the seeds are not preground, they will exit the body whole without bestowing any of their benefits.

# Essential Fat Needs

If you slash fat to miniscule levels or cut it out altogether, you risk developing an essential fat deficiency. This is not a widespread problem, because Americans get their fill of fat. Even so, I have seen many athletes, bodybuilders in particular, go to extremes in cutting fat. When this happens, the body has trouble absorbing the fat-soluble vitamins A, D, E, and K. Furthermore, the health of cell membranes is jeopardized because low-fat diets are low in vitamin E. Vitamin E is an antioxidant that prevents disease-causing free radicals from puncturing cell membranes, and it also helps in the muscle repair process that takes place after exercise. Men who go on low-fat diets put their bodies in hormonal jeopardy, because fat is required to make the male hormone testosterone. Women who slash their fat feel terrible in general, and even start to crave processed carbohydrate.

You can also go overboard on fat. Too much dietary fat causes weight gain and gradually leads to obesity and related health problems. Excessive saturated fat in the diet can also elevate cholesterol, particularly the dangerous type (LDL). On the other hand, polyunsaturated and monounsaturated fats have been shown to cut cholesterol levels. However, polyunsaturated fat may also lower the protective type of cholesterol (HDL). Very high intakes of polyunsaturated fat have been linked to higher risks of cancer.

So where's the happy medium between too much fat and too little? According to the American Heart Association, the maximum amount of fat considered healthy in your daily diet is 30 percent or less, based on the number of calories you eat over several days (such as a week). Saturated fat should be 7 to 10 percent or less of your total daily calories; polyunsaturated fat should also be at 10 percent or less; and monounsaturated fat should make up to 15 percent of your total calories. A diet that contains these amounts is considered a good target for managing depression, anxiety, and stress. Dietary cholesterol should be kept to a daily maximum of 300 milligrams, according to the AHA. To be more specific, here are some recommendations:

### DRIs for Essential Fats

Linoleic acid: 12 grams daily for women; 17 grams daily for men

Alpha-Linolenic acid: 1.1 grams daily for women; 1.6 grams daily for men

EPA and DHA combined: 2 grams daily, based on a 2,000-calorie diet (This is a United Kingdom recommendation because there is no EPA and DHA DRI for the United States.)

## Fat Recommendations for Active People

If you're an exerciser, bodybuilder, or strength trainer trying to stay lean, you should control your total fat intake to control your total calorie intake. Keep your fat intake at 25 to 30 percent of calories each day. Your diet should contain much more unsaturated than saturated fat: 5 percent saturated, 10 to 15 percent monounsaturated, and 7 to 10 percent polyunsaturated.

One way to monitor your fat intake is by counting the grams of fat in your diet each day. You can calculate your own daily fat intake by using the following formulas:

### Total Fat

Total calories × 30% = daily calories from fat / 9 = g total fat

Example: 2,000 calories × 0.3 = 600 / 9 = 67 g total fat

**Saturated Fatty Acids (SFA)**

Total calories × 5% = daily calories from SFA / 9 = g SFA

Example: 2,000 calories × 0.05 = 100 / 9 = 11 g SFA

Following the Power Eating plan, first determine your protein and carbohydrate needs. All of your leftover calories are fat calories—most of which should be monounsaturated and polyunsaturated fats. Be sure to read food labels for the fat content per serving of the foods you buy in the supermarket. The grams of fat are listed on any food package that provides a nutrition label.

## Fat Substitutes and Fat Replacers

Many low-fat foods replace the fat with starch, fiber, protein, and other forms of fat. But why even bother with fat substitutes and fat replacers when you need the right kinds of fat in your diet? Go ahead and continue to enjoy healthy fat in foods such as olive oil, nuts, avocados, and nut and seed oils. Your body needs and deserves them.

What's more, we don't yet know what effect artificial fat has on health. Some nutritionists and other health advocates are concerned that consumers may get so carried away with eating fat-free foods that they won't obtain enough of the healthy fat their bodies truly need.

# Reducing Bad Fat in Your Diet

Saturated fat, trans fat, and cholesterol in your diet can lead to high cholesterol in your blood, which in turn clogs blood vessels, contributing to heart disease and stroke. You should be vigilant about reducing these fats in your diet.

The major sources of saturated fat are meats and whole-milk dairy products. However, fat from animals is not necessarily bad in and of itself. The real problem with animal fat may be the industrial farming methods used to raise animals. Caged animals fed corn develop very different, and harmful, fat composition compared to wild animals that eat grasses. Meat and dairy from wild animals may not have unhealthy levels of fat, and in fact may have healthy fatty acid profiles. In addition, most farming chemicals such as pesticides and herbicides are fat soluble. So when you are eating foods that have fat in them on a regular basis, it's wise to choose organic. However, because research is ongoing on this topic, you should limit your consumption of animal-based saturated fats in general. When no nutrition information is available for a particular food, remember these helpful hints about the sources of saturated fat, trans fat, and cholesterol in foods.

- Choose lean cuts of select meat such as round, sirloin, and flank, and eat portions that are no larger than the palm of your hand. Chicken, turkey, and fish are always leaner meat choices. To give an example, a 3-ounce (90 g) portion of beef has at least 2 grams of saturated fat; skinless chicken has 0.5 gram of saturated fat. Chicken breast with skin is equal to beef, at about 2 grams of saturated fat.

- When preparing and eating meat, make sure to trim all visible fat and skin. Use cooking racks when baking, broiling, grilling, steaming, or microwaving the meat to avoid melting the fat back into the meat.

- When eating lunch meat, select low-fat chicken or turkey breast rather than high-fat bologna or salami.

- Dairy foods are very important in your diet, including for weight control. To cut the fat in dairy foods, choose low-fat products rather than whole-milk products, and include them in your diet two or three times each day.

- Cholesterol is found only in animal products, and egg yolk is a concentrated source. Substitute two egg whites for one yolk, or use an egg substitute. Limit your intake to one egg yolk per day.

- Processed and prepared foods, especially snack foods, can be concentrated sources of fat. Hydrogenated vegetable fat contains trans-fatty acids that promote heart disease, so pay the most attention to the types and total amounts of fat in the food you eat. Read labels carefully, even if the packaging says that the product is light, to determine whether products really are low in fat. Be aware, also, that legally any product that has 0.5 gram of trans fat or less can be labeled trans fat free. So you probably are eating plenty of trans fats if you are eating a lot of packaged baked goods that say 0 trans fats per serving. Each serving may have up to 0.5 gram of trans fat.

All of the accumulated sport nutrition information tells us that the right kinds of dietary fat have profound effects on weight management, mood, and overall health. If we cut out all the fat in our diets, we eliminate not only the bad saturated fat, but also the good unsaturated fat. In today's world, the effective message is that the wrong fat can hurt, and the right fat can help. As long as you balance your calories, a diet high in lean protein, good carbohydrate, and good fat will leave little room for unhealthy foods to creep in. Keep your sight on all the good foods you need to eat every day and then the bad foods won't get you down.

## Sport Nutrition Fact Versus Fiction: Is Chocolate Healthy or Harmful?

Answer: Healthy! Chocolate is a healthy choice in prudent amounts. First, when you're feeling low or run-down, a bit of chocolate not only pampers you, but it actually works with your brain chemistry to lift your mood and make you feel better. The combination of sugar and fat in chocolate elevates two key neurotransmitters, serotonin and endorphins. Low levels of these brain chemicals are linked with depression and anxiety. By raising them, you feel calmer, more relaxed, and happier. Not bad for a few hundred calories!

Second, eating chocolate may actually make you healthier. This finding originated with the research on dietary saturated fat and its association with an increased risk of developing heart disease. Over a decade ago, the discovery that stearic acid, the predominant saturated fat in chocolate, actually has a neutral effect on blood cholesterol levels exonerated chocolate, removing it from the list of foods that are bad for your heart. Even feeding subjects one whole chocolate bar a day didn't change their levels of blood cholesterol.

What's more, scientists have discovered that chocolate is full of antioxidants, including flavonols and flavonoids. These compounds appear to have cardioprotective effects, including antioxidant properties, the ability to reduce the stickiness of blood cells, and the ability to help the lining of blood vessels remain dilated, allowing blood to pass more freely and keeping blood pressure at normal levels.

The richest source of flavonols is natural, non-Dutched (no alkali) cocoa powder. It is also the healthiest source because it is devoid of sugar and very low in fat and calories. Next on the list are baking chocolate and dark chocolate. Dark chocolate has twice the amount of flavonols as milk chocolate.

Curious about the antioxidant content of cocoa compared with wine and tea, Dr. Chang Yong Lee of Cornell University tested the antioxidant content of the following beverages: 1 cup (240 ml) of hot water containing 2 tablespoons of pure cocoa powder, 1 cup (240 ml) of water containing a standard-size bag of green tea, 1 cup (240 ml) of black tea, and a 5-ounce (150 ml) glass of California merlot (red wine). On a per-serving basis, the antioxidant concentration in cocoa was the highest. Its concentration was almost two times stronger than the concentration in red wine, two to three times stronger than in green tea, and four to five times stronger than in black tea. Dr. Lee also found that hot cocoa triggers the release of more antioxidants than cold cocoa.

Dr. Mary Engler and colleagues of the University of California at San Francisco investigated the effects of a flavonoid-rich dark chocolate on endothelial function (the function of the cells lining blood vessels), oxidative stress, blood lipids, and blood pressure in 21 healthy adults. The subjects were assigned to eat either a daily high-flavonoid or low-flavonoid dark chocolate bar for two weeks. There were no obvious differences between the two bars. The subjects were instructed to keep their diets the same as usual, except to eliminate all other foods and beverages high in flavonoids, alcohol, vitamin supplements, and nonsteroidal anti-inflammatory drugs. The results showed that endothelial function improved with the consumption of the high-flavonoid chocolate bars. Blood vessels were more dilated and blood flow was freer. Other biochemical measures indicated a strong association with the intake of flavonoids. No differences in oxidative stress or lipid profiles were seen between the two groups.

Deciding which side of the line chocolate falls on goes back to two major tenets of nutrition: variety and moderation. To be sure, chocolate bars, whether they contain dark or milk chocolate, are high in calories, sugar, and fat. When searching for sources of antioxidants in your diet, remember that fruits, vegetables, fish, nuts, seeds, and tea are rich sources of many important nutrients and antioxidants. Flavonol-rich cocoa is available in candy bars, cocoa powder, and even desserts. On a regular basis it is probably best to get your flavonols from a cup of cocoa that is lighter in fat and calories. Then, when you can really enjoy it, savor your piece of dark chocolate as you would a glass of fine wine.

# 5

# Burning Fat

Why do you want to lose body fat? To compete in a lower weight class? Get ready for a bodybuilding contest? Improve your performance? Look better in your clothes? All are admirable goals for fat loss, and there are umpteen ways to reach them. Two of the most widely used and unhealthy methods are crash dieting and fad dieting.

Crash dieting involves a drastic reduction in calories, usually to about 800 calories or fewer a day, and results in equally drastic consequences, such as the following:

- **Muscle and fluid losses along with fat loss.** If you lost 20 pounds (9 kg) in 20 days, the first 6 to 10 pounds (2.7 to 4.5 kg) would be fluid; the rest would be fat and muscle. You are not gaining anything by dropping a lot of weight in a short period of time.

- **Loss of aerobic power.** Your body's capacity to take in and process oxygen, or $\dot{V}O_2$max, will decline significantly. As a result, less oxygen will be available to help your muscle cells combust fat for fuel.

- **Loss of strength.** This is a major handicap if you need strength and power for competition or to get through a workout without fizzling out.

- **Metabolic slowdown.** Crash dieting slows your metabolic rate to a crawl. Your metabolic rate is the speed at which your body processes food into energy and bodily structures. It is made up of two interrelated factors: basal metabolic rate (BMR) and resting metabolic rate (RMR). Your BMR represents the energy it takes just to exist; it is the energy required to keep your heart beating, your lungs breathing, and your other vital internal functions going strong. Basal metabolic needs must be met. If you're a woman, for example, you expend as many as 1,200 to 1,400 calories a day just fueling the basic work of your body's cells. Imagine the harm you are doing to your life processes by subsisting on a diet of 800 calories a day!

RMR includes your BMR plus additional energy expenditures required for the light activities of waking up, getting dressed, sitting up, and walking around. Your RMR accounts for about 60 percent of the energy you expend daily. The higher this rate is, the more efficient your body is at burning fat.

Specifically, it is your RMR that slows down when you restrict calories. In a one-year study of overweight men, those who cut calories to lose weight (as opposed to those who exercised) experienced a significant drop in their RMR. One reason was that they lost muscle tissue, and RMR is closely linked to how much muscle you have. The moral of the story is that following restrictive diets for an extended period will decelerate your RMR, and you can kiss the muscle you worked so hard to build good-bye.

Crash dieting is a losing proposition all the way around. There is nothing to be gained—except more weight! About 95 to 99 percent of all people who go on such diets regain their weight plus interest within a year.

Fad diets—eating plans that eliminate certain foods and emphasize others—are just as bad as crash diets. A major problem with fad diets is that they are nutritionally unbalanced, and you could be missing out on some of the key nutrients you need for good health. An analysis of 11 popular diets revealed deficiencies in one or more essential nutrients, several of the B-complex vitamins, calcium, iron, and zinc. One diet derived 70 percent of its calories from fat. Such dangerously high levels of fat can lead to heart disease.

But there are other problems, too. Take the mostly protein diet (with hardly any carbohydrate), one of the most popular fad diets among strength trainers. And no wonder it's popular! At first, it works great. You get on the scale, see a huge weight loss, and feel wonderful—until you go off the diet. Then the weight comes back as fast as it left. That is because mostly protein diets are dehydrating; they flush water right out of your system to help the body get rid of excess nitrogen. Dehydration is dangerous, too, potentially causing fatigue, lack of coordination, heat illnesses such as heat stress and heatstroke, and in extreme cases (a loss of 6 percent or more of body fluid), death. Even with a mere 2 percent drop in body weight as fluid, your performance will diminish. That is the equivalent of 3 pounds (1.4 kg) of water loss in a 150-pound (68 kg) person.

Enough said about what doesn't work. There are antifat exercise and diet strategies that do work—namely a fat-burning training program and an individualized, nutritionally balanced eating plan that emphasizes a balanced combination of carbohydrate, protein, and the right kinds of fat. Before beginning, though, you should set some physique goals.

## Go for Your Goal

Whether you realize it or not, you already know what your goal is. Just ask yourself: At what weight, or body-fat percentage, do I look, feel, or perform the best? The answer to that question is your goal.

The first step is to figure out how close to the mark you are. There are lots of ways to figure this out, including height and weight charts, body mass index (BMI) calculations, and bathroom scales. But the problem with most of these is that they are not very accurate for people who strength train. None of these methods takes into account the amount of muscle you have on your body; they might even indicate that you are overweight!

Bathroom scales tempt you to step on them every morning. That can be a downer, because your weight goes up and down daily as a result of normal fluid fluctuations. It can be easy to get obsessed with the numbers you see on the scale, especially because when you begin a program to lose fat by following the proper diet, exercising, and drinking enough water, you may often gain weight before you lose it. Here's why: For every molecule of glycogen stored in your muscles, you store an additional three molecules of water inside your muscles, which lie there ready to assist in metabolism. When you step on the scale, you may see a gain that is the result of water weight.

A better measurement technique is body-composition testing, which determines how much of your weight is muscle and how much is fat. Several methods are in use. One is underwater weighing, considered the gold standard and very accurate if done properly with the right equipment. But it is not convenient (I certainly don't have a water tank in my office), and it can be rather expensive.

Another method that is rapidly improving in reliability and validity is bioelectrical impedance analysis (BIA), which involves passing a painless electrical current through the body by means of electrodes placed on the hands and feet. Fat tissue won't conduct the current, but fat-free tissue (namely, water found in muscle) will. Thus, the faster the current passes through the body, the less body fat there is. Readings obtained from the test are plugged into formulas adjusted for height, gender, and age to calculate body-fat and fat-free mass percentages.

You can now purchase bathroom scales on which you can weigh yourself while measuring your body composition with BIA at the same time. These scales are not necessarily accurate, but as long as you follow the weigh-in instructions, you can see trends in your body-composition changes. You should be well hydrated, because if you are dehydrated even a little, as most people are, you won't get an accurate reading. Also, don't eat within four hours of weighing, and don't drink any alcohol or exercise intensely within 12 hours of weighing. When instructions are followed, these scales are fairly reliable in showing whether your body-fat percentage is increasing or decreasing. If you want to keep tabs on your body composition, it is a good idea to check it only once every few weeks because it takes time for this change to occur.

Another accurate method of checking body composition is the skinfold technique, which measures fat just under the skin and uses those measurements to calculate body composition, including body-fat percentage. One of the keys to getting accurate and reliable measurements with the skinfold method is to use the same technician, time after time, month after month. That way, you don't get as much variability in the measurements.

I use another strategy with strength trainers and athletes, one that can be a real motivator as they progress toward their goals. I have them take circumference measurements (with a cloth tape measure) of selected widths on the upper arm, chest, waist, hips, thighs, and calves. You should take these measurements every four to six weeks to see the evidence of the positive changes that strength training, combined with the right diet, makes in your body. Because it is the easiest method, it can also be the most motivating!

## Your Optimal Body-Fat Percentage

Exactly what is optimal in terms of body fat? Healthy ranges of body fat are 20 to 25 percent for women and 15 to 20 percent for men. But if you are a strength trainer or bodybuilder, it is desirable to have even lower percentages: 10 to 18 percent for women and 5 to 15 percent for men.

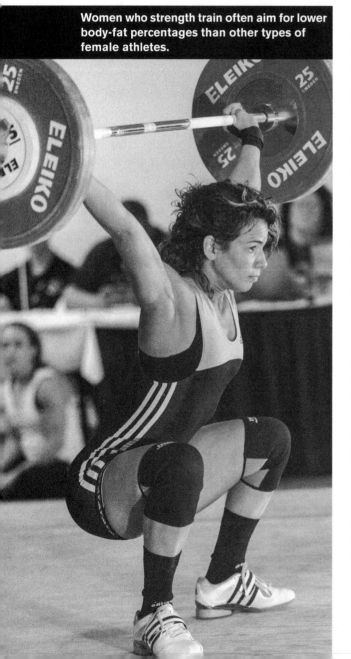

Women who strength train often aim for lower body-fat percentages than other types of female athletes.

### The Female Athlete Triad

Many elite female athletes have less than 10 percent body fat. Female competitive runners, for example, may have as little as 5 or 6 percent body fat, according to some studies. A low percentage of body fat may be perfectly normal and desirable for some female athletes because it enhances sport performance. As long as you don't consciously restrict calories while training for a sport, there is nothing unhealthy about having a naturally lean figure. However, calorie restriction combined with overexercising depletes body-fat stores to unhealthy levels, which elevates the risk of a syndrome known as the female athlete triad.

The female athlete triad refers to three interrelated health problems seen in women: disrupted eating habits, menstrual irregularities, and weak bones. If you have the female athlete triad, you may suffer from an eating disorder such as anorexia or bulimia, or you may have reduced energy because your food intake is too low for your exercise level. Also, your menstrual periods have ceased, and you may also have the beginnings of osteoporosis, a disease that makes your bones thin and weak.

You are at the highest risk for the female athlete triad if you

- are a competitive athlete;
- are involved in sports such as gymnastics or bodybuilding that require you to check your weight often;
- exercise more than you need to, without taking in enough calories;
- constantly diet for performance, appearance, or both;
- have perfectionist personality traits;
- have stopped eating with your family and friends; and
- have the attitude that amenorrhea (loss of your period), excessive exercise, and weight loss are positive attributes in athletics.

Some symptoms of the female athlete triad are weight loss, absent or irregular periods, fatigue and stress fractures, and increase in illness due to a weakened immune system. I have occasionally encountered the female athlete triad in my practice. For example, I once worked with a woman who was an ultraendurance athlete and did an extreme amount of exercise. She had begun to experience bone fractures all over her body, along with various illnesses. Her periods had become very irregular. Once we talked, it was apparent that she was consuming fewer calories than her body required to carry out all its activity. We corrected this situation through a higher-calorie diet with the correct percentages of protein, carbohydrate, and fat. Ultimately, she had to cut back on her exercise to regain her health. Once she was healthy again, she was able to return to her sport in much better shape than she left it.

What typically happens is that women deliberately try to lose weight to improve their performance or appearance, and so body fat is drastically reduced. In response, the ovaries cut back production of estrogen. When estrogen is reduced, menstrual periods become irregular or cease altogether. With poor diet and low calcium intake along with low estrogen levels, osteoporosis becomes a serious concern that can result in fracture risk.

To prevent the female athlete triad, as well as treat it,

- follow a healthy, energy-rich diet adequate for the demands of your sport;
- increase your caloric intake and make sure you get adequate calcium and vitamin D to help guard against osteoporosis;
- cut back on your training intensity; and
- see a sports medicine physician, who may prescribe hormone replacement therapy temporarily to replace lost estrogen and to stop your body from losing any more bone strength.

For more information and resources on the female athlete triad, visit www.femaleathletetriad.org.

## *Body Dysmorphia in Men*

Women aren't the only ones who obsess about their weight and appearance; men can be just as preoccupied. Body dissatisfaction in men has nearly tripled over the last three decades. An obsessive dissatisfaction with one's body is termed body dysmorphia; it is seen largely in men and tends to manifest in athletes. Whereas women tend to believe that their bodies are bigger than they really are, men with this disorder tend to falsely believe that their bodies or their muscles are too small. They may have a poor body image and an obsessive desire to build muscle and avoid gaining fat.

Following are some of the signs of body dysmorphia:

- Excessive strength training (spending countless hours in the gym) and other compulsive exercising that interferes with work and life
- Body checking (looking in mirrors and other reflections) or avoiding mirrors altogether
- Obsessive weighing
- Spending less time with family or friends
- Using anabolic steroids

If you find that you're training excessively and you're worried about it interfering with your daily life, and if your joy in life has diminished at the same time, seek counseling, because this disorder is psychiatric. It does not respond to aesthetically oriented interventions such as exercise programs, diets, or plastic surgery to correct perceived bodily flaws. Some research indicates that antidepressants may help. See a qualified psychologist if you or someone you love may be suffering from this disorder.

## Your Weight-Loss Goal Formula

Once you have determined your body composition through an appropriate method, you can figure out how much weight you need to lose to reach a lower body-fat percentage with the following formula:

1. Present body weight × present body-fat % = fat weight
2. Present body weight – fat weight = fat-free weight
3. Fat-free weight / desired % of fat-free mass = goal weight
4. Present body weight – goal weight = weight-loss goal

As an illustration, let's say you weigh 140 pounds (63.5 kg), with a present body-fat percentage of 12 percent. Your goal is to achieve 7 percent body fat. Your body-composition goal, then, is 7 percent fat and 93 percent fat-free mass. How many pounds do you need to lose?

Here's the calculation:

$$140 \text{ lb } (63.5 \text{ kg}) \times 0.12 = 16.8 \text{ lb } (7.6 \text{ kg}) \text{ fat weight}$$

$$140 \text{ lb } (63.5 \text{ kg}) - 16.8 \text{ lb } (7.6 \text{ kg}) = 123.2 \text{ lb } (55.9 \text{ kg}) \text{ fat-free weight}$$

$$123.2 \text{ lb } (55.9 \text{ kg}) / 0.93 = 132.5 \text{ lb } (60.1 \text{kg})$$

$$140 \text{ lb } (63.5 \text{ kg}) - 132.5 \text{ lb } (60.1 \text{ kg}) = 7.5 \text{ lb } (3.4 \text{ kg})$$

To arrive at 7 percent body fat, you need to lose 7.5 pounds (3.4 kg). Naturally, you want those 7-plus pounds to be fat pounds. Here's a look at how to maximize fat loss and minimize muscle loss.

# Exercise and Fat Loss

Your objective is to lose body fat without losing muscle mass. You don't want to lose strength or endurance, either, and you don't want your performance to suffer. So how can you keep on the losing track? Forget about diet for a moment; the other key is exercise.

When it comes to burning fat, exercise is your best friend in three ways:

1. **The more exercise you do, the less you have to worry about calories.** By burning 300 to 400 calories a day through exercise, you enhance the rate of fat burning. As I noted previously, these caloric deficits have been tested in research and proven accurate.

2. **Exercise hikes your RMR.** After you exercise, your RMR stays elevated for several hours, and you burn extra calories even at rest. If you strength train, you get even more of a metabolic boost: The muscle you develop is calorie-burning, metabolically active tissue. Having more muscle tissue cranks your metabolic rate even higher.

   At Colorado State University, researchers recruited 10 men, aged 22 to 35, to see what effect strength training had on metabolism. At various times in the study, the men participated in strength training, aerobic exercise, or a control condition of quiet sitting. During the experiment, the subjects followed controlled diets with a composition of 65 percent carbohydrate, 15 percent protein, and 20 percent fat.

   In the strength-training portion of the experiment, the men performed a fairly standard, yet strenuous, routine: five sets of 10 different upper- and lower-body exercises for a total of 50 sets. They worked out for about 100 minutes. For aerobic exercise, the men cycled at moderate intensities for about an hour.

   The researchers reported these findings: Strength training produced a higher rate of oxygen use than either aerobic exercise or quiet sitting, meaning that it was a better elevator of RMR. The men's RMR stayed elevated for about 15 hours after working out. Clearly, strength training stood out as a metabolic booster and a calorie burner. With strength training, it is easy to keep fat off and control your weight.

3. **Exercise preserves muscle.** If you lose 10 pounds (4.5 kg) of body weight, you may be lighter, but if 5 pounds (2.3 kg) of that loss are muscle, you sure won't be stronger, and your performance can suffer. Appearance-wise, you can still look flabby when muscle tissue is lost. Exercise is one of the best ways to make sure you are shedding weight from fat stores rather than from muscle stores.

Researchers have put this principle to the test. In a study of 10 overweight women, half of the women were placed in a diet-plus-exercise group and half of the women, in an exercise-only group. The women in the first group followed a diet that reduced their calories by 50 percent of what it took to maintain their weight, and they worked out aerobically six times a week. The women in the exercise-only group followed the same aerobic exercise program but followed a diet designed to stabilize their weight.

After 14 weeks, it was time to check the results. Here is what happened: Both groups lost weight. But the composition of that loss was vastly different between the groups. In the group that dieted and exercised, the weight lost was 67 percent fat and 33 percent lean mass. In the group that only exercised, the women lost much more fat—86 percent fat and only 14 percent lean mass! Not only that, but RMR declined by 9 percent among the dieters, whereas it was maintained in those who only exercised.

What does all this tell us? Sure, you can lose weight by low-calorie dieting. But you risk losing muscle. Also, your metabolic rate can plummet, sabotaging your attempts at successful weight control. With exercise and a nonrestrictive diet, you preserve calorie-burning muscle and keep your metabolism in gear.

## High-Intensity Interval Training Counts

If you want to get totally lean for competition or looks, but without sacrificing precious muscle, get familiar with high-intensity interval training, otherwise known as HIIT.

With HIIT, your workouts will be shorter, but you'll actually be working out harder than anyone on the cardio machines at your gym. Basically, you work out in intervals—bouts of all-out effort at a rate of 80 to 90 percent of your maximal heart rate (MHR) alternated with short stretches of active recovery. You can do any kind of high-intensity exercise to meet the guidelines of HIIT all-out effort training (e.g., sprinting outside on a track or working out inside on a rowing machine, using a stationary bike or treadmill, or even performing plyometrics) for one to two minutes. On a 1 to 10 scale of perceived exertion, your high-intensity training should exceed a level of 7. Active recovery can be the same activity but at a lower intensity (e.g., from a sprint on a track to a jog, from a two-minute hill climb on an indoor bike to a three-minute flat at a level of 4 or 5, or from intense plyometrics to squats, sit-ups, and push-ups). This cycle is repeated for about 20 minutes. Plenty of research shows that HIIT is a super-effective way to burn fat. Following are some cases in point.

An early study, done by researchers at Laval University (Quebec, Canada), used two groups in a months-long experiment. One group followed a 15-week program using HIIT, while the other performed only regular cardio exercise. The regular cardio folks burned 15,000 calories more than their HIIT counterparts did, but the HIIT trainers lost more body fat.

A 2001 study from East Tennessee State University found similar results with exercisers who did HIIT for eight weeks. Again, HIIT turned out to be a superior fat burner (the participants shed 2 percent of their body fat over the course of the trial). The regular cardio exercisers didn't lose an ounce of fat.

An Australian study found that a group of women who followed a 20-minute HIIT program consisting of 8-second sprints followed by 12 seconds of rest lost an amazing six times more body fat than a group that followed a typical 40-minute cardio program performed at a constant intensity of 60 percent maximum heart rate (MHR).

And here's something else: HIIT is a great way to burn belly fat. In a study from the University of Virginia, researchers recruited 27 middle-aged, obese women with the metabolic syndrome (a prediabetic condition) and had them complete one of three 16-week aerobic exercise interventions: (1) no exercise training (control); (2) low-intensity exercise training (LIET); and (3) HIIT. At the end of the experimental period, HIIT had significantly reduced total abdominal fat, and there were no such changes in the control or LIET groups.

The reason HIIT works so well is that it cranks up your metabolism—an effect supported by research. Generally, HIIT results in a caloric "afterburn," meaning that your body continues to burn a lot of calories in the 24 hours after exercise. HIIT appears to be tougher on your body, which means that your body needs more calories to repair itself. Oh—and that Laval study mentioned earlier found that the HIIT exercisers' muscle fibers had significantly higher markers for fat oxidation (fat burning) than those of the subjects in the regular cardio group. Translation: HIIT seems to turn your body into a true fat-burning factory. Another plus is that shorter exercise sessions let you preserve muscle.

So if you're looking for a way to burn fat without losing muscle, HIIT is it.

## Other Intensity Strategies for Fat-Burning

If you don't do HIIT, there are other ways to burn fat through exercise. For example, try to work out at a level hard enough to raise your heart rate 70 to 85 percent of MHR. MHR can be calculated by subtracting your age from the number 220. During low-intensity exercise (20 minutes or longer at around 50 percent of MHR), fat supplies as much as 90 percent of your fuel requirements. High-intensity aerobic exercise at roughly 75 percent of MHR burns a smaller percentage of fat (around 60 percent), but results in more total calories burned overall, including more fat calories.

To illustrate this concept, here's a comparison based on studies of aerobic intensity. At 50 percent of MHR, you burn 7 calories a minute, 90 percent of which come from fat. At 75 percent of MHR, you burn 14 calories a minute, 60 percent from fat. So at 50 percent intensity, at which 90 percent of the calories are from fat, you are burning only 6.3 fat calories per minute ($0.9 \times 7$ calories per minute), but at 75 percent intensity, at which only 60 percent of the calories are from fat, you are burning as much as 8.4 fat calories per minute ($0.6 \times 14$ calories per minute). In short, you burn more total fat calories at higher intensities.

Intensity in strength training refers to how much weight you lift. For your muscles to respond—that is, get stronger and better developed—you have to challenge them to handle heavier weights. That means continually putting more demands on them than they're used to, progressively increasing the weight you lift from workout to workout. The more muscle you can develop, the more efficient your body becomes at fat burning, because muscle is the most metabolically active tissue in the body.

If you have difficulty exercising at a high intensity, try increasing your duration—how long you exercise. You can burn just as much fat working out longer at a lower intensity as you can exercising at a higher intensity for a shorter duration.

To increase your rate of fat loss, gradually increase your aerobic exercise sessions from 30 to 60 minutes, or strive for longer distances. For example, running a mile (1.6 km) expends about 100 calories. Run 5 miles (8 km), and you will burn 500 calories.

Another option related to duration is frequency—working out more times a week to obtain a greater caloric expenditure. Perhaps you could add spinning, a cardiorespiratory step class, kickboxing, or aerobic dance to your aerobic program for some variety as well as for some extra calorie burning.

With these strategies—lots of quality calories and lots of intense exercise—Mike was able to reduce his body fat from 9 percent to a contest-sharp 6.9 percent, without sacrificing muscle.

You don't have to start working out five hours a day (unless perhaps you are a professional bodybuilder training for a contest). But there is a connection between exercise and diet to burn body fat. You don't necessarily have to cut calories; you can actually keep them high. Exercising at moderate to high levels of intensity will take care of the fat.

## Competitive Strategy of a Professional Bodybuilder

Years ago, a group of researchers at Arizona State University studied the diet and exercise strategies of Mike Ashley, known in bodybuilding circles as "Natural Wonder," because he does not use anabolic steroids. During an eight-week precontest period, Mike did the following:

- Consumed roughly 5,000 calories daily–3,674 calories from food plus a carbohydrate-rich sport drink–and an amino acid supplement.

- Took in an additional 1,278 calories a day from supplemental MCT oil (see chapter 8 for more about MCTs). This meant that 25.5 percent of his calories came from a fat source, not including food intake. However, MCTs are not metabolized the way conventional fat is; the body uses them immediately for energy rather than storing them as fat. (Although MCTs represent a more compact source of energy–9 calories per gram versus 4 calories per gram for carbohydrate–this approach is not recommended for everyone. The nutrition plan outlined in chapter 13 has wider application and will work for more people.)

- Trained on a stair-climbing machine for a full hour, six days a week.

- Weight trained six days a week, dividing his routine into two or three workouts a day. In total, Mike worked out five to six hours a day at a high level of intensity.

# Antifat Diet Strategies

The old-fashioned way of figuring out how many calories you should eat to lose weight is to just chop off 500 to 1,000 calories from your current diet. One pound (0.5 kg) of fat is equivalent to 3,500 calories. According to the laws of thermodynamics, if you feed yourself 500 calories fewer than you need each day for seven days, theoretically you should lose 1 pound (0.5 kg) by the end of the week. Double that amount and you should lose 2 pounds (0.9 kg). But dietitians have known for years that it never works this way, and this strategy becomes more frustrating as the weeks of dieting wear on.

At Georgia State University, Dr. Dan Benardot wondered why these seemingly clear laws of physics don't hold true within the human body. His research has shown that once food enters the biological system of the body, there are more variables at work than the simple number of calories that are given off by a pound of fat when measured directly in a science lab. The human body is a living organism, and the drive for survival allows the rules of the system to change based on thousands of years of adaptation to the environment. Dr. Benardot tested two groups of female gymnasts and runners: One group ate a diet of 500 fewer calories than they needed to maintain their weight each day, and the other group ate 300 fewer calories. What he found was astounding: The group that ate 300 fewer calories had a lower percentage of body fat than the group that actually ate less food. His theory is that when too few calories are eaten, resting energy expenditure (REE) slows down to meet the energy available to the body.

The ability of the body to slow metabolic rate to meet available energy has long been understood by scientists. Called starvation adaptation, it is induced in extreme circumstances of famine to allow the body to survive far longer than would be predicted based on normal metabolic rates of energy use. Dr. Benardot proposed for the first time that even under mild states of energy deficit, energy use slows down. There is no benefit to eating far fewer calories than your body needs. In fact, he called a 300-calorie deficit the ideal metabolic window for women to lose the most amount of fat in the shortest amount of time.

So forget low-calorie dieting. When you reduce your caloric intake by 300 calories (women) or 400 calories (men), you can keep your metabolic rate high enough to continue to burn fat at a good clip. Additionally, you want to have enough energy to perform at peak levels both physically and mentally. Here's how to eat to give yourself the best chance at losing fat and saving muscle:

## Don't Starve Yourself

Because you strength train and probably do aerobics as well, you actually need more food, not less. Researchers at Tufts University found that when older men and women began a strength-training program, they needed 15 percent more calories just to maintain their body weight. This finding is not so surprising, really. With strength training, the exercisers began to expend more calories. Plus, their RMR increased because they had built more muscle.

You can figure out exactly how many calories you need to lose fat. Based on my research with competitive bodybuilders, I have concluded that an intake of 35 to 38 calories per kilogram of body weight a day is reasonable for fat loss and muscle preservation in someone training five or more days per week. The minimum is 29 to 32 calories per kilogram for a rapid cut for the same level of training. If you are training only three or four days per week, then of course, your calories will be lower. Anything less than that is too restrictive, and you won't be well nourished.

Let's say you are a man exercising five or more days per week and you weigh 180 pounds (82 kg). Here's how to figure your calorie requirements to lose fat: 82 kg × 38 calories/kg = 3,116 calories. For maintaining body weight, you should eat up to 42 calories per kilogram of body weight a day, or 3,444 calories a day. If you want to build muscle and you increase your exercise intensity, duration, or frequency, go even higher—to 52 calories per kilogram of body weight or more, or 4,264 calories a day.

If you still need a calorie deficit to continue losing fat or to break a plateau, get that deficit by increasing your activity level and modifying your calories slightly. For example, restrict your calories by about 300 to 400 calories a day and increase your aerobic exercise. This deficit, again, is the ideal metabolic window for weight loss.

## Correct Your Dietary Fat

Be sure to include the right kinds of fat in your diet, including omega-3 fat from fish and monounsaturated fat from olive oil, avocados, nuts and seeds, and nut and seed oils. A recent Australian study showed that diets rich in monounsaturated fat helped premenopausal women preserve muscle while losing weight. Diets high in omega-3 fat may actually protect against obesity; many studies have observed the fat-burning effect of omega-3 fat. Include up to five fish meals in your diet each week. The more muscle you maintain while losing fat, the greater your chance of keeping the weight off for good.

## Preserve Muscle With Protein

To lose mostly fat and keep your metabolism running in high gear with muscle mass preserved, you must have adequate protein in your diet. Protein also helps control your appetite. If you go on a diet that is too low in calories, there is a good chance that your dietary protein will not be used to build tissue but instead will be broken down and used for energy much like carbohydrate and fat are. As a reminder, for losing body fat, the nutrient profile of your diet should be 30 percent protein, 40 percent carbohydrate, and 30 percent fat.

## Lower Body Fat With Less Carbohydrate

In the past, I've hesitated to recommend lower-carbohydrate diets to highly active groups of people. I didn't think an active person or athlete could exercise hard under conditions of low-carbohydrate intake. However, several new lines of research reveal that a low-carbohydrate diet with adequate vegetables, dairy, and small amounts of nuts and seeds can provide fuel for workouts, while still triggering weight loss. These days, I now endorse the right kind of lower-carbohydrate dieting as an effective way to get lean.

The fat-loss diet I recommend is not painful; nor will it make you feel deprived. I've organized the plan to precisely time and combine foods to maximize your mood, mental focus, and physical energy. I also make sure that you have the right amount of calories and nutrients in a targeted way throughout the day to put all the necessary nutrients to work for you. Check out chapters 15 and 16 for menu plans that will support your training, physique, and fat-loss goals.

## Reach for Veggies and Whole Foods

The best dietary strategy for weight loss and fat loss and shaping your body is to eat an abundance of vegetables. Ideally, these vegetables should be grown using sustainable methods with the smallest carbon footprint, and not be genetically modified organisms (GMOs). I believe these methods will make you feel good about what you're eating.

Although the research is ongoing as to whether organically raised foods are nutritionally healthier than those grown with pesticides and herbicides, or even do the least damage to you or to the environment, it is most likely that they are better for the health of the farmworkers in the fields. What we do know is that when you shop at a farmers' market, or you meet the farmer who raised your food, you have a direct connection to the person who put time and effort into creating the food you eat. By buying local produce, you contribute to the livelihood of your community and to the physical care of your environment. Research shows that these positive connections enhance immune function, overall health, and quality of life.

Whole foods are infinitely healthier than processed foods. Despite all of the science that has given us functional, engineered foods, we still have not outdone Mother Nature. Individual vitamins and minerals, phytonutrients and food factors, fatty acids, amino acids, and fibers never work as well as supplements as they do when combined in their natural form in whole food. Supplements are helpful, but only for convenience, for targeted action, and as extra nutritional insurance. I certainly use products and supplements in my diet and suggest them to my clients. But supplements, whether in food or pill form, will never replace whole foods.

Even though an athlete's life can be busy, hectic, and demanding, the choice to use whole foods makes a huge difference in physical and mental performance. It may take a little extra effort, but the effort is worth it. You'll need to plan ahead by creating shopping lists, meal plans, and recipes. If you travel, you'll need to think ahead and purchase the kinds of foods that stay fresh and are appropriate for an on-the-go lifestyle. You'll also have to scope out restaurants and grocery stores that can meet your needs. And you'll have to understand food well enough to make adjustments to your food plan and still stay on track to meet your goals.

Remember, it is far more important to eat a diet abundant in vegetables and fruits than to avoid them because you can't find or can't afford organically raised produce. Whether conventional or organic, always wash your produce well.

Throughout the day you should eat plenty of nonstarchy vegetables. This results in a diet rich in anti-inflammatory nutrients, fluids, and fiber. These characteristics make vegetables filling, which helps when you're cutting back on calories and trying to control your appetite. The fibers from most nonstarchy vegetables are not gas forming, either; they create little to no discomfort and bloating in athletes.

## Monitor Added Sugar in Your Diet

Added sugar in your diet promotes fat gain by reducing the sensitivity of your cells to insulin so that insulin cannot shuttle sugar into your muscles. It then heads to the liver, which turns the sugar into fat. When you eat low-glycemic foods, you avoid this situation entirely.

Case in point: Researchers at Indiana University analyzed the diets of four groups of people: lean men (average body fat of 15 percent), lean women (average body fat of 20 percent), obese men (average body fat of 25 percent), and obese women (average body fat of 35 percent). The obese men and women ate more of their calories from fat (as high as 36 percent of total calories) and refined sugars, such as candy, doughnuts, and ice cream (which are also high in fat) than the lean men and women did. In other words, there was a link between high-fat, high-sugar diets and obesity.

The lesson is this: Change the composition of your diet to keep the fat off. This means cutting down on high-fat, sugary foods. If you have a sweet tooth, choose dark chocolate or combine the sweet food with a protein and a healthy fat so that you slowly absorb the food and slowly release sugar and, ultimately, insulin into your bloodstream. Stay away from beverages and foods sweetened with high-fructose corn syrup, which has been linked to the high incidence of obesity.

If you are considering using artificially sweetened foods, proceed with caution. See the section on artificial sweeteners later in this chapter for more on the controversy over their use.

## Don't Fast Prior to Exercise if Performance Is Your Goal

Fasting prior to exercise has been rumored to boost fat burning. This strategy is still controversial. While some studies confirm that there is no difference in fat loss between exercising on an empty stomach and exercising after having eaten, others disagree. In reality, fasting prior to exercise may slightly boost fat burning but will not improve exercise performance!

Additionally, if you exercise after fasting, your body doesn't have enough muscle glycogen for fuel—a precarious situation. The fact is, inadequate glycogen causes muscle protein breakdown, which is not the state you want to achieve for building muscle, strength, and power.

My advice is to always go into exercise well fueled. If you train early in the morning and feel that you can't eat a full breakfast prior to training, then have a small snack at least. Ideally, your snack would have 20 to 25 grams of protein and at least 35 grams or more of carbohydrate, depending on your own total carbohydrate needs, but even half of that is better than nothing. You might find that a liquid shake made from whey protein and a carbohydrate source such as fruit, juice, or a carbohydrate supplement is your best strategy. Yogurt is often well tolerated and is a natural carbohydrate–protein combo. Then have a full breakfast after your training. Timing for any preworkout meal or snack is highly individualized based on what you can tolerate. Some can eat and train; others need up to 60 or even 90 minutes before exercise. Experiment on your own, and remember that liquids empty most quickly from your stomach.

If you train later in the day, you'll have already been feeding yourself and fueling your muscles. So make sure that you have eaten within 90 minutes to two hours prior to exercise. Find the foods that work for you. Yogurt is a good choice; so are liquid shakes. If you're someone who enjoys a burger prior to training hard, that is fine too. Do what works best for you.

But keep your fat intake to a minimum in your preworkout snacks and meals. It will slow digestion and make you feel fuller for longer. Avoid high-fiber foods around exercise for the same reasons.

## Don't Skip Breakfast

Skipping breakfast is not a good way to lose body fat; in fact, it could even make you fatter! Most people who skip breakfast make up those calories, with interest, throughout the day. In Madrid, Spain, researchers found that overweight and obese people spent less time eating breakfast and ate smaller quantities and less varied types of food at breakfast compared with normal-weight people. Eating breakfast stokes your metabolic fires for the day. By contrast, going hungry in the morning is just another form of fasting, which slows down your metabolism. Plus, your physical and mental performance suffers when you are running on empty.

If you're like me, you're rushed in the morning, with barely enough time to shower and dress, let alone eat breakfast. If that is the case, eat what you can. Even on my busiest mornings, I plan ahead and never skip breakfast. Something is better than nothing. A study done in England found that because ready-to-eat cereals are high in vitamins and minerals and low in fat, they make a great choice for breakfast. When choosing cereals, those made from whole grains with low sugar and high fiber are the best bets.

The best breakfasts include a combination of carbohydrate, protein, and fat. If you are always on the go, you need some nutritious breakfasts that take minutes to fix. There are several breakfast recipes in chapter 17 to help you. Some of these can even go on the road with you—so there is no excuse to skip breakfast!

## Limit Alcohol Intake

If your goal is to perform at peak levels, be aware that alcohol consumption will limit your progress. The data are quite clear that alcohol, a central nervous system depressant, diminishes athletic performance not only within hours but also within days of consumption. Alcohol also increases appetite and caloric intake, both of which are detrimental to losing body fat.

There is a broad misconception that calories from alcohol are not recognized by the body and so don't count. This is false. The calories are absolutely recognized by the body and metabolized. Just like protein, carbohydrate, and fat, alcohol calories are stored as fat when caloric consumption is above caloric needs. Current research shows that alcohol calories add to all of the other calories that you eat in the day, yet they are considered "empty" calories because they provide virtually no nutrients. And because alcohol lowers your inhibitions, when you drink and eat, all of your best intentions go out the window.

Alcohol consumed before or with meals tends to increase food intake both by lowering inhibitions and enhancing the short-term rewarding effects of food. It is true that moderate alcohol intake may protect against obesity, particularly in women; however, increased alcohol consumption and dependence, as well as binge drinking, may increase risks of obesity. Most likely, you want to avoid obesity and stay as lean as possible. Except on special occasions, alcohol has no regular place in the diet of someone trying to achieve physique and performance goals.

## Sport Nutrition Fact Versus Fiction: Do Sugar Substitutes Have a Place in a Fat-Loss Program?

Sugar substitutes are either natural or synthetic. For instance, the sugar substitute stevia is natural, but the sugar substitute saccharine is artificial. Some sugar substitutes such as agave nectar and rice syrup are considered high-intensity sweeteners, because they are many times sweeter then sucrose or common table sugar. Because of the intensity of sweetness, only very small amounts are needed.

Most sugar substitutes approved for use by the FDA are artificially synthesized, but there are some natural compounds, including stevia, sorbitol, and xylitol. Despite FDA oversight of these food additives, sugar substitutes remain controversial, and some question whether they pose health risks.

The most common reason people use sugar substitutes is to reduce calorie consumption to control body weight and body fat. Recent scientific studies indicate that this may not be quite so simple. Animal studies have shown that a sweet taste in the mouth induces an insulin response, causing increased fat storage from circulating carbohydrate. When a sugar substitute leads to this insulin response without an increase in blood sugar, there can be an increase in hypoglycemia or hyperinsulinemia as the result. These conditions lead to increased food intake, no weight loss, and possible weight gain. Additionally, the body's usual response to sugar consumption in small amounts is to increase heat production and energy usage, and to blunt the appetite later in the day. With sugar substitutes, these responses never happen.

Population studies in humans have shown that increased consumption of artificially sweetened beverages leads to weight gain. Randomized controlled trials are very limited, however, and there is no strong clinical evidence to show a cause-and-effect relationship. My advice about all sugar substitutes is to keep these factors in mind and limit any use of added sweeteners in the diet, natural or otherwise.

# Best Fat-Burning Foods

A decade ago, all kinds of foods and supplements were sold with promises to burn fat. None of them, however, had any scientific data to support the claims. This has all changed. Scientists are now beginning to understand how certain foods actually do rev up metabolism or enhance hormones to help us burn fat. The best of these foods are discussed in this section.

## Protein

In addition to helping build muscle, lean protein helps stoke the fat-burning fires. Its thermogenic effect is 20 to 30 percent compared with an anemic 3 to 12 percent for carbohydrate. This basically means that it takes many more calories to digest, absorb, and use protein than carbohydrate. When you include protein in every meal and snack all day long, you raise your fat-burning potential.

Make sure to choose lean protein sources such as eggs, chicken, turkey, fish, lean red meat, low-fat or nonfat dairy (such as Greek yogurt), and vegetable protein. If you don't already have a blender and some protein powder, buy them. When you crave a high-fat or high-carbohydrate snack, reach for a protein shake instead.

## Fish

For many years, nutritionists assumed that people lost weight when they ate fish because it has fewer calories, pound for pound, than red meat. Now, however, it appears that the reasons go above and beyond calories. Most important, the type of fat found in fish appears to enhance the efficiency of the hormone leptin. This protein circulates in your bloodstream and, like the hormone insulin, is key in the weight-management equation. Leptin regulates your food intake as well as your body's energy expenditure. When cells in your brain sense a rise in leptin, they signal other parts of your nervous system to turn down your appetite and turn up your metabolism.

I recommend that all my clients eat five fish meals a week. Omega-3 fat supports a healthy heart, brain, and nervous system, and possibly enhances the efficiency of leptin in boosting your metabolism and controlling your appetite. It hardly gets better than this. Although all fish have more omega-3 fat than a hot dog, the fatty fish such as salmon, black cod, herring, sardines, mackerel, halibut, fresh tuna, and shellfish are highest in omega-3 fat.

## Probiotics

Your digestive system is home to between 10 trillion and 100 trillion bacteria, many of them friendly and health enhancing. The friendly bacterial cultures in your gut are called probiotics. Scientists believe that people with certain kinds of unfriendly microbes may get more calories from their food and therefore pack on more fat than people with a different type of microbes. As a result, manipulating these bacteria by diet or supplements may be a way to fight obesity. How could you do this? One way is to take prebiotics, which enhance the growth of certain healthy microbes. Prebiotics act as food for the probiotic cultures and are found in foods such as whole grains, flaxseed, onions, bananas, garlic, honey, leeks, and artichokes; probiotics are found in certain yogurts and kefir that contain live bacteria, as well as in supplements. It is believed that these friendly microbes digest excess calories. The net effect is that fewer calories are stored as fat. In a Canadian study published in the *American Journal of Clinical Nutrition*, 48 over-weight people took either a placebo or a prebiotic (oligofructose) for 12 weeks. Without consciously making any lifestyle changes, those taking the prebiotic lost an average of 2.27 pounds (1 kg), whereas those on the placebo gained nearly 1 pound (0.5 kg). Researchers found that the prebiotic also reduced hunger and improved blood sugar and insulin function. One of the easiest strategies for adding a healthy prebiotic every day is to include 1 to 2 tablespoons of ground flaxseed meal at breakfast in cold or hot cereal, or in yogurt. It can also easily be added to salads at lunch or dinner.

## Olive Oil

The kinds of fat you eat can influence your energy expenditure and body weight. Energy is released through heat production in a process called nonshivering thermogenesis, which is controlled by uncoupling proteins (UCP) in the cells of brown fat, white fat, and muscle. Researchers interested in finding out whether diet can influence this process investigated possible dietary enhancements of thermogenesis in rats. They found that olive oil, which is high in monounsaturated fat, increased the activity of UCPs, and hence metabolic rates. Because of the short duration of the study, published in the *American Journal of Clinical Nutrition*, no differences in body weight were recorded between the rats fed olive oil and those fed other forms of fat. However, international studies have shown that Mediterranean-style diets higher in olive oil are associated with weight maintenance and little weight gain over time compared with diets lower in olive oil. However, overall fat consumption still does add many calories to the diet, and those subjects with a very high fat consumption were overweight compared to those who controlled their total fat intake.

## Green Tea

Certain natural chemicals called catechins are abundant in green tea. Animal and human studies show that these chemicals appear to increase fat burning and stimulate thermogenesis, and the combination with caffeine in tea appears to boost the effect. The amount that you need to consume isn't absolutely clear. In a 1999 study in Maryland, subjects drank 6 quarter-cups (1,500 ml) of tea per day for four days. A more recent Japanese study found successful results from 2 1/2 cups (600 ml) every day for 12 weeks. A recent study from the UK demonstrated increased fat burning in exercising young men who ingested three capsules a day of a green tea extract (containing a total of 890 +/− 13 mg polyphenols and 366

+/– 5 mg EGCG [the catechins]). Because the amount of catechins is difficult to control with brewing, many practitioners recommend using a green tea extract for better dose control.

## Milk

Milk ranks high on the list of fat-burning foods. No doubt you've read about or heard the commercials for how milk can help you lose weight. The high calcium content of milk helps it turn off a key obesity gene, keeping your body from turning up the fat-making machinery to high, and helping your fat-burning metabolism run smoothly. At the same time, milk is the primary source of whey protein, shown in studies to enhance fat burning and limit the turnover of calories into fat storage by the liver. Subjects on a calorie-reduced diet given 20 grams of whey protein supplement every day after an exercise bout lost significantly more fat and maintained significantly more muscle mass compared to subjects given a placebo. Milk is a natural source of whey protein, and you will also benefit from adding a whey protein supplement to your diet.

## Chili Peppers

Studies have shown a thermogenic effect of capsaicin, a compound found in chili peppers. Subjects fed chili-containing meals regularly for four weeks had an attenuation of high blood insulin levels after the meals. Although weight loss was not studied, a lowering of blood insulin levels in overweight subjects may ultimately lead to weight loss. Other studies using a capsaicin supplement have been shown to be effective, but the dosage must be strictly followed. One Danish study of overweight and obese men using a supplement combining green tea extract, capsaicin, tyrosine, and calcium for seven days showed a 2 percent increase in energy expenditure. The researchers found that only the capsules that were not enterocoated were effective. The coating, which inhibits digestion in the stomach, inactivated the efficacy of capsaicin. (A new supplement containing a variant of capsaicin, capsinoid, has eliminated the spicy side effect and is more well tolerated than capsaicin supplements. This is discussed further in chapter 9.)

## Sport Nutrition Fact Versus Fiction: Cheat on Your Diet and Still Lose Weight

One of the most typical diet questions that I'm asked while standing at the buffet table at a party is, "What do you think about having a cheat day?" Here's my answer (a little more detailed than you'd get at the party).

The idea of the cheat day came out of the world of bodybuilding. Although notorious for their ability to follow a very restricted diet before competitions, male bodybuilders observed that on the day after their competition they looked much better than when they were on stage for the event. Not surprisingly, although they were eating only tuna and chicken breast to get cut before competition, immediately after the competition the nearest ice cream parlor was packed with competitors. After the late afternoon indulgence, they'd awake the next morning to an incredibly buff body, showing more cuts and definition than the day before. It didn't take long for the cheat day to be incorporated into the standard dieting regimes of male bodybuilders.

But what about female bodybuilders? By self-report, the women I work with find that adding a cheat day every once in a while is fine. However, unlike their male counterparts, who seem to be able to return to their diet regimens with great control, women tend to have less restraint during the week following a cheat day.

Pamela Peeke, MD, MPH, confirms this idea in her book, *Body-for-LIFE for Women* (Rodale, 2005). According to Dr. Peeke, women are more likely to binge during a cheat day. She recommends incorporating balance into your everyday diet to promote healthy relationships with food that can lead to successful weight loss.

Until recently, the concept of a cheat day was based on theory and anecdote. Now, however, there are data on what happens behaviorally and the outcome of that behavior. In 2005, a study published by researchers at the Center for Human Nutrition at the University of Colorado examined the common characteristics of successful long-term weight-loss maintainers on the National Weight Control Registry (NWCR). The NWCR lists over 4,800 people who have been successful in long-term weight-loss maintenance. Although the NWCR does not represent a random sample of all dieters, it does have value in identifying strategies that may help others become successful in keeping weight off.

One of the key results was that participants who maintained a consistent diet across the week were 1.5 times more likely to maintain their weight within 5 pounds (2.3 kg) over the subsequent year than were participants who allowed themselves a cheat day during the week. The same was true for people who allowed themselves more flexibility during holidays and traveling. Both groups that had free time outside their diet plans had a greater risk of regaining their lost weight.

To my way of thinking, the whole concept of cheating exemplifies a negative approach toward food. Cheating, whether planned or not, implies guilt for a bad deed done. Because we experience ourselves as living through a week of deprivation during which our favorite foods are off limits, all we do is crave them while working hard at avoiding them. Then comes our cheat day, and rather than eating a normal serving size of chocolate cake, we binge and eat half the cake. Then the guilt sets in, and there goes the other half of the cake. What a waste of time and emotion!

Get rid of the idea of cheating. Build a positive approach to food and dieting by daily balancing your food with your exercise, and your favorite foods with all the foods that you eat to maintain your health.

The easiest way to maintain balance in your diet is to start with the big picture. What are your favorite foods that you think you should avoid, and which days are your most active days? By plugging in sweet treats after exercise, you put the sugar to work for you. Not only do you not feel guilty about eating it, but your body benefits from the sugar after exercise. You can feel good about rewarding yourself for a hard, sweaty workout. Whatever that sweet treat is, make sure to include a source of milk protein at the same time, to get the biggest bang for your buck. Is a sweet, blended milk-based drink at your neighborhood latté stand or smoothie bar a sweet? Or maybe a cookie and a glass of milk? What about a latté and a bagel? All of these contain the right ingredients to help your muscles recover, build, and refuel after exercise. Of course, keeping your serving sizes small will help contain your calories, but it will seem like plenty when you've never before allowed yourself to eat anything after exercise!

Is your weakest moment in the evening? Are you dying for chocolate? Plan to have a hot cocoa to help you relax and get you over the hump. The high tryptophan levels in milk combined with the few grams of carbohydrate will raise your serotonin levels and help your mind and body get ready for sleep. Non-Dutched, natural cocoa powder, or bittersweet chocolate containing at least 70 percent cacao, will do the same. This is a way to plan something good for you into your days.

What about the unplanned splurge? There will always be very special moments in life when we do something, or eat something, just because we feel like it at the moment. I say, celebrate those moments; don't disparage them. Don't ruin your wedding because the cake isn't in your plan for the day. Don't avoid the champagne toast on your birthday. And definitely don't forgo sharing food during a special moment with a loved one. Food plays a very intimate role in our lives, and restricting food during tender moments, happy occasions, and celebrations can make you feel left out. I'm talking about really special occasions that happen very infrequently—not every holiday or day off from work.

When the day is done, look back on it with fondness. I hope the food and the moment were as good as you had hoped. Then tomorrow, go back to your plan. Cheating included; no guilt allowed!

# 6

# Hydrating for Heavy-Duty Workouts

Quick: What's the most critical nutrient for growth, development, and health?

If you guessed water, congratulations! People frequently overlook the importance of water in their diet, and most don't even consider water an essential nutrient. Without enough water and other fluids, though, you'd die within a week.

Although water does not provide energy in the same way carbohydrate and fat do, it plays an essential role in energy formation. As the most abundant nutrient in your body, water is the medium in which all energy reactions take place. Thus, you need ample fluids for fuel and stamina. You get those fluids from a variety of sources—the foods you eat; the beverages you consume; and the plain, pure water you drink. Here's a closer look at the importance of water and other fluids in the diet.

## Water: An Essential Nutrient

The fluids in your body form a heavily trafficked river through your arteries, veins, and capillaries that carries nutrients to your cells and waste products out of the body. Fluids fill virtually every space in your cells and between cells. Water molecules not only fill space, but they also help form the structures of macromolecules such as protein and glycogen. The chemical reactions that keep you alive occur in water, and water is an active participant in those reactions.

It's hard to say enough good things about water. It makes up about 60 percent of the body's weight in adults. As the primary fluid in your body, water serves as a solvent for minerals, vitamins, amino acids, glucose, and many other nutrients. Without water, you can't even digest these essential nutrients, let alone absorb, transport, and use them.

In addition to carrying nutrients throughout the body, water transports waste products out of the body. It is a part of the lubricant in your joints that keeps them moving. And when your body's temperature begins to rise, water acts as the coolant in your radiator. Enough said! You can see why water is so vital to health.

## Temperature Regulation

Your body produces energy for exercise, but only 25 percent of that energy is actually used for mechanical work. The other 75 percent is released as heat. The extra warmth produced during exercise causes your body to heat up, raising your core temperature. To get rid of that extra heat, you sweat. As sweat evaporates, your blood and body cool. If you couldn't cool off, you would quickly succumb to heat stress caused by the increase in your body's core temperature.

## Fat Burning

Drinking more water can actually help you stay lean. Your kidneys depend on water to do their job of filtering waste products from the body. In a water shortage, the kidneys need backup, so they turn to the liver for help. One of the liver's many functions is mobilizing stored fat for energy. By taking on extra assignments from the kidneys, the liver can't do its fat-burning job as well. Fat loss is compromised as a result.

In addition, water can help take the edge off hunger so that you eat less, and it has no calories. If you are on a high-protein diet, water is required to detoxify ammonia, a by-product of protein energy metabolism. And, as you burn off stored fatty acids as energy, you release any fat-soluble toxins that have been benignly stored in your fat cells. The more fluid you drink, the more you dilute the toxins in your bloodstream, and the more rapidly they exit the body.

## Muscle Strength and Control

Ever wonder why some days you're so pooped you can't pump iron? One reason may be dehydration. To move your muscles, you need water. Of all the places in the body, water is found in highest concentrations in metabolically active tissues such as muscle and is found in lowest concentrations in relatively inactive tissues such as fat, skin, and some parts of bone. Muscles are controlled by nerves. The electrical stimulation of nerves and contraction of muscles occur as a result of the exchange of electrolyte minerals dissolved in water (sodium, potassium, calcium, chloride, and magnesium) across the nerve and muscle cell membranes.

If you're low on water or electrolytes, muscle strength and control are weakened. A water deficit of just 2 to 4 percent of your body weight can cut your strength-training workout by as much as 21 percent—and your aerobic power by a whopping 48 percent. Your body's thirst mechanism kicks in when you've lost 2 percent of your body weight in water. But by that time, you're already dehydrated. To prevent dehydration, you must get yourself on a scheduled plan to drink often throughout the day.

If gaining muscle is your goal, you should care about cell volumization, or the hydration state of your muscle cells. In a well-hydrated muscle cell, protein synthesis is stimulated and protein breakdown is decreased. On the other hand, dehydration of muscle cells promotes protein breakdown and inhibits protein synthesis. Cell volume has also been shown to influence genetic expression, enzyme and hormone activity, and metabolism.

## Joint Lubrication

Water forms the makeup of synovial fluid, the lubricating fluid between your joints, and cerebrospinal fluid, the shock-absorbing fluid between vertebrae and around the brain. Both fluids are essential for healthy joint and spine maintenance. If your diet is water deficient, even for a brief period, less fluid is available to protect these areas. Strength training places tremendous demands on the joints and spine, and the presence of adequate protective fluid is essential for optimum performance and long-term health.

## Mental Performance

Whether at the office or in competition, your hydration state affects your performance. Dehydration, in particular, decreases mental energy; causes fatigue, lethargy, light-headedness, and headaches; and can certainly make you feel down. In a study of subjects' abilities to perform mental exercises after dehydration induced by heat stress, a fluid loss of only 2 percent of body weight caused reductions of up to 20 percent in arithmetic ability, short-term memory, and the ability to visually track an object. With that powerful proof, you should be motivated to stay well hydrated to keep your mental energy high and your focus sharp.

## Disease and Illness Prevention

Probably the most surprising fact about water is the effect that chronic, mild dehydration has on health and disease. It was a practice of Hippocrates to recommend large intakes of water to increase urine production and decrease the recurrence of urinary tract stones. Today, approximately 12 to 15 percent of the general population will form a kidney stone at some time in life. Many factors can modify the risk factors for developing stones. Of these, diet—especially fluid intake—is the only one that can be easily changed and that has a marked effect on all aspects of urinary health.

A little-known fact is that low water intake is a risk factor for certain types of cancers. One study found that patients with urinary tract cancer (bladder, prostate, kidney, and testicle) drank significantly smaller quantities of fluid compared with healthy controls.

In another study, researchers discovered that women who drank more than five glasses of water a day had a 45 percent lower risk of colon cancer compared with those who consumed two or fewer glasses a day. For men, the risk was cut by 32 percent when they drank more than four glasses a day versus one or fewer glasses a day.

Why does adequate water intake appear to have an anticancer effect? One theory holds that the more fluid you drink, the faster you flush the toxins and carcinogenic substances out of your body, and the less chance there is for them to be resorbed into the body or to be concentrated long enough to cause tissue change.

Even more fascinating, a pilot study reported that the odds of developing breast cancer were reduced by 79 percent, on average, among water drinkers. In this case, maintaining a dilute solution within the cells possibly reduces the potency of estrogen and its ability to cause hormone-related cancers, according to the theory proposed by the authors of this research.

Mild dehydration can also be a factor in the occurrence of mitral valve prolapse, a defect of one of the heart valves that controls the flow of blood between the chambers of the heart. Mitral valve prolapse is a relatively harmless condition, but in a small percentage of cases, it causes rapid heartbeat, chest pain, and other cardiac symptoms. In a study of 14 healthy women with normal heart function, mitral valve prolapse was induced by mild dehydration and resolved with rehydration.

## How Much Water Do You Need?

Nearly all the foods you eat contain water, which is absorbed during digestion. Most fruits and vegetables are 75 to 90 percent water. Meats contain roughly 50 to 70 percent water. And beverages such as juice, milk, and glucose–electrolyte solutions are more than 85 percent water. On average, you may consume about 4 cups (1 L) of water daily from food alone, but this is true only if you're eating an abundance of fruits and vegetables, which are the major food sources of water.

Most people are walking around in a moderately dehydrated state. You need 9 to 12 cups (2 to 3 L) of total fluids daily—even more to replace the fluid you lose during exercise. Of these 9 to 12 cups, make sure at least 5 of them (1 L) are pure water.

You lose about a quart (4 cups, or 1 L) of water per hour of exercise, depending on your size and perspiration rate. When you're working out moderately in a mild climate, you are probably losing 1 to 2 quarts (or liters), or 2 to 4 pounds (0.9 to 1.8 kg), of fluid per hour through perspiration. That means that a 150-pound (68 kg) person can easily lose 2 percent of body weight in fluid (3 lb, or 1 kg) within an hour. If exercise is more intense or the environment is more extreme, fluid losses will be greater. Thus, you can see how easily you become dehydrated.

If you don't replenish fluid losses during exercise, you will fatigue early and your performance will be diminished. If you don't replenish fluid after exercise, your performance on successive days will decay, and your long-term health may be at risk.

Moreover, according to the National Athletic Trainers' Association (NATA), dehydration

- impairs your physical performance in less than an hour of exercise—or sooner if you start working out in a dehydrated state,
- cuts your performance by as much as 48 percent, and
- increases your risk of developing symptoms of heat illness, such as heat cramps, heat exhaustion, and heatstroke.

In addition to exercise, many other factors increase water requirements, including high heat, low humidity, high altitude, high-fiber foods, illness, travel, and pregnancy.

What about you? Are you dehydrated? Table 6.1 lists the early and severe warning signs of dehydration and heat stress.

### TABLE 6.1    Signs of Dehydration and Heat Stress

| Early signs | Severe signs |
| --- | --- |
| Fatigue | Difficulty swallowing |
| Loss of appetite | Stumbling |
| Flushed skin | Clumsiness |
| Heat intolerance | Shriveled skin |
| Light-headedness | Sunken eyes and dim vision |
| Dark urine with strong odor | Painful urination |
| Dry cough | Numb skin |
| Burning sensation in stomach | Muscle spasm |
| Headache | Delirium |
| Dry mouth |  |

Following are easy actions you can take to monitor yourself for early signs of dehydration:

- Pay attention to how well hydrated you are going into exercise. If you were already dehydrated when you began your training session, then your fluid losses may be greater at the end of exercise. You will need to compensate for this every time it happens.

- Check your hydration status by observing how frequently you void, how much urine you pass, and the color of your urine. If you're urinating less frequently, the volume is markedly diminished, or the color is darker than usual, then you are dehydrated. The color should be no darker than straw; it should not be colorless, and it should not be as dark as brewed tea.

- Weigh yourself without clothing before and after exercise. For every pound (0.5 kg) lost during exercise, you've lost 2 to 3 cups (480 to 720 ml) of fluid. Any weight lost during exercise is fluid loss and should be replaced by drinking fluids as soon after exercise as possible.

- Take note of a sore throat, dry cough, or hoarse voice, which are all signs of dehydration.

- Be aware that a burning sensation in your stomach can signal dehydration.

- Be aware of muscle cramps. No one knows for sure what causes muscle cramps, but a shortfall of water may be an important factor. Muscle cramps are more apt to occur when you're doing hard, physical work in the heat and don't drink enough fluids. You can usually alleviate the cramps by moving to a cool place, drinking fluids, and replacing electrolytes with a glucose–electrolyte solution.

- If you're a "salty sweater," you may need to drink saltier beverages during exercise and eat more salt throughout the day. You can check whether you are a salty sweater by wearing a dark or black T-shirt during exercise. If you see salt stains on the chest and under the armpits of the T-shirt where sweat has evaporated after exercise, then you are losing significant amounts of salt. This can lead to increases in muscle cramps. Replace salt lost during exercise by drinking beverages with slightly higher salt contents during exercise and consuming salt with foods at meals and snacks.

# Drinking Schedule for Strength Trainers

You usually can't rely on thirst to tell you when to drink fluids. By the time your thirst mechanism kicks in during exercise, you've already lost 1 to 2 percent of your body weight as sweat. You need to drink water at regular intervals whether you're thirsty or not, and you need to do so every day. Remember, if you fail to drink enough fluids one day, your body can't automatically rehydrate itself the next. You'll be doubly dehydrated and possibly begin to show some signs of dehydration.

For workouts, here's a schedule that will keep you well hydrated. If you are an athlete, you can also refer to the recommendations from the NATA in table 6.2.

## Before Exercise

Drink at least 16 ounces (2 cups, or 480 ml) of fluid two to three hours before exercise. Then, drink 8 ounces (1 cup, or 240 ml) of fluid immediately before exercise to make sure the body is well hydrated. In very hot or cold weather, you need even more water: 12 to 20 ounces (1.5 to 2.5 cups, or 360 to 600 ml) of fluid 10 to 20 minutes before exercise. Exercising during cold weather elevates your body temperature, and you still lose water through perspiration and respiration.

## During Exercise

Drink 7 to 10 ounces (210 to 300 ml) every 10 to 20 minutes during exercise, and more in extreme temperatures. Although this might seem tough at first, once you schedule it into your regular training routine, you'll quickly adapt to the feeling of fluid in your stomach. In addition, the fuller your stomach is, the faster it will empty. Dehydration slows the rate at which your stomach empties. Make regular water breaks part of your training.

## After Exercise

This is the time to replace any fluid you've lost. Weigh yourself before and after exercise; then drink 2 to 3 cups (480 to 720 ml) of fluid within two hours after exercise for every pound (0.5 kg) of body weight you've lost. Continue to drink an additional 25 to 50 percent more fluid for the next four hours.

## TABLE 6.2  Fluid Replacement for Athletes: Practical Applications

| Fluid guidelines |
|---|
| **Before exercise** |
| 2-3 h before, drink 17-20 oz (510-600 ml) of water or sport drink. |
| 10-20 min before, drink 7-10 oz (210-300 ml) of water or sport drink. |
| **During exercise** |
| Athletes benefit from drinking fluid with carbohydrate in many situations. |
| If exercise lasts more than 45 min or is intense, fluid with carbohydrate (sport drink) should be provided during the session. |
| A 6-8% carbohydrate solution maintains optimal carbohydrate metabolism. |
| During events in which a high rate of fluid intake is necessary to sustain hydration, carbohydrate composition should be kept low (less than 7%) to optimize fluid delivery. |
| Fluids with salt (sodium chloride) are beneficial for increasing thirst and voluntary intake of fluids as well as offsetting losses of salt. |
| Cool beverages at temperatures of 10-15 degrees C (50-59 degrees F) are recommended. |
| Every 10-20 min, drink 7-10 oz (210-300 ml) of water or a sport drink. Athletes should be encouraged to drink beyond their thirst. |
| **After exercise** |
| Within 2 h, drink enough to replace any weight loss from exercise; drink approximately 20 oz (600 ml) of water or sport drink per pound (0.5 kg) of weight loss. |
| Within 6 h, drink an additional 25-50% more than weight loss from exercise. |

# Best Sources of Water

The easiest way to get water is right from your faucet. But reports of contaminated tap water are of concern to many people—and with good reason. The water supply in some areas contains contaminants such as lead, pesticides, and chlorine by-products that exceed recommended limits. A good move is to buy a water purifier, which filters lead and other contaminants from tap water. Some filters attach right to the tap; others can be installed as part of the entire water system. One of the most convenient and economic filtering methods is the pour-through filter you can place in a special pitcher and put right in your refrigerator. If you use a filtration product that removes fluoride from your water, discuss this concern with your dentist, because fluoride can support good dental health.

Another option is to purchase bottled water. There are hundreds of brands, the most popular of which offer spring water and mineral water. Spring water is taken from underground freshwater springs that form pools on the surface of the earth. Mineral water comes from reservoirs located under rock formations. It contains a higher concentration of minerals than most sources. Well water is another type of bottled water, which is tapped from an aquifer. Spring, mineral, and well waters still may contain some contaminants. For this reason, federal regulations are tightening on the bottled water industry. Although bottled water is not the most environmentally friendly option, it is an option for regular hydration. Once you get in the habit of drinking water regularly, buy your own personal reusable water bottle that you can fill at home with pure water and take with you to support hydration.

Distilled water, also labeled as purified water, is another type of bottled water. It has been purified through vaporization and is then condensed. A drawback of distilled water is that it does not contain any minerals. In addition, fluoride is missing from many bottled waters. However, several brands now add back a mineral package, making it more nutritious and usually better tasting.

Some people like seltzer water. This is a sparkling water that is bubbly because of the addition of pressurized carbon dioxide. Many of these products are flavored and contain sucrose or fructose. Although carbonated waters are fine to drink throughout the day, they are not desirable during exercise. The gas from the bubbles takes up space in your stomach and makes you feel fuller, decreasing the amount of total fluid you will drink during and after exercise.

Regardless of what type of water you drink, be sure to drink the 9 to 12 cups (2 to 3 L) or more of fluids you need daily to stay well hydrated, and make at least 5 of these cups (1 L) pure water.

## Designer Waters

Water now comes in more varieties than ever before. Today, there's fortified water, fitness water, herbal water, oxygen-enriched water, electrolyzed water—the list goes on. Welcome to the world of designer waters. Although they may taste great, watch out for unsubstantiated claims on the labels, and for what I call "clear soda pop" masquerading as water. Some sweetened waters have almost as much sugar as soda. I'm concerned not only about the amount of sugar added to many of these so-called waters, but also about the amount of sugar substitutes. If you're drinking more than two of these beverages a day—namely, any that use sugar substitutes for sweetening—while consuming sugar substitutes in other foods, then you're pumping your body with too many sugar substitutes.

One problem, too, is that you're training your palate to be satisfied with only very sweet flavors. And quite possibly, you're stimulating your appetite even though you're taking in low-calorie food and beverages. So, while drinking water, try to limit or eliminate altogether a need for sweetness in that water.

With any of the waters that include herbs, botanicals, or any ingredients that companies claim are functional, try to determine what the active ingredients are and how much the beverage contains. If the manufacturer won't list what is in the beverage, don't drink it. The reason for not listing ingredients is most likely either that manufacturers don't know the exact amount of ingredients because there is no serious quality control, or there's really nothing special about their ingredients, and they don't want you to know that their marketing claims are overblown. If you can't find that information, you can probably conclude that the dose is not effective. Otherwise, they'd be eager to tell you that they have an effective dose. Always read ingredient and nutrition labels to make informed choices.

## Fortified Water

Featuring a splash of flavor and sweetness, these waters are fortified with predissolved vitamins and minerals. Some are formulated for people who want to drink their supplements; others, for active people who drink water during workouts and want a little more flavor than plain water provides.

Fortified waters are not to be confused with sport drinks or glucose–electrolyte solutions, which are packed with more carbohydrate energy and higher amounts of electrolytes than specialty waters contain.

## Fitness Water

These designer waters contain some vitamins, but with only 10 calories per serving. They are meant to be used when you want some flavor in your water but don't need a glucose–electrolyte solution or extra calories.

## Herbal Water

Fairly new on the water front are herb-enhanced waters. You can now swill water containing such popular herbs as echinacea, ginkgo biloba, Siberian ginseng, ginger, or Saint-John's wort. These beverages are a good option if you want the benefits of medicinal herbs without popping pills. Generally, herb-enhanced waters have a hint of flavor without sugar, calories, or carbonation.

Be aware of how many servings you consume of herbal or fortified waters, along with other sources of the same herbs, vitamins, and minerals. You might easily take in too much of these substances. And because the herbal part of the food industry is yet to be regulated, there's no guarantee that you're getting the ingredients listed on the label.

## Oxygen-Enriched Water

These beverages are said to be enhanced with up to 40 times the normal oxygen concentration found naturally in water. Available flavored or unflavored, they claim to boost energy by increasing oxygen saturation in the red blood cells. To date, though, no published medical evidence has validated such claims. There appears to be no value in them other than as another good source of water.

## Electrolyzed Water

This category describes water that has been separated into alkaline and acid fractions. The alkaline fraction is bottled for drinking with a pH of about 9.5, compared with other bottled waters in which pH ranges from 6 to 8. The process removes contaminants and most of the total dissolved solids but leaves in electrolytes such as calcium, magnesium, potassium, sodium, and bicarbonates. Claims for electrolyzed water include smoother taste, healthier water, improved hydration ability, electrolyte availability, and antioxidant properties. Aside from smoother-tasting water, the scientific research into most of these claims is in its infancy. Keep an eye on this research.

## What About Coconut Water?

Coconut water—the liquid that sloshes around in coconuts—is positioned as a healthy alternative to sport drinks. One reason is that it is packed with 15 times the amount of potassium as the leading sport drink, plus it contains no fat, dyes, or added sugar. What's more, coconut water is a natural "isotonic" beverage, meaning that it contains the same levels of electrolytes as your blood.

But how does coconut water stack up against plain water and sport drinks for rehydration after exercise? A study published in 2002 looked into this. It evaluated the effects of three fluids: water, a carbohydrate–electrolyte drink, and coconut water. The researchers found that coconut water basically worked as well as a carbohydrate–electrolyte beverage and performed better than water for rehydration.

Another study regarding this issue, which appeared in 2007 in the *Southeast Asian Journal of Tropical Medicine and Public Health,* reached a similar conclusion after comparing the effects of plain water, sport drink, fresh coconut water, and sodium-enriched fresh coconut water on rehydration. The findings? The most effective rehydration occurred with the sport drink and the sodium-enriched coconut water.

To date, these are the only two studies published on coconut water and exercise. Other health claims made by manufacturers about coconut water are absolutely unsubstantiated. These include claims that coconut water prevents cancer, slows aging, gives you smoother skin, normalizes blood pressure, lowers unhealthy cholesterol, and cures a number of kidney and digestive disorders. As for the cancer claim, some of the substances in coconut water, such as selenium, are antioxidants and fight cancer in the lab, but many fruits, vegetables, nuts, and whole grains contain the same cancer-fighting compounds. So far, only animal studies have hinted that coconut water may lower cholesterol and blood pressure. Honestly, no single food substance can do all these things, and we just don't have enough research to make such claims about coconut water.

Even so, coconut water can be a good choice for rehydration. Compared to other beverages, it is a healthy option, thanks to its content of potassium, vitamin C, antioxidants, and phytochemicals.

## Are Sport Drinks Superior to Water?

In some cases, yes. For general types of exercise lasting less than one hour, water is still the best sport drink around. The nutrient you most need to replace during and after these types of workouts is water.

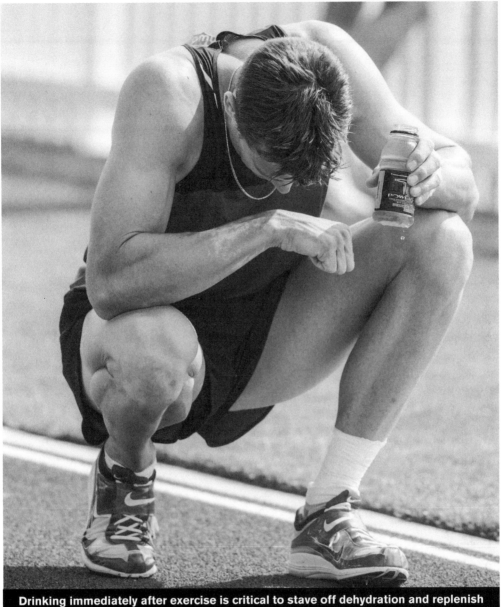

**Drinking immediately after exercise is critical to stave off dehydration and replenish depleted nutrients.**

Glucose–electrolyte solution drinks (also known as sport drinks) do have their place, mostly during high-intensity intermittent exercise and exercise lasting more than 45 minutes, and they are especially useful for endurance and ultraendurance athletes. These products are a mixture of water, carbohydrate, and electrolytes. Electrolytes are dissolved minerals that form a salty soup in and around cells. They conduct electrical charges that let them react with other minerals to relay nerve impulses, make muscles contract or relax, and regulate the fluid balance inside and outside cells. In hard workouts or athletic competitions lasting 45 minutes or longer, electrolytes can be lost through sweat.

Where glucose–electrolyte solutions may have an edge over water is in their flavor. A lot of people don't drink much water because it doesn't taste good to them. Soldiers participating in a study at the U.S. Army Research Institute of Environmental Medicine were given the choice of drinking plain chlorinated water, flavored water, or lemon-lime glucose–electrolyte solution drinks. Most soldiers chose the glucose–electrolyte solutions or flavored water over plain water. If you don't need the extra carbohydrate and electrolytes, one way to sneak more water in and still get the flavor is to dilute your glucose–electrolyte solution or use one of the new flavored fitness waters. But remember, you will not get the performance-enhancement effect for exercise over one hour if you do this.

If you're an avid water drinker and really like water, you'll benefit just as much from water as you will from using a glucose–electrolyte solution, unless you're exercising an hour or more. But if you don't like water or tend to avoid it during exercise, try filtered or bottled water, which tastes different than regular water. Or try a glucose–electrolyte solution that contains less than 8 percent carbohydrate and some sodium. Another idea is to put some powdered sport drink mix into your water, although the powdered mixes sometimes don't taste as good as their premixed counterparts. At the very least, if a glucose–electrolyte solution encourages you to drink more, it has done its job.

## Is Juice a Good Sport Drink?

Juices are a source of fluids. Orange juice, for example, is nearly 90 percent water and is full of vitamins and minerals. Although juices count as part of your fluid requirement, you'll feel at your best if you base your daily fluid plan on at least 5 cups (1 L) of water and use small servings of juice to help you attain your minimum 9 to 12 cups (2 to 3 L) of total fluids.

There are some cautions to consider regarding juice as a fluid in your training diet. In recent years, there has been a lot of hype surrounding the health benefits of fruit and vegetable juices. The makers of commercial juicing machines claim that fresh juices are a panacea for all kinds of ills, from digestive upsets to cancer. But is it better to drink your five servings of fruits and veggies every day rather than eat them? No way!

In most juices, the pulp has been removed from the fruit or vegetables to make the juice. That means that the all-important fiber has also been subtracted, because the pulp is where you find the fiber. Granted, some juice machines boast that their process keeps the pulp in the juice to retain the important fiber and concentrate the nutrients. These products are excellent choices for a once-a-day juice. But they still do not replace whole fruit.

Freshly squeezed juice is often touted as a better source of nutrients than commercial juices. But commercially prepared juices that are frozen and refrigerated properly are only slightly lower in nutrients than fresh juice. If you don't buy fresh produce, don't store it properly at home, and don't drink your freshly squeezed juice immediately, your homemade juice may even be lower in nutrients than a well-made frozen or refrigerated brand.

Whether they are cooked, squeezed, dried, or raw, fruits and vegetables need to be a big part of your diet. If using a juice machine is one way of eating more fruits and vegetables and is enjoyable for you, go for it. But remember the drawbacks, and don't use juice as your only source of fruits and vegetables.

If you want to drink juice to rehydrate your body, dilute it with water by at least twofold. A cup (240 ml) of orange or apple juice plus 2 cups (480 ml) of water will provide a 6 to 8 percent carbohydrate solution, similar to a sport drink formulation. Don't use this combination during exercise, however, because of its fructose content. The body doesn't use fructose as well as the combination of sugars in a regular sport drink. In addition, some people are fructose sensitive and may experience intestinal cramping after drinking juice. As noted earlier, juice may interfere with fluid absorption if consumed during exercise. Instead, drink your juice–water mix as part of your fluids an hour or more after exercise. The addition of water will speed the emptying of the fluid from your stomach and thus rehydrate your body more rapidly, and the carbohydrate will help replenish glycogen.

# Hydration Danger Zones

It's hard to imagine that water could be bad for you, but just like everything else, too much water at the wrong time can actually be harmful. Moderation is the key, even when we're talking about water.

## Overhydration

When considering your water intake, you must also consider overhydration. Hydration is a delicate balance between fluids and minerals. The concentration of sodium and other minerals (collectively known as electrolytes) in the bloodstream must fall within a very narrow range, or it can affect muscle contractions. That includes those of the most important muscle: your heart.

When you take in too much water relative to the amount of electrolytes in your body, the result will eventually be a condition called hyperhydration or hyponatremia. The problem is that the blood has become too dilute, which is just as dangerous as dehydration. During dehydration there are high levels of electrolytes without enough fluids. Surprisingly, the symptoms of dehydration and hyperhydration are basically the same.

Hyperhydration occurs more frequently than you might think, particularly in endurance events such as marathons and triathlons. Not nearly as well documented is the possibility of bodybuilders hyperhydrating as a result of high intakes of purified water combined with very low food and sodium intakes during a cutting diet. Although no occurrences of hyponatremia have been documented in strength trainers not participating in another sport, you should be aware that very high intakes of purified water over an extended period of time may put you at risk. Whether you're training for an endurance event or preparing for a strength-training competition, you can avoid hyponatremia with a few simple precautions.

If you're training for your first marathon or triathlon, don't cut all salt out of your diet (though, as a general rule, most of us could get away with a lot less than we currently take in). If the day is cooler or less humid than you expected, compensate by drinking less than you'd planned during the event.

Go for sport drinks over pure water, especially if you're competing in endurance competitions. A 2006 study published in the *British Journal of Sports Medicine* looked into the fluid-intake behaviors of runners competing in ultraendurance events. The researchers concluded that they could finish their competitions relatively dehydrated and hypernatremic—and that it was detrimental to performance to overdrink water. They also stated that the best way to prevent hyponatremia was to consume electrolyte-containing sport drinks.

If you're not an endurance athlete, don't think you have to match those more highly trained competitors drink for drink. Their sweat is different from yours; it contains more water and fewer electrolytes. Your body is leaking sodium, while theirs are holding onto it. If you see pretzels being handed out along the course of a distance race, help yourself, assuming you're not sodium sensitive and you don't have high blood pressure. The extra sodium will prevent you from becoming hyperhydrated.

When you are dieting to make weight prior to a competition, don't overdo the water. Drink water with minerals in place of purified water, or don't remove all the sodium from your diet. As long as you are eating, your risk of hyponatremia is remarkably diminished.

## Water, Body Weight, and Competition

For years sport nutritionists, myself included, have recommended that athletes drink before they get thirsty and make sure that they don't lose more than 2 percent of their total body weight during an exercise session or race event. The assumption was that any body weight lost during exercise is completely fluid, and that these losses hamper performance.

A new study published in the *Journal of Sports Medicine* refutes that assumption. The researchers found that, in two races, athletes drinking only in response to thirst lost more body mass than total body water. The researchers speculated that this loss in body mass confers a competitive advantage. If you can lose body mass during the race and weigh less, yet stay adequately hydrated, you have a better chance of winning.

In this study, the athletes stayed adequately hydrated. Thirst mechanisms appeared to be triggered to maintain electrolyte status, and sodium and potassium concentrations remained within healthy ranges. Therefore, the researchers recommended that athletes not drink based on body weight losses, but allow their natural thirst mechanisms to drive their hydration practices.

As for sodium, many athletes wonder whether they should supplement with this electrolyte to boost performance. The researchers of the preceding study examined this issue too with athletes competing in an Ironman Triathlon in South Africa. A third of the subjects received sodium tablets to use freely for the 12 hours of the race; another third received a placebo starch tablet to use freely throughout the race; and the final third did not supplement at all.

At the end of the race there was absolutely no difference in performance or the concentration of sodium and other electrolytes in the athletes' bodies. The researchers concluded that the Institute of Medicine recommendation of 1.5 grams of sodium per day for the general population is adequate to maintain serum sodium concentrations during a 12-hour ultraendurance event. Although some people may have increased needs, in general eating a standard Western diet should offer adequate amounts of sodium. On the other hand, do not reduce your sodium intake when preparing for an endurance event.

## What Not to Drink

Certain types of beverages should be shunned during exercise, according to the NATA in its position paper on fluid replacement for athletes. These beverages include fruit juices, carbohydrate gels (always consume these with extra water), sodas, and glucose–electrolyte solutions with carbohydrate levels greater than 8 percent. Such beverages slow fluid absorption and may cause gastrointestinal problems. The NATA also discourages the consumption of beverages containing high amounts of caffeine, alcohol, and carbonation, because they stimulate excess urine production and thus dehydrate your body.

## Alcohol

It has been a long time since a client has asked me whether drinking beer is a good way to replenish fluids and carbohydrate. But clients frequently ask whether alcohol will hurt their exercise performance, and even more frequently, they want to know whether drinking a little bit of alcohol may actually be heart healthy. Thanks to an ever-growing body of scientific research and knowledge, here are some answers to those questions and more:

### What's in Alcohol?

Alcohol is a carbohydrate, but it's not converted to glucose as other kinds of carbohydrate are. Instead, it is converted into fatty acids and thus is more likely to be stored as body fat. So if you drink and train, alcohol puts fat burning on hold. It's not your friend if you're trying to stay lean.

Pure alcohol supplies 7 calories per gram and nothing else. In practical terms, a shot (1.5 oz, or 45 ml) of 90-proof gin contains 110 calories, and 100-proof gin contains 124 calories. Beer has a little more to offer, but not much. On the average, a 12-ounce (360 ml) can of beer contains 146 calories, 13 grams of carbohydrate, traces of several B-complex vitamins, and, depending on the brand, varying amounts of minerals. Light beer and nonalcoholic beer are lower in calories and sometimes carbohydrate. All table wines have similar caloric content. A 3.5-ounce (105 ml) serving of table wine contains about 72 calories, 1 gram of carbohydrate, and very small amounts of several vitamins and minerals. Sweet or dessert wines are higher in calories, containing 90 calories per 2-ounce (60 ml) serving.

## What Are Alcohol's Side Effects?

Today, alcohol is the most abused drug in the United States. Ten percent of users are addicted, and 10 to 20 percent are abusers or problem drinkers. Alcohol is a central nervous system depressant. Compared with other commonly used substances, alcohol has one of the lowest effective dose–lethal dose ratios. In other words, there's a small difference in the amount of alcohol that will get you drunk and the amount that will kill you. The reason more people don't die from alcohol intoxication is that the stomach is alcohol sensitive and rejects it by vomiting.

Acute alcohol intoxication results in tremors, anxiety and irritability, nausea and vomiting, decreased mental function, vertigo, coma, and death. In large amounts, alcohol causes the loss of many nutrients from the body, including thiamin, vitamin $B_6$, and calcium. Furthermore, chronic alcohol abuse has negative effects on every organ in the body, particularly the liver, heart, brain, and muscle, and can lead to cancer and diseases of the liver, pancreas, and nervous system.

Don't drink alcohol in any form if you're pregnant. It can cause birth defects. Drinking alcohol in large amounts can also lead to accidents, as well as social, psychological, and emotional problems.

## How Does Alcohol Affect Exercise Performance?

Because alcohol depresses the central nervous system, it impairs balance and coordination and decreases exercise performance. Strength and power, muscle endurance, and aerobic endurance are all zapped with alcohol use. Alcohol also dehydrates the body considerably.

To be a little more specific, if you knock down a few alcoholic beverages after a strength-training workout, you're likely to increase damage to your muscles, experience greater muscle soreness, and diminish strength and power. These effects have been observed in research.

As for endurance athletes, a study of trained cyclists given a small amount of alcohol after 60 minutes of cycling showed a significant decrease in average cycling power output, oxygen consumption, carbon dioxide production, and glucose oxidation. Their heart rates increased and they felt more fatigued and less energetic when they consumed alcohol. So basically, drinking alcohol has a negative effect on endurance performance. Also, alcohol use increases the risks of sport injuries.

The bottom line: Alcohol will clearly put your training on the skids. It has no place during tournament play, when training occurs the day after a game, or when several games or events are played weekly. Although celebrating with alcohol may appear to be fun, it puts you and your teammates at risk.

## Is Alcohol Really Heart Healthy?

Research has found that daily consumption of one drink per day can do your heart good by positively affecting the levels of good cholesterol (HDL) in your blood. The higher your HDL levels, the lower your risk of heart disease.

However, excessive alcohol intake increases your chance of developing heart disease. More than two drinks a day can raise your blood pressure and contribute to high triglycerides, a risk factor for heart disease. Drinking large amounts of alcohol on a habitual basis can also cause heart failure and lead to stroke.

Alcohol consumption contributes to obesity, another major risk factor in the development of heart disease. Extra pounds are hard on your heart, and the higher your weight climbs, the greater your risk. Being overweight also raises blood pressure and cholesterol, which are risk factors themselves.

### Is a Drink a Day Good Prevention?

The risks of alcohol outweigh its positives. If you drink alcoholic beverages, do so in moderation, with meals, and when consumption does not put you or others in harm's way. Moderation is defined as no more than one drink per day for women and no more than two drinks per day for men. One drink is 12 ounces (360 ml) of regular beer, 5 ounces (150 ml) of wine, and 1.5 ounces (45 ml) of 80-proof distilled liquor. However, exercising, quitting smoking, and lowering your blood cholesterol with a healthy diet are better ways to prevent heart disease without any added risks.

## Sport Nutrition Fact Versus Fiction: Do Soft Drinks Rehydrate the Body?

If given the option, many people would choose a soft drink over water to rehydrate themselves following workouts. And who can blame them? Soft drinks taste good, seem to quench thirst, and are generally refreshing.

But soft drinks are among the worst choices for rehydration. Soft drinks are laced with huge amounts of sugar—roughly the equivalent of 10 teaspoons per can. Because of their sugar content, soft drinks are absorbed less rapidly than pure water. The sugar in them keeps the fluid in your stomach longer, so less water is available to your body. Rather than rehydrating your system, soft drinks can make you feel even thirstier. Also, the sugar can trigger a sharp spike in insulin, followed by a fast drop in blood sugar. This reaction can leave you feeling tired and weak. In addition, the sugar in soft drinks is high-fructose corn syrup, which does not replenish glycogen as rapidly as other forms of carbohydrate. Fructose also can cause cramps in people who are sensitive to it.

What about sugar-free soft drinks? These beverages contain artificial sweeteners, which remain controversial. Furthermore, all soft drinks are, of course, carbonated, and carbonation produces gas. Who wants a gassy stomach, which will limit the amount that you drink and fully rehydrate?

Diluting a soft drink isn't a good option either. Even diluted, soft drinks have nothing beneficial to offer. As far as rehydration is concerned, no fluids—including artificially sweetened soft drinks—have yet been proven to do a better job than plain old water or a good glucose–electrolyte solution.

# Supplements

Now that you've built your nutrition foundation and have your diet down to a science, it's time to consider supplements. Of course, supplements are just that—extras you can add to your well-designed food plan. In the past decade, the science of nutritional anthropology has shown us that our ancestors evolved consuming an average of 3,500 to 5,000 calories a day, both males and females. The food they ate was nutrient dense but not calorically dense, meaning that they had to eat a large volume of food to take in that many calories each day. Their diets were diverse and plant based, whenever seasonally possible, and therefore rich in antioxidants and the anti-inflammatory factors found predominantly in plant foods. Successful hunting allowed for intermittent days of eating protein-rich wild game, which was rich in omega-3 fat not found in the meat of present-day corn-fed animals. Today, most people can't eat that many calories and still balance their body weight. Even if you could train hard enough to need that many calories, you would probably not take the time your body needs to recover, or have the time to prepare food equal in quality to that of our ancestors. As a result, supplements have come to play an essential role in boosting our nutritional intake.

In addition, supplements are convenient for our busy lives. Consider the following:

- Perhaps there are critical foods that you can't eat or don't like. Supplements can fill in the nutritional gaps left by excluding such foods.
- Or, perhaps your schedule is so hectic that you don't have time to prepare food immediately after exercise when your body really needs it for muscle growth. If so, supplements to the rescue!
- And maybe you want to gain just a little competitive edge. A few supplements work powerfully to give you that edge.

Part II reviews the most popular supplements used by strength-training athletes. Using the most current scientific research, I evaluate the usefulness of these supplements as well as any potential for harm. Use my rating system to decide for yourself which products meet their marketing claims, which have promise and which fall flat, and which are potentially harmful.

# 7

# Vitamins and Minerals for Strength Trainers

Want to get ripped, shredded, striated, and vascular? Every supplement company says it's got the product for you. You have probably stood in the supplement aisle for hours, reading ingredients and wondering which ones really work. Ads for supplements certainly promise dramatic results. However, scientists have only begun to research the nutritional requirements of muscle building in the last two decades, which isn't very long. The research is promising, but the whole story on what works and what doesn't is not in yet.

Among the many pills and potions on store shelves are vitamins and minerals. Quite possibly, you may need extra amounts of both. Research shows that most Americans fall short of the requirements for many key nutrients, including vitamins C, E, and $B_{12}$; folic acid; zinc; and magnesium, which is why a growing number of Americans are turning to supplements. A survey by the Centers for Disease Control and Prevention (CDC) shows that more than 60 percent of the general population takes supplements daily.

Some data even suggest that taking supplements may help you live longer. A study published in 2009 in the *American Journal of Clinical Nutrition* analyzed data from 586 older women. The researchers drew the women's blood and assessed the length of telomeres, which are pieces of DNA on chromosomes. As we age, our telomeres shorten. So the longer they are, the better our bodies are at maintaining our youth. In women who took multivitamins, telomeres were longer, indicating that these basic supplements may promote longevity.

The American Medical Association (AMA) recommends that everyone take a multivitamin and mineral supplement daily; doing so has been shown to help prevent chronic illnesses such as cancer, heart disease, and osteoporosis. Even people who eat five daily servings of fruits and vegetables may not get enough of certain vitamins for optimum health. Most people, for instance, cannot get the healthiest levels of folate and vitamin D and E from their diets.

Hard workouts increase your nutritional needs, as does dieting. That's why you may want to add certain vitamins and minerals to your nutritional arsenal. From a sport science perspective, if you are deficient in vitamins and minerals, your performance can suffer. Research shows that if you've taken in less than one third of the daily required amounts of certain B vitamins ($B_1$, $B_2$, and $B_6$) and vitamin C, you can lose aerobic power and strength in a matter of weeks. Taking a multivitamin and mineral supplement isn't going to help you lift more, run faster, or build more muscle, but it will help prevent deficiencies that could impair your performance.

Keep in mind that vitamin and mineral supplements should not replace food. With the right planning, your body can get almost all the nutrients it needs from a balanced diet. Notice that I said *almost*. What's more, your body absorbs nutrients best from food. However, if you would like the insurance of closer to 100 percent nutritional coverage, a good move is to take a daily antioxidant multivitamin mineral containing at least 100 percent of the daily values for vitamins and minerals. These formulations help you cover your nutritional bases and contain nutrients that have special value to strength trainers.

## Choosing the Right Supplement

Following are the three most important issues to consider when selecting a vitamin or mineral supplement (or both):

1. **Is the supplement safe to take?** Purchase products that are tested and certified for purity by third-party, independent agencies. This is the best way to be certain that what is listed on the label is actually in the product, *and* that there is nothing contaminating the product that is not on the label.

2. **Does the supplement get absorbed?** Supplements can pass through the digestive tract partially or completely unabsorbed. Make sure that the supplement meets USP standards for potency, uniformity, disintegration, and dissolution to ensure that you are getting all that you expect from it.

3. **Is the formulation science based, and is the company credible?** Expect to see studies proving the quality and research of the product. Look for studies that are done by a credible and independent third-party source. The company should manufacture the products itself, rather than outsourcing the production. It should voluntarily meet the highest manufacturing standards known as Pharmaceutical Good Manufacturing Practices (Pharma GMP).

Finally, don't believe everything you hear or read in the media about supplements. The media try to interpret scientific studies, and they are not trained to do so. When looking for specific information on how to take care of your own personal health and needs, turn to the nutritional experts for advice.

# Daily Reference Intake (DRI)

A new way of rating the amounts of the nutrients we need for good health is the DRI. It expands on and includes the familiar RDA (recommended daily allowance), but whereas the RDAs target nutrient deficiencies, the DRIs aim to prevent chronic diseases (refer to chapter 1).

Applied to vitamins, minerals, and protein taken by men and women in specific age groups, the DRIs contain three rating sets appropriate for discussion here: the RDAs, a set of values that help us maintain our health; the tolerable upper intake levels (UL), which establish ceilings to help us avoid taking too much of a nutrient; and adequate intakes, or AIs, which are estimates of average intakes that seem healthy and won't harm health. For the purposes of this book, I place all nutrient recommendations under the heading of DRIs.

# Antioxidants

There has been a lot of research done in strength sports about antioxidants—beta-carotene, vitamin C, and vitamin E and the minerals selenium, copper, zinc, and manganese. Antioxidants help fight free radicals, chemicals that are produced naturally by the body and that cause irreversible damage (oxidation) to cells. Free radical damage can leave your body vulnerable to advanced aging, cancer, cardiovascular disease, and degenerative diseases such as arthritis. The exercise-related functions of the key antioxidants are summarized in table 7.1.

Certain environmental factors such as cigarette smoke, exhaust fumes, radiation, excessive sunlight, certain drugs, and stress can increase free radicals. And, ironically, so can the healthy habit of exercise. During respiration, cells pick off electrons from sugars and add them to oxygen to generate energy. As these reactions take place, electrons sometimes get off course and collide with other molecules, creating free radicals. Exercise increases respiration, which produces more free radicals. Scientists are still studying why this happens and how to better defend against it; however, exercise also induces the production of enzymes that fight free radicals.

Body temperature, which tends to rise during exercise, may be another factor in generating free radicals. A third possibility is the increase in catecholamine production during exercise. Catecholamines are hormones released in response to muscular effort. They increase heart rate, let more blood get to muscles, and provide the muscles with fuel, among other functions.

Another source of free radical production is the damage done to the muscle cell membrane after intense exercise, especially eccentric exercise such as putting down a heavy weight or running downhill. In a domino-like series of chemical reactions, free radicals hook up with fatty acids in cell membranes to form substances called peroxides. Peroxides attack cell membranes, setting off a chain reaction that creates many more free radicals. This process is called lipid peroxidation and can lead to muscle soreness. The point is, several complex reactions occur with exercise, and each one may accelerate free radical production.

## TABLE 7.1 Key Antioxidants

| Vitamins | |
|---|---|
| **Beta-carotene** | |
| Exercise-related function | May reduce free radical production as a result of exercise and protect against exercise-induced tissue damage; complements antioxidant function of vitamin E. |
| Best food sources | Carrots, sweet potatoes, spinach, cantaloupe, broccoli, any dark green leafy vegetable, and orange vegetables and fruits. |
| Side effects and toxicity | None known because the body carefully controls its conversion to vitamin A. Daily intakes of 20,000 IU from either food or supplements over several months may cause skin yellowing. This disappears when the dosage is reduced. |
| DRIs for adults | No established limits. 2,500 IU daily from supplements is safe. You can get the same amount from a large carrot. |
| **Vitamin C** | |
| Exercise-related function | Maintains normal connective tissue; enhances iron absorption; may reduce free radical damage as a result of exercise and protect against exercise-induced tissue damage. |
| Best food sources | Citrus fruits and juices, green peppers, raw cabbage, kiwi fruit, cantaloupe, and green leafy vegetables. |
| Side effects and toxicity | The body adapts to high dosages. Dosages between 5,000 and 15,000 mg daily may cause burning urination or diarrhea. |
| DRIs for adults | Women, 75 mg; pregnant women, 85 mg; lactating women, 120 mg; men, 90 mg. Also, 110 mg for female smokers and 130 mg for male smokers. |
| *UL for adults | 2,000 mg. |
| **Vitamin E** | |
| Exercise-related function | Involved in cellular respiration; assists in the formation of red blood cells; scavenges free radicals; protects against exercise-induced tissue damage. |
| Best food sources | Nuts, seeds, raw wheat germ, polyunsaturated vegetable oils, and fish liver oils. |
| Side effects and toxicity | None known. |
| DRIs for adults | 15 mg; lactating women, 19 mg. |
| UL for adults | 1,000 mg. |

### Selenium

| | |
|---|---|
| Exercise-related function | Interacts with vitamin E in normal growth and metabolism; preserves the elasticity of the skin; produces glutathione peroxidase, an important protective enzyme. |
| Best food sources | Cereal bran, brazil nuts, whole-grain cereals, egg yolk, milk, chicken, seafood, broccoli, garlic, and onions. |
| Side effects and toxicity | 5 mg a day from food has resulted in hair loss and fingernail changes. Higher dosages are linked to intestinal problems, fatigue, and irritability. |
| DRIs for adults | Women, 55 mcg; pregnant women, 60 mcg; lactating women, 70 mcg; men, 55 mcg. |
| UL for adults | 400 mcg. |

### Copper

| | |
|---|---|
| Exercise-related function | Assists in the formation of hemoglobin and red blood cells by aiding in iron absorption; required for energy metabolism; involved with superoxide dismutase, a key protective antioxidant enzyme. |
| Best food sources | Whole grains, shellfish, eggs, almonds, green leafy vegetables, and beans. |
| Side effects and toxicity | Toxicity is rare. |
| DRIs for adults | Women and men, 900 mcg; pregnant women, 1,000 mcg; lactating women, 1,300 mcg. |
| UL for adults | 10,000 mcg. |

### Zinc

| | |
|---|---|
| Exercise-related function | Involved in energy metabolism and immunity. |
| Best food sources | Animal protein, oysters, mushrooms, whole grains, and brewer's yeast. |
| Side effects and toxicity | Dosages higher than 20 mg a day may interfere with copper absorption, reduce HDL cholesterol, and impair the immune system. |
| DRIs for adults | Women, 8 mg; pregnant women, 11 mg; lactating women, 12 mg; men, 11 mg. |
| UL for adults | 40 mg. |

> *continued*

TABLE 7.1 *> continued*

### Manganese

| | |
|---|---|
| Exercise-related function | Involved in metabolism; involved with superoxide dismutase, a key protective antioxidant enzyme. |
| Best food sources | Whole grains, egg yolks, dried peas and beans, and green leafy vegetables. |
| Side effects and toxicity | Large dosages can cause vomiting and intestinal problems. |
| DRIs for adults | Women, 1.8 mg; pregnant women, 2.0 mg; lactating women, 2.6 mg; men, 2.3 mg. |
| UL for adults | 11 mg. |

### Lipids

### Coenzyme Q10

| | |
|---|---|
| Exercise-related function | A coenzyme for mitochondrial enzymes of the oxidative phophorylation pathway essential for ATP production; a potent antioxidant that decreases oxidative damage to tissues. |
| Best food sources | Organ meats, beef, soy oil, sardines, mackerel, and peanuts. |
| Side effects and toxicity | None known. |
| DRIs for adults | No established limits. Doses of 30-300 mg per day have been used in clinical studies of heart failure patients. |
| UL for adults | No established limits. |

*UL refers to tolerable upper intake levels, which have been established for vitamins and minerals. These levels represent the maximum intake of a nutrient that is likely to pose no health risks.

## Antioxidants and Inflammation

Antioxidants also help guard against inflammation in the body. But here's the rub: Scientists have lately questioned whether it is beneficial to tamp down training-induced inflammation. Some inflammation, it turns out, is necessary for muscle building. Australian researchers looked into this issue by analyzing an assortment of studies.

In essence, exercise causes stress and damage to the muscle. This creates free radicals and leads to inflammation. The inflammation is a defense mechanism that actually supports muscle building. It does so by causing the body to build bigger and stronger muscle tissue as protection against further assault. Without this inflammatory response, the muscle won't rebuild to the same level. Thus, you won't get as great a training effect from a hard workout.

This review study concluded that to get the best results from training, you should limit antioxidant supplementation. However, researchers caution that if you're involved in very intense competition such as endurance sports, supplementing with antioxidants is a good idea, because these sports can severely deplete the body's natural supply of antioxidants, compromising health. However, never rely on antioxidant supplements alone. Get your antioxidants through a whole-foods diet that is rich in these nutrients.

My own recommendation is to eat in a Power Eating style while supplementing with antioxidants in a conservative way (no megadosing), at least until more is known about the effects of inflammation and antioxidants on training and performance.

## Beta-Carotene

Beta-carotene is a member of a group of substances known as carotenoids. There are hundreds of carotenoids in nature, found mostly in orange and yellow fruits and vegetables and dark green vegetables.

Once ingested, beta-carotene is converted to vitamin A in the body on an as-needed basis. As an antioxidant, beta-carotene can destroy free radicals after they're formed, and it has been shown to reduce muscle soreness by minimizing exercise-induced lipid peroxidation. With less soreness, you may be able to work out more times a week.

However, most clinicians now advise against supplementing with beta-carotene. Here is why: People who took supplemental beta-carotene while enrolled in a large cancer-prevention trial called the Carotene and Retinol Efficacy Trial, or CARET, continued to have increased rates of lung cancer six years after the trial was stopped early and the supplements discontinued, according to a long-term follow-up of trial participants. The results add to earlier evidence from this study and a second large prevention trial that, contrary to earlier expectations, not only do beta-carotene supplements not prevent lung cancer in people at high risk for the disease, but they also appear to increase rates of the disease, particularly among smokers. These findings hint that some adverse reaction is going on in the body. Therefore, it is wise to get your beta-carotene from vegetables instead.

## Vitamin C

Vitamin C, or ascorbic acid, is a nutrient that can be synthesized by many animals, but not by humans. It's an essential component of our diets and functions primarily in the formation of connective tissues such as collagen. Vitamin C is also involved in immunity, wound healing, and allergic responses. As an antioxidant, vitamin C keeps free radicals from destroying the outermost layers of cells. When paired with a plant-based iron source, vitamin C enhances the absorption of this hard-to-absorb form of nonheme iron. Adding lemon juice to your spinach can give a better boost to your iron stores.

If you work out regularly or train for athletic competition, you know that a cold or respiratory infection can sideline you pretty fast. Fortunately, researchers have found that supplementing with 500 milligrams daily of vitamin C appears to cut the risk of upper respiratory tract infections. This benefit may be due to the antioxidant effect of vitamin C or to its overall immune-boosting capability.

Supplementing with vitamin C will improve your performance, but only if you are deficient in this nutrient. Supplementation does not enhance performance if you already eat a healthy, nourishing diet that is high in citrus fruits (which are high in vitamin C) and other fruits and vegetables.

## Vitamin E

Many studies on antioxidants and exercise have focused on vitamin E, which resides in muscle cell membranes. Part of its job is to scavenge the free radicals produced by exercise, saving the tissues from damage. There is so much research in this area that I'd like to summarize some of the findings for you. A few studies on vitamin E have found the following benefits to supplementation:

- A daily 800-milligram vitamin E supplement protected against muscle damage and free radical production in subjects aged 55 and older who exercised by walking or running downhill.
- Supplementation appears to prevent the destruction of oxygen-carrying red blood cells. That means that your muscles benefit from improved or sustained oxygen delivery during exercise.
- Supplementation may improve exercise performance at high altitudes; however, this benefit has not been observed at sea level.

Other studies on vitamin E have not shown benefits. Consider the following:

- Two months of vitamin E supplementation at 800 IU a day actually increased oxidative stress and levels of homocysteine (a protein in the blood that can have heart-damaging effects) in triathletes.
- Supplementation with vitamin E (1,200 IU daily) was not effective at preventing muscle damage or oxidative stress in untrained men who performed strength training for the first time. Several studies have found the same results.
- A review study of relevant research conducted on vitamin E since 1985 concluded that vitamin E supplementation does not appear to decrease exercise-induced lipid peroxidation.

Beyond sport performance, vitamin E has been widely studied as a nutrient that may help prevent chronic disease, which is why it has been recommended so widely and in such high doses. Recent findings, however, have reversed these recommendations. In one long-running study involving some 7,000 volunteers taking 400 IU daily, vitamin E supplementation failed to reduce the risk of heart disease and cancer and actually may have increased the risk of heart disease in people with diabetes or preexisting heart problems. In a second study, the same dose of vitamin E nearly tripled the risk of new cancers among 540 patients undergoing cancer treatment.

Sounds pretty grim, but the better news is that taking 200 IU of vitamin E appears safe. This is the dosage now being recommended. Some people can get the recommended daily intake of 30 IU by eating foods rich in vitamin E, including nuts, sunflower seeds, and vegetable oils.

If you supplement your diet with vitamin E, choose a natural form of the nutrient over a synthetic version. Labeled as d-alpha tocopherol, natural vitamin E is isolated from soybean, sunflower, corn, peanut, grapeseed, and cottonseed oils. Synthetic vitamin E, labeled as dl-alpha tocopherol, is processed from substances found in petrochemicals. A recent review of 30 published studies on vitamin E concluded that the natural version is absorbed better by the body than the synthetic version.

Avoid taking supplemental vitamin E if you are taking anticlotting drugs such as low-dose aspirin or Coumadin, because vitamin E can further thin your blood.

## Coenzyme Q10

Coenzyme Q10 (CoQ10) is actually a lipid that acts like a vitamin and is an essential component in the body's production of energy. But it is also an antioxidant that has been widely studied. CoQ10 is present in every cell in the body and is found in the greatest concentration in the heart muscle, where it probably improves oxygen uptake at the cellular level. CoQ10 supplementation has been effective in the treatment of heart failure.

Because of its role in energy production and oxygen uptake, CoQ10 has been theorized to improve aerobic performance. A few new studies have examined this connection. I'll summarize what we currently know: Supplementation helps reduce oxidative stress (which occurs when free radicals start outnumbering antioxidants) in sedentary men who start strength training; and it may slightly improve performance in untrained men. The dosage was 90 milligrams, as recommended by the supplement manufacturer on the package label.

The amount of supplemental CoQ10 for the treatment of disease is often 150 to 200 milligrams daily, but also can vary within a range of 90 to 390 milligrams.

## Antioxidant Supplements and Exercise

An antioxidant cocktail may help prevent oxidative stress, a condition in which free radicals outnumber antioxidants and that may result in damage to muscle tissues, according to a study from the Washington University School of Medicine in St. Louis. For one month, unexercised medical students took high doses of antioxidants daily: 1,000 IU of vitamin E, 1,250 milligrams of vitamin C, and 37.5 milligrams of beta-carotene. The doses were divided into five capsules a day. Some of the subjects took placebos.

Before supplementation, the students ran at a moderate pace on a treadmill for about 40 minutes, followed by 5 minutes of high-intensity running to exhaustion. The same exercise bout was repeated after supplementation.

The researchers discovered that oxidative stress caused by exercise was high before supplementation. In other words, there was a lot of tissue damage going on. With antioxidants, there was still some oxidative stress caused by exercise, but it wasn't as great. The researchers concluded that taking antioxidants offered protection against tissue damage. When you can reduce this damage, you might be able to optimize competitive sport performance. But like much research with supplements, other studies have come up with different results; namely, that antioxidant supplementation does not appear to prevent exercise-induced muscle tissue damage.

Much of the research in antioxidant supplementation has been done with endurance athletes. But what about strength trainers? If you work out consistently, you are tearing down a lot of tissue, and muscles generate free radicals during and after exercise. For these reasons, there may be some benefit to taking antioxidant supplements; they may help protect against the potential onslaught of free radicals.

Most of the people I have worked with follow diets that are deficient in vitamin E and other antioxidants. One of the reasons is that active, health-conscious people typically go on diets that are low in fat, but dietary fat from vegetable oils, nuts, and seeds is one of the best sources of vitamin E. What's more, some active people, particularly strength trainers, limit their intake of fruit. They incorrectly believe that the fructose in fruit will end up as body fat. But by cutting out fruits, they cut out foods that are loaded with beta-carotene and vitamin C.

## Antioxidant Supplements and Performance

If you take antioxidants, will you be able to work out longer and harder? Whether antioxidant supplementation really improves performance hasn't been adequately nailed down by research. If you are undernourished—that is, you have a vitamin deficiency—you will definitely feel better and perform better by correcting that deficiency. But if your diet is already high in antioxidants, supplementing with extra antioxidants may not make much of a difference in your performance.

The amounts of vitamin C and beta-carotene that seem to be protective are easily obtained from food. To get enough of these two vitamins, follow my Power Eating recommendations in chapters 12 through 16 and throughout the book. Strive to eat three or more servings of vegetables and two or more servings of fruits every day.

As for vitamin E, a supplement of 100 to 200 IU per day is safe and adequate. To boost your intake of the other antioxidants, be sure your daily vitamin and mineral supplement contains antioxidants.

# B-Complex Vitamins

There are nine major B-complex vitamins—thiamin, riboflavin, niacin, vitamin $B_{12}$, folic acid, pyridoxine, pantothenic acid, biotin, and choline—that work in accord to ensure proper digestion, muscle contraction, and energy production. Although these nutrients do not enhance performance, training and diet do alter the body's requirement for some of them. If you are active and you restrict your calories, or if you make poor nutritional choices, then you put yourself at risk for deficiencies, particularly of thiamin, riboflavin, and pyridoxine. Table 7.2 summarizes the exercise-related functions of the B-complex vitamins.

## Thiamin

Thiamin helps release energy from carbohydrate. Thiamin, along with pyridoxine and vitamin $B_{12}$, is believed to be involved in the formation of serotonin, a feel-good

## TABLE 7.2   B-Complex Vitamins

### Thiamin (B$_1$)

| | |
|---|---|
| Exercise-related function | Carbohydrate metabolism; maintenance of nervous system; growth and muscle tone. |
| Best food sources | Brewer's yeast, wheat germ, bran, whole grains, and organ meats. |
| Side effects and toxicity | None known. |
| DRIs for adults | Women, 1.1 mg; pregnant women, 1.4 mg; lactating women, 1.4 mg; men, 1.2 mg. |

### Riboflavin (B$_2$)

| | |
|---|---|
| Exercise-related function | Metabolism of carbohydrate, protein, and fat; cellular respiration. |
| Best food sources | Milk, eggs, lean meats, and broccoli. |
| Side effects and toxicity | None known. |
| DRIs for adults | Women, 1.1 mg; pregnant women, 1.4 mg; lactating women, 1.6 mg; men, 1.3 mg. |

### Niacin

| | |
|---|---|
| Exercise-related function | Cellular energy production; metabolism of carbohydrate, protein, and fat. |
| Best food sources | Lean meats, liver, poultry, fish, peanuts, and wheat germ. |
| Side effects and toxicity | Liver damage, jaundice, skin flushing and itching, nausea. |
| DRIs for adults | Women, 14 mg; pregnant women, 18 mg; lactating women, 17 mg; men, 16 mg. |
| UL for adults | 35 mg. |

### Vitamin B$_{12}$

| | |
|---|---|
| Exercise- related function | Metabolism of carbohydrate, protein, and fat; formation of red blood cells. |
| Best food sources | Meats, dairy products, eggs, liver, and fish. |
| Side effects and toxicity | Liver damage, allergic reactions. |
| DRIs for adults | Women, 2.4 mg; pregnant women, 2.6 mg; lactating women, 2.8 mg; men, 2.4 mg. |

### Folic acid

| | |
|---|---|
| Exercise-related function | Regulation of growth; breakdown of protein; formation of red blood cells. |
| Best food sources | Green leafy vegetables and liver. |
| Side effects and toxicity | Gastric problems; can mask certain anemias. |

> continued

TABLE 7.2 > *continued*

**Folic acid, *continued***

| | |
|---|---|
| DRIs for adults | Women, 400 mcg; pregnant women, 600 mcg; lactating women, 500 mcg; men, 400 mcg. |
| UL for adults | 1,000 mcg. |

**Pyridoxine (B$_6$)**

| | |
|---|---|
| Exercise-related function | Protein metabolism; formation of oxygen-carrying red blood cells. |
| Best food sources | Whole grains and meats. |
| Side effects and toxicity | Liver and nerve damage. |
| DRIs for adults | Women aged 19-30, 1.3 mg; women aged 31-70, 1.5 mg; pregnant women, 1.9 mg; lactating women, 2 mg; men aged 19-30, 1.3 mg; men aged 31-70, 1.7 mg. |
| UL for adults | 100 mg. |

**Pantothenic acid**

| | |
|---|---|
| Exercise-related function | Cellular energy production; fatty acid oxidation. |
| Best food sources | Found widely in foods. |
| Side effects and toxicity | None known. |
| DRIs for adults | Women, 5 mg; pregnant women, 6 mg; lactating women, 7 mg; men, 5 mg. |

**Biotin**

| | |
|---|---|
| Exercise-related function | Breakdown of fat. |
| Best food sources | Egg yolks and liver. |
| Side effects and toxicity | None known. |
| DRIs for adults | Women, 30 mcg; pregnant women, 30 mcg; lactating women, 35 mcg; men, 30 mcg. |

**Choline**

| | |
|---|---|
| Exercise-related function | May lessen fatigue and improve performance in aerobic sports. |
| Best food sources | Egg yolks, nuts, soybeans, wheat germ, cauliflower, and spinach. |
| Side effects and toxicity | None known. |
| DRIs for adults | Women, 425 mg; pregnant women, 450 mg; lactating women, 550 mg; men, 550 mg. |
| UL for adults | 3,500 mg. |

chemical made in the brain. Serotonin helps elevate mood and induce relaxation. Large doses of these vitamins (60 to 200 times the daily requirement) have been shown to help fine motor control and performance in pistol shooting. It remains to be seen whether supplementation with these vitamins would affect performance in precision sports that depend on fine motor control.

A study published in 2011 looked into supplementation with dietary thiamin and riboflavin in college swimmers (men and women) undergoing intensive training. The study found that during intensive training, swimmers had an increased need for thiamin but not for riboflavin.

The amount of carbohydrate and calories in your diet determines your dietary requirement for thiamin. By eating a well-balanced, carbohydrate-dense diet, you generally get all the thiamin you need. The best food sources of thiamin are unrefined cereals, brewer's yeast, legumes, seeds, and nuts.

There is one possible exception, however. Are you taking a carbohydrate supplement to increase calories? If so, you may need extra thiamin, particularly if your carbohydrate formula contains no thiamin. For every 1,000 calories of carbohydrate you consume from a formula, you need to add 0.5 milligram of thiamin to your diet.

Dieting and erratic eating patterns can leave some nutritional gaps, too. To be on the safe side, be sure to take a daily multivitamin that contains 100 percent of the DRI for thiamin or up to 1.2 milligrams of the nutrient. It is not a good idea to exceed the upper limit (UL) recommendation for any B vitamins.

## Riboflavin

Like thiamin, riboflavin helps release energy from foods. Also as with thiamin, your dietary requirement of riboflavin is linked to your caloric and carbohydrate intake. As a strength trainer, you need to consume at least 0.6 milligram of riboflavin for every 1,000 calories of carbohydrate in your diet, and some athletes may need even more. Riboflavin is easily lost from the body, particularly in sweat. In a study of older women (aged 50 to 67), researchers at Cornell University discovered that exercise increases the body's requirement for riboflavin. An earlier study at Cornell found that very active women required about 1.2 milligrams of riboflavin a day. However, increasing riboflavin intake did not improve performance.

Foods rich in riboflavin include dairy products, poultry, fish, grains, and enriched and fortified cereals. A daily multivitamin containing 100 percent of the DRI, or up to 1.3 milligrams, of riboflavin will help prevent a shortfall.

## Niacin

Like the previously mentioned B-complex vitamins, niacin is involved in releasing energy from foods. Supplementing with too much extra niacin is not a good idea and may be harmful, according to a great deal of research. For example, supplementation with extra niacin may block the release of fat from fat tissue, causing a premature reliance on the use of stored carbohydrate and depletion of muscle glycogen. It may also impair aerobic performance. Excessive amounts of niacin could also contribute to liver damage.

The amount of niacin you need each day is linked to your caloric intake. For every 1,000 calories you eat daily, you need 6.6 milligrams of niacin, or 13 milligrams for every 2,000 calories. If you are using a carbohydrate formula that contains no niacin, make sure you take 6.6 milligrams of niacin for every 1,000 calories that you supplement. The best food sources of niacin are lean meats, poultry, fish, and wheat germ. Taking a multivitamin every day will help you guard against deficiencies.

## Vitamin B$_{12}$

Vital to healthy blood and a normal nervous system, vitamin B$_{12}$ is the only vitamin found primarily in animal products. It works in partnership with folic acid to form red blood cells in the bone marrow.

If you are a vegetarian who eats no animal foods, you must be sure to get enough vitamin B$_{12}$. Fermented and cultured foods such as tempeh and miso contain some B$_{12}$, as do vegetarian foods fortified with the nutrient. The safest approach is to supplement with a multivitamin containing 3 to 10 micrograms of vitamin B$_{12}$.

If you are over 50 years old, your ability to absorb vitamin B$_{12}$ from food may be limited. The Institute of Medicine recommends that you consume foods fortified with B$_{12}$ or take a vitamin B$_{12}$ supplement.

## Folic Acid

Folic acid is the vitamin that, with B$_{12}$, helps produce red blood cells in the bone marrow. Found in green leafy vegetables, legumes, and whole grains, it also helps reproducing cells to synthesize proteins and nucleic acids.

Folic acid first attracted attention for its role in pregnancy. During pregnancy, folic acid helps create red blood cells for the increased blood volume required by the mother, fetus, and placenta. Because of folic acid's role in the production of genetic material and red blood cells, a deficiency can have far-reaching consequences for fetal development. If the fetus is deprived of folic acid, birth defects can result. Folic acid intake is so important to women in their childbearing years that foods are now being fortified with it. The most recent findings is that pregnant women should take a multivitamin supplement to ensure that they get enough folic acid.

There is renewed excitement about folic acid because of its protective role against heart disease and cancer. It reduces homocysteine, a proteinlike substance, in the tissues and blood. High homocysteine levels have been linked to heart disease. Scientists predict that as many as 50,000 premature deaths a year from heart disease can be prevented if we eat more folic acid.

Recent scientific experiments have revealed that folic acid deficiencies cause DNA damage resembling the DNA damage in cancer cells. This finding has led scientists to suggest that cancer could be initiated by DNA damage caused by a deficiency in this B-complex vitamin. Other studies show that folic acid suppresses cell growth in colorectal cancer. It also prevents the formation of precancerous lesions that could lead to cervical cancer, a discovery that may explain why women who don't eat many vegetables and fruits (good sources of folic acid) have high rates of this form of cancer.

Stress, disease, and alcohol consumption all increase your need for folic acid. You should make sure that you're getting 400 micrograms a day of this vitamin, a level that is found in most multivitamins.

## Pyridoxine

Pyridoxine, also known as vitamin $B_6$, is required for the metabolism of protein. It's also vital in the formation of red blood cells and the healthy functioning of the brain. The best food sources of pyridoxine are protein foods such as chicken, fish, and eggs. Other good sources are brown rice, soybeans, oats, and whole wheat.

Researchers in Finland found that exercise alters pyridoxine requirements somewhat. They learned this by testing the blood levels of various nutrients in a group of young female university students who followed a 24-week exercise program.

Ever feel anxious before an athletic competition? If so, try supplementing with a cocktail of pyridoxine, thiamin, and vitamin $B_{12}$. By increasing levels of serotonin—a mood-elevating chemical in the brain—this trio has been found to reduce anxiety and thus improve competitive performance.

The DRI for pyridoxine in women aged 19 to 50 is 1.3 milligrams; for women aged 51 and older, 1.5 milligrams; for pregnant women, 1.9 milligrams; for lactating women, 2 milligrams; for men aged 19 to 50, 1.3 milligrams; and for men aged 51 and older, 1.7 milligrams. If you're wondering whether your own requirement for pyridoxine falls within safe bounds, rest assured that it probably does. A training diet that contains moderate amounts of protein will give you all the pyridoxine you need. In other words, there's no need to supplement. Besides, large doses (in excess of 50 milligrams a day) can cause nerve damage.

## Pantothenic Acid

Pantothenic acid participates in the release of energy from carbohydrate, fat, and protein. Because this vitamin is so widely distributed in foods (particularly meats, whole grains, and legumes), it is rare to find a deficiency without a drop in other B-complex vitamins. They all work as a team.

The safe range of intake for pantothenic acid is 4 to 7 milligrams a day. Exercise does affect pantothenic acid metabolism, but only to a slight degree. By following my strength-training nutrition plan in chapters 12 to 16, you'll take in plenty of this vitamin, enough to cover any extra needs you might have as a result of exercise.

## Biotin

Biotin is involved in fat and carbohydrate metabolism. Without it, the body can't burn fat. Biotin is also a component of various enzymes that carry out essential biochemical reactions in the body. Some good sources of biotin are egg yolks, soy flour, and cereals. Even if you don't get the 30 to 100 micrograms you need daily from food, your body can synthesize biotin from intestinal bacteria. So there's no reason to supplement with extra biotin.

Together with choline and inositol, two other B-complex members, biotin is often found in lipotropic (prevents or reduces fat accumulation in the liver) supplements promoted as fat burners. However, there is no credible evidence that biotin or any other supplemental nutrient burns fat.

Some research shows that biotin levels are low in active people. No one is sure why, but one explanation is that it may have to do with exercise. Exercise causes lactic acid, a waste product, to build up in working muscles, and biotin is involved in the process that breaks down lactic acid. The more lactic acid that accumulates in muscles, the more biotin is needed to break it down. But don't rush out to buy a bottle of biotin. There is no need to supplement with this vitamin, because your body can make up for any marginal deficiencies on its own.

Some strength trainers are in the habit of concocting raw-egg milkshakes. Raw egg white contains avidin, a protein that binds with biotin in the intestine and prevents its absorption. Eating raw eggs on a consistent basis can thus lead to a biotin deficiency. But once eggs are cooked, the avidin is destroyed, and there is no danger of blocking biotin absorption.

## Choline

Present in all living cells, choline is another B-complex vitamin. It is synthesized from two amino acids, methionine and serine, with help from vitamin $B_{12}$ and folic acid. Choline works with inositol, another lipotropic dietary factor, to prevent fat from building up in the liver and to shuttle fat into cells to be burned for energy.

Choline is involved in the formation of acetylcholine in the body. Acetylcholine is a neurotransmitter, a chemical that sends messages between nerves and between nerves and muscles. If acetylcholine is reduced in the nervous system, fatigue may set in. Because acetylcholine is the most abundant neurotransmitter in the body, acting every time we think or move, it's not surprising that low levels would lead to fatigue.

Choline plays a central role in many other physiological pathways, including the cell membrane signaling involved in brain function and the methyl-group metabolism involved in hormone and energy metabolism.

Researchers at MIT studied runners before and after the Boston Marathon and found a 40 percent drop in their plasma choline concentrations. They don't know why this happened; however, they speculated that choline is used up during exercise to produce acetylcholine. Once choline is depleted, there's a corresponding drop in acetylcholine production, and when production falls off, the ability to do muscular work falls off.

A 2008 study published in the *International Journal of Sport Nutrition and Exercise Metabolism* pointed out that strenuous and prolonged physical activity may decrease circulating choline stores. Supplementing with choline prevents this, and may even improve endurance. Endurance activity stresses many of the pathways in which choline performs. The longer and harder you train, the more choline you use, and possibly use up. There is no research published on choline and strength training, but we do know that low choline levels will absolutely limit exercise performance.

Choline is best absorbed when taken as phosphatidylcholine (PC), which is the body's natural reservoir of choline and is also available as a supplement. PC is the major building block for all cell membranes, and it supports cell, tissue, and organ functions. Supplementing with PC helps maintain sufficient choline reserves for good health.

You can also boost absorption by taking PC with phosphatidylserine (PS), another key membrane building block for cells. PS dietary supplements also may help you improve your athletic performance by suppressing cortisol, a potent, catabolic (breakdown) stress hormone. Too much cortisol in the body, which can result from intense workouts, may have negative effects on your training, performance, and physique. Research has shown that short-term oral supplementation of 750 milligrams per day of phosphatidylserine for 10 days improves exercise capacity during high-intensity cycling and increases running performance. Supplementing with PS is a natural, drug-free choice for athletes who want to overcome the effects of exercise-induced stress.

PS and PC have both been shown to play an important role in brain cell health and memory function. These two phospholipids are required to create the channels in brain cell membranes that allow nutrients to pass into the cells and toxins to pass out. Research from the National Institutes of Mental Health has shown that supplementing with PS and PC may slow the rate of progression of degenerative diseases of the brain. These are critical compounds to have in our diets.

Most Americans are low in choline. The best food sources of phosphatidylcholine and phosphatidylserine are soy lecithin and egg yolks. Concern over cholesterol in egg yolks caused a lot of us to stop eating yolks—thus, the drop in choline in our diets. But guess what: Several studies have revealed that an egg yolk a day does not raise blood cholesterol levels if you're healthy with no signs of cardiovascular disease. I recommend to all of my clients to include one whole egg in their diets each day. This increases choline consumption by 50 percent. It also significantly increases phosphatidylserine consumption.

Most vitamin supplements contain choline, and you should make sure to consume at least the DRI for choline daily. The effective dosage in sport studies is 0.2 gram of phosphatidylcholine per kilogram of body mass. This does not need to be any kind of loading strategy, but can just be a maintenance program. The effective dosages for phosphatidylserine in exercise studies range from 300 to 800 milligrams per day for 10 to 15 days. Studies that investigated cognitive function and memory, and support during periods of mental stress associated with physical stress, suggested a range from 100 to 300 milligrams of phosphatidylserine per day.

## Other Vitamins

The fat-soluble vitamins A, D, and K are rarely promoted as exercise aids, most likely because they're toxic in large doses. Vitamin A, or retinol, is found primarily in animal sources such as liver, fish, liver oils, margarine, milk, butter, and eggs. Vitamin A is involved in the growth and repair of tissues, the maintenance of proper vision, and resistance against infection. It also helps maintain the health of the skin and mucous membranes. Massive doses in excess of the DRI can cause nausea, vomiting, diarrhea, skin problems, and bone fragility, among other serious problems.

Including beta-carotene, also known as previtamin A, is a safe way to ensure good vitamin A status and boost your antioxidant consumption. You have a natural governor in your body controlling vitamin A production: You will manufacture vitamin A from beta-carotene only if your body needs it. The best food sources of beta-carotene are orange, red, yellow, and dark green vegetables and fruits.

## Vitamin D

Contrary to what most people believe, vitamin D is not a vitamin, but a steroid hormone. It is produced in various parts of the body but exerts its influence elsewhere in the body—which is what hormones do. Your body can manufacture vitamin D on its own when your skin is exposed to sunlight. Just 10 to 15 minutes a day in the sun without sunscreen a few days a week supplies sufficient amounts of vitamin D. If you can't get out in the sun, live in northern climates where there is not too much sunlight, or frequently wear sunscreen, you may need to take supplements. The form of vitamin D manufactured by the liver and measured in the bloodstream is called calcidiol, or 25 hydroxyvitamin D-2. The activated vitamin D steroid hormone is processed by the kidneys and is known as calcitriol, or 25 hydroxyvitamin D-3. Calcitriol circulates as a hormone in your body regulating the amounts of calcium and phosphate in your bloodstream and maintaining the health of your bones.

As a steroid hormone, vitamin D regulates more than 1,000 vitamin D–responsive human genes and may influence athletic performance, particularly if an athlete is deficient in this nutrient, Numerous studies over many decades have revealed that physical and athletic performance peaks when 25 hydroxyvitamin D levels peak in the summertime, and declines as the steroid hormone declines in the body, in the wintertime. Athletes tend to have low vitamin D levels in winter, according to a number of studies. If you're an older athlete, make sure you get enough vitamin D from food and supplements, because elderly people are typically deficient in this nutrient. Supplements with vitamin D have been shown in numerous studies to boost performance in older adults.

Although it is well recognized that vitamin D plays a critical role in bone health, emerging evidence is revealing that vitamin D also reduces the risk for certain conditions that are important to athletes, such as stress fractures, total body inflammation, infections, and muscular function.

There is also a connection between vitamin D and weight management. Vitamin D helps your body better absorb calcium, which has a fat-burning effect. So for calcium to assist in fat burning, your body requires sufficient vitamin D. On the other hand, if the calcium levels in your body are low, a hormone called parathyroid hormone (PTH) and vitamin D increase in response to the shortage and trick your body into thinking it is starving. Consequently, you may pack away more calories in the form of fat and put on extra weight when this imbalance occurs.

To get enough vitamin D, don't rely on supplements alone. Instead, get at least 10 to 15 minutes of sun exposure daily. Also, include vitamin D–rich foods in your diet: fatty fish and fortified milk products. And, include vitamin D supplements as part of your daily routine. Each of us absorbs vitamin D differently, but the current recommendation for supplementation is 600 to 2000 IU of the nutrient daily.

## Eight Reasons to Pump Up Your Vitamin D

1. Supports bone health
2. Bolsters immunity
3. Boosts mood when taken with the omega-3 fatty acid DHA
4. Assists in neuromuscular control
5. Helps regulate body weight
6. Helps prevent aging-related inflammation
7. Lengthens telomeres (a factor in longevity)
8. Decreases the risk of many chronic and degenerative diseases

## Vitamin K

The primary function of vitamin K is to assist in the process of normal blood clotting. It is also required for the formation of other kinds of body protein found in the blood, bone, and kidneys. However, research has revealed another side to vitamin K that most people were not aware of: It is vital for building healthy bones, which is why a number of calcium supplements are now being formulated with vitamin K. With a shortfall of vitamin K, bone can become weakened because of insufficient levels of osteocalcin, a protein involved in bone hardening. In one study with female athletes, 10 milligrams daily of vitamin K decreased the process of bone breakdown and increased bone formation. These improvements were measured by looking at the amount of osteocalcin (an indicator of bone formation), as well as at by-products of bone breakdown, in the bloodstream and urine.

A vitamin K deficiency is extremely rare, and there's usually no need for supplementation unless recommended by your physician. The best food sources are dairy products, meats, eggs, cereals, fruits, and vegetables. The functions of vitamins A, D, and K and their possible roles in exercise performance are summarized in table 7.3.

### TABLE 7.3　Vitamins A, D, and K

| Vitamin A | |
| --- | --- |
| Exercise-related function | Growth and repair of tissues, including muscles; building of body structures. |
| Best food sources | Liver, egg yolks, whole milk, and orange and yellow vegetables. |
| Side effects and toxicity | Digestive system upset, damage to bones and certain organs. |
| DRIs for adults | Women, 700 mcg; pregnant women, 770 mcg; lactating women, 1,300 mcg; men, 900 mcg. |
| Tolerable upper intake level | 3,000 mcg. |
| **Vitamin D** | |
| Exercise-related function | Normal bone growth and development. |
| Best food sources | Sunlight, fortified dairy products, and fish oils. |
| Side effects and toxicity | Nausea, vomiting, hardening of soft tissues, kidney damage. |
| DRIs for adults | Women aged 19-50, 5 mcg; women aged 51-70, 10 mcg; women aged 70+, 15 mcg; pregnant women, 5 mcg; lactating women, 5 mcg; men aged 19-50, 5 mcg; men aged 51-70, 10 mcg; men aged 70+, 15 mcg. |
| Tolerable upper intake level | 4,000 IU; 600 IU for pregnant and lactating women; 800 IU for men and women older than 70. |
| UL for adults | 50 mcg. |
| **Vitamin K** | |
| Exercise-related function | Involved in glycogen formation, blood clotting, and bone formation. |
| Best food sources | Vegetables, milk, and yogurt. |
| Side effects and toxicity | Allergic reactions, breakdown of red blood cells. |
| DRIs for adults | Women, 90 mcg; men, 120 mcg. |

# Minerals and Performance

Minerals found naturally in food are particularly important to exercisers and athletes because of their involvement in muscle contraction, normal heart rhythm, oxygen transport, transmission of nerve impulses, immune function, and bone health. If you are not adequately nourished with minerals, a deficiency could harm your health, and this in turn could adversely affect your performance. What follows is a look at various minerals that can have a bearing on your performance. The functions of major and trace minerals are summarized in table 7.4.

## TABLE 7.4   Major Minerals and Trace Minerals

| Major | |
|---|---|
| **Calcium** | |
| Exercise-related function | A constituent of body structures; plays a part in muscle growth, muscle contraction, and nerve transmission. |
| Best food sources | Dairy products and green leafy vegetables. |
| Side effects and toxicity | Excessive calcification of some tissues, constipation, mineral absorption problems. |
| DRIs for adults | Women aged 19-50, 1,000 mg; women aged 51-70+, 1,200 mg; pregnant women, 1,000 mg; lactating women, 1,000 mg; men aged 19-50, 1,000 mg; men aged 51-70+, 1,200 mg. |
| UL for adults | 2,500 mg. |
| **Phosphorus** | |
| Exercise-related function | Metabolism of carbohydrate, protein, and fat; growth, repair, and maintenance of cells; energy production; stimulation of muscular contractions. |
| Best food sources | Meats, fish, poultry, eggs, whole grains, seeds, and nuts. |
| Side effects and toxicity | None known. |
| DRIs for adults | 700. |
| UL for adults | Women and men aged 19-70, 4,000 mg; aged 70+, 3,000 mg. |
| **Potassium** | |
| Exercise-related function | Maintenance of normal fluid balance on either side of cell walls; normal growth; stimulation of nerve impulses for muscular contractions; conversion of glucose to glycogen; synthesis of muscle protein from amino acids. |
| Best food sources | Potatoes, bananas, fruits, and vegetables. |
| Side effects and toxicity | Heart disturbances. |
| DRIs for adults | No DRI, but a minimum requirement of 1,600 mg for sedentary adults and 3,500 mg for active adults. |
| **Sodium** | |
| Exercise-related function | Maintenance of normal fluid balance on either side of cell walls; muscular contraction and nerve transmission; keeps other blood minerals soluble. |
| Best food sources | Found in virtually all foods. |
| Side effects and toxicity | Water retention and high blood pressure. |
| DRIs for adults | No DRI; a recommended safe minimum intake is 2,400 mg daily. |

> continued

TABLE 7.4 > *continued*

## Chloride

| | |
|---|---|
| Exercise-related function | Helps regulate the pressure that causes fluids to flow in and out of cell membranes. |
| Best food sources | Table salt (sodium chloride), kelp, and rye flour. |
| Side effects and toxicity | None known. |
| DRIs for adults | No DRI; a recommended safe minimum intake is 500 mg daily. |

## Magnesium

| | |
|---|---|
| Exercise-related function | Metabolism of carbohydrate and protein; assists in neuro-muscular contractions. |
| Best food sources | Green vegetables, legumes, whole grains, and seafood. |
| Side effects and toxicity | Large amounts are toxic. |
| DRIs for adults | Women aged 19-30, 310 mg; women aged 31+, 320 mg; pregnant women aged 19-30, 350 mg; pregnant women aged 31+, 360 mg; lactating women aged 19-30, 310 mg; lactating women aged 31+, 320 mg; men aged 19-30, 400 mg; men aged 31+, 420 mg. |
| UL for adults | 350 mg from supplements alone. |

## Trace

## Iron

| | |
|---|---|
| Exercise-related function | Oxygen transport to cells for energy; formation of oxygen-carrying red blood cells. |
| Best food sources | Liver, oysters, lean meats, and green leafy vegetables. |
| Side effects and toxicity | Large amounts are toxic. |
| DRIs for adults | Women aged 19-50, 18 mg; women aged 51+, 8 mg; pregnant women, 27 mg; lactating women, 9 mg; men, 8 mg. |
| UL for adults | 45 mg. |

## Iodine

| | |
|---|---|
| Exercise-related function | Energy production; growth and development; metabolism. |
| Best food sources | Iodized salt, seafood, and mushrooms. |
| Side effects and toxicity | Thyroid enlargement. |
| DRIs for adults | 150 mcg. |
| UL for adults | 1,000 mcg. |

## Chromium

| | |
|---|---|
| Exercise-related function | Normal blood sugar; fat metabolism. |
| Best food sources | Corn oil, brewer's yeast, whole grains, and meats. |
| Side effects and toxicity | Liver and kidney damage. |
| DRIs for adults | Women aged 19-50, 25 mcg; women aged 51+, 20 mcg; pregnant women, 30 mcg; lactating women, 45 mcg; men aged 19-50, 35 mcg; men aged 51+, 30 mcg. |

## Fluoride

| | |
|---|---|
| Exercise-related function | None known. |
| Best food sources | Fluoridated water supplies. |
| Side effects and toxicity | Large amounts are toxic and can cause mottling of teeth. |
| DRIs for adults | Women, 3 mg; men, 4 mg. |
| UL for adults | 10 mg. |

## Molybdenum

| | |
|---|---|
| Exercise-related function | Involved in the metabolism of fat. |
| Best food sources | Milk, beans, breads, and cereals. |
| Side effects and toxicity | Diarrhea, anemia, and depressed growth rate. |
| DRIs for adults | 45 mcg. |
| UL for adults | 2,000 mcg. |

## Boron

| | |
|---|---|
| Exercise-related function | No clear biological function in humans has been identified. |
| Food sources | Fruit-based beverages and products, potatoes, legumes, milk, avocados, peanut butter, and peanuts. |
| DRIs for adults | None established. |

## Vanadium

| | |
|---|---|
| Exercise-related function | No clear biological function in humans has been identified. |
| Food sources | Mushrooms, shellfish, black pepper, parsley, and dill seed. |
| Side effects and toxicity | Large doses are extremely toxic and may cause excessive fatigue. |
| DRIs for adults | None established. |

Other important minerals that can affect your performance include zinc and selenium, which are included in table 7.1.

## Electrolytes

The tissues in your body contain fluids both inside cells (intracellular fluid) and in the spaces between cells (extracellular fluid). Dissolved in both fluids are electrolytes, which are electrically charged minerals or ions. The electrolytes work in concert, regulating water balance on either side of the cell membranes. Electrolytes also help make muscles contract by promoting the transmission of messages across nerve cell membranes. Electrolyte balance is critical to optimal performance and overall health. The two chief electrolytes are sodium and potassium. Sodium regulates fluid balance outside cells, whereas potassium regulates fluids inside cells.

Sodium is obtained mostly from salt and processed foods. On average, Americans eat 2 to 3 teaspoons (12 to 18 g) of salt every day—far too much for good health. A healthier sodium target is 500 milligrams (the minimum requirement) to 2,400 milligrams per day, or no more than 1 1/4 teaspoons (1.6 g) of table salt each day.

Although some sodium can be lost from sweat during exercise, you don't have to worry about replacing it with supplements. Your usual diet contains enough sodium to replace what was lost. What's more, the body does a good job of conserving sodium on its own.

Severe sodium depletion, however, can occur during ultraendurance events such as triathlons that last more than four hours. Consuming 1/2 to 3/4 of a cup (120 to 180 ml) of sport drink every 10 to 20 minutes, along with adding salty foods to the diet, is enough to replenish an endurance athlete's need for sodium. Thus, during an endurance event lasting longer than three hours, you want to have a sport drink containing 200 to 300 milligrams of sodium per 8 ounces (240 ml). To restore fluid balance during recovery after endurance exercise, you need sodium in your beverage because it lets water enter your cells.

Drinking too much plain water (overhydration), however, can cause sodium and other electrolytes to become overly diluted. This imbalance can negatively affect performance.

Potassium works inside cells to regulate fluid balance. Potassium is also involved in maintaining a regular heartbeat, helping muscles contract, regulating blood pressure, and transferring nutrients to cells.

In contrast to sodium, potassium is not as well conserved by the body, so you should be sure to eat plenty of potassium-rich foods such as bananas, oranges, and potatoes. You need between 1,600 and 2,000 milligrams of potassium a day, which can be easily obtained from a diet plentiful in fruits and vegetables.

To get cut, some competitive bodybuilders use diuretics, drugs that increase the formation and excretion of urine in the body. This is a dangerous practice because diuretics can flush potassium and other electrolytes from the body. Life-threatening mineral imbalances can occur, and some professional bodybuilders have died during competition as a result of diuretic abuse. I can see no rational reason for taking diuretics for competitive purposes. The potential damage just isn't worth it.

# Soda and Phosphate Loading

For many years, strength trainers and other athletes have put their faith in the alkaline power of sodium bicarbonate (better known as baking soda) by soda loading. The idea behind soda loading is that it neutralizes lactic acid in the blood. Lactic acid accumulation makes muscles burn and eventually brings them to a point of fatigue. Soda loading may offset burn and fatigue.

Soda loading affects the alkalinity of your diet, and a more alkaline diet is favorable for repair, recuperation, and growth. Research has also found that alkaline diets may have some health benefits, including preserving muscle mass in older men and women and younger unhealthy patients; correcting growth hormone secretion to improve bone health; decreasing cardiovascular risk factors; improving body composition, memory, and cognition; and decreasing chronic low back pain. Foods that promote alkalinity are vegetables, fruits, legumes, and most plant foods.

But back to soda loading. A lot of research has been done recently on soda loading. I'm going to give you a very brief synopsis of the data, to help you decide whether soda loading would be helpful for you.

In one study rowers supplemented with sodium bicarbonate and simulated a 2,000-meter race by using ergometer testing. They did see a buffering effect against lactic acid buildup, but no enhancement in rehydration or performance during the study.

Rugby players who tried soda loading (at the standard 0.3 g/kg of body weight mixed into water) experienced a lot of gastrointestinal discomfort during and after competition. This hampered their physical performance. (An Australian study done in 2011 discovered that soda loading with a high-carbohydrate meal can minimize these stomach troubles.)

In a study of BMX elite cyclists, soda loading at the standard dose had no effect on performance, although it did reduce lactic acid buildup.

A 2011 study published in *Medicine & Science in Sports & Exercise* found that cyclists who supplemented with beta-alanine and soda loaded improved their performance significantly.

The studies on soda loading are far from conclusive. If you want to experiment with it to see if it works for you (it may, because individual responses do vary), do it during training and not during competition.

Although soda loading and phosphate loading both depend on salts, their actions are completely different. For a long time, athletes have experimented with phosphate loading as a way to extend performance. Phosphate is a type of salt made from phosphorus, the second most abundant mineral in the body. The supplement is usually taken in large doses several times daily a few days before competition. By some indications, phosphate loading increases oxygen availability from the blood and makes more glucose available to the working muscles—two advantages if you're a competitive athlete. One study found that phosphate supplementation improved oxygen uptake and improved performance on a bicycle ergometer. In addition, phosphate loading improves certain respiratory and circulatory factors, making phosphate useful for endurance athletes. The recommended dosage is generally 4 grams a day. But be forewarned: Phosphate loading can cause vomiting, upset the body's electrolyte balance, and lead to other untoward reactions.

Phosphates are constituents of some natural weight-loss supplements, too, because they may prevent a drop in metabolism by preserving thyroid hormone levels during severe dieting. A Polish study found that phosphate supplementation may even increase RMR in women on a diet of 1,000 calories a day, suggesting a fat-burning effect. More research is needed in this area, however.

## Other Vital Minerals

Several other minerals could be low in your diet, particularly if you're a competitor and you frequently follow restrictive cutting diets.

### Calcium

Ninety-nine percent of the calcium in the body is stored in the skeleton and teeth. The other 1 percent is found in blood and soft tissues. Calcium is responsible for building healthy bones, conducting nerve impulses, helping muscles contract, and moving nutrients in and out of cells. Exercise helps your body better absorb calcium. At the same time, high-intensity endurance exercise may cause your body to excrete calcium.

The chief sources of calcium in the diet are milk and other dairy products. However, almost every strength trainer and bodybuilder I have ever counseled has avoided dairy products like the plague during precompetition dieting. They believe that these foods are high in sodium, but I say that's nonsense. One cup (240 ml) of nonfat milk contains 126 milligrams of sodium and 302 milligrams of calcium. Two egg whites, a popular food in the diet of strength trainers and bodybuilders, contain 212 milligrams of sodium and only 12 milligrams of calcium. Sodium hardly seems to be a problem here, and there is no better low-fat source of calcium than nonfat milk.

So are milk and dairy products really your enemy? Absolutely not. As I pointed out earlier, milk in particular contains two proteins (whey and casein) that are involved in muscle building, fat burning, and recovery. (See chapter 2 for more information on these important milk proteins and how to use them.)

There's more to this story, however, and it has to do with the calcium in milk and dairy products. A number of studies show that this mineral may help you manage your weight. How? Calcium may assist the body in the breakdown of body fat. It appears that the more calcium a fat cell contains, the more fat the cell will burn.

In one widely publicized study, 32 obese adults were randomly assigned to one of the following diets for 24 weeks: (1) a standard diet containing 400 to 500 milligrams per day of calcium plus a placebo supplement; (2) a standard diet supplemented with 800 milligrams per day of calcium; or (3) a diet containing three servings per day of dairy products, providing 1,200 to 1,300 milligrams per day of calcium, plus a placebo supplement. Each diet cut calories by 500 calories a day. By the end of the experimental period, the average weight loss was 14.5 pounds (6.6 kg) with the standard diet, 19 pounds (8.6 kg) with the calcium-supplemented diet, and about 24.5 pounds (11 kg) with the high-dairy diet. Fat loss from the trunk region represented 19 percent of the total fat loss on the standard diet, 50 percent of total fat loss on the calcium-supplemented diet, and 66.2 percent of total fat loss on the high-dairy diet.

In sum, dietary calcium intake clearly enhanced weight loss and fat loss in obese subjects who followed a reduced-calorie diet. Interestingly, higher calcium intake increased the percentage of fat lost from the trunk region. Finally, consuming calcium in the form of dairy products was significantly more effective than taking calcium supplements. I have to add here, however, that the last finding, though significant, should be interpreted cautiously, because the study was funded by the National Dairy Council.

No one knows yet whether calcium from other foods such as leafy greens has the same effect. Additional research needs to be conducted to ascertain similar benefits. The take-home message is that if you're trying to drop weight, don't drop dairy products, and be sure to select low-fat products.

Overall, the calcium in dairy foods is essential to maintaining good health. With plenty of high-calcium foods, your diet provides the calcium needed to maintain healthy blood calcium levels. If you don't have enough in your diet, your body will draw calcium from bones to maintain blood calcium levels. As more and more calcium is removed from bones, they become brittle and break. The most susceptible areas are the spine, hips, and wrists. An exit of calcium from the bones can lead to the bone-weakening disease osteoporosis. In women who develop the female athlete triad (disordered eating, menstrual irregularities, and weakened bones), low calcium intakes are common.

Female athletes, particularly those in weight-control sports, are often at risk of losing bone calcium. In a study I conducted at the 1990 National Physique Committee (NPC) USA Championships in Raleigh, North Carolina, female bodybuilders recorded their diets; were weighed and had their fat measured; and answered questions about their training, nutrition, and health. None of the women ate or drank any dairy products for at least three months before the competition, and most of them never used dairy products at all. None of them took calcium supplements, either.

Of these women, 81 percent reported that they did not menstruate for at least two months before a contest. The physical stress of training, the psychological stress of competition, the low-calorie diet, and the loss of body fat can all lead to a decrease in the body's production of estrogen. As in menopause, without enough estrogen, a woman stops menstruating. What's worse, no calcium can be stored in the bone when estrogen levels are low. Of course, these women were very lean, too. On average, they had 9 percent body fat. Extremely low body fat is another risk factor for loss of calcium from bones.

If your dietary practices regarding calcium mirror any of these, you must get calcium back into your diet by eating calcium-rich foods—namely, nonfat milk and dairy products. If for some reason you cannot or will not drink milk, try nonfat yogurts. They are equally high in calcium, and they often do not cause the intestinal problems that some people experience from milk. You can also obtain calcium from alternative sources if you are on a milk-free diet. Table 7.5 lists those sources.

### TABLE 7.5 Alternative Sources of Calcium for Milk-Free Diets

| Food | Amount | Calcium (mg) | Calories |
|---|---|---|---|
| Collards, frozen, cooked* | 1/2 cup (95 g) | 179 | 31 |
| Soy milk (fortified) | 1 cup (240 ml) | 150 | 79 |
| Mackerel, canned | 2 oz (56 g) | 137 | 88 |
| Dandelion greens, raw, cooked* | 1/2 cup (53 g) | 74 | 17 |
| Turnip greens, frozen, cooked* | 1/2 cup (72 g) | 125 | 25 |
| Mustard greens, frozen, cooked* | 1/2 cup (75 g) | 76 | 14 |
| Kale, frozen, cooked* | 1/2 cup (65 g) | 90 | 20 |
| Tortillas, corn | 2 | 80 | 95 |
| Molasses, blackstrap | 1 tbsp (21 g) | 176 | 48 |
| Orange | 1 large | 74 | 87 |
| Sockeye salmon, canned, with bone, drained | 2 oz (60 g) | 136 | 87 |
| Sardines, canned, with bone, drained | 2 medium | 92 | 50 |
| Boston baked beans (navy or pea bean), vegetarian, canned | 1/2 cup (127 g) | 64 | 118 |
| Pickled herring | 2 oz (60 g) | 44 | 149 |
| Soybeans, cooked | 1/2 cup (90 g) | 88 | 149 |
| Broccoli, cooked | 1/2 cup (78 g) | 36 | 22 |
| Rutabaga (Swedish or yellow turnip), cooked, mashed | 1/2 cup (120 g) | 58 | 47 |
| Artichoke, cooked | 1 medium | 54 | 60 |
| White beans, cooked | 1/2 cup (90 g) | 81 | 124 |
| Almonds, blanched, whole | 1/4 cup (36 g) | 94 | 222 |
| Tofu | 2 oz (60 g) | 60 | 44 |

* Frozen, cooked vegetable greens are higher in calcium than fresh, cooked greens If you eat the fresh variety, you need to double your portion to get the same amount of calcium.

Some people are lactose intolerant and can't digest milk. They lack sufficient lactase, the enzyme required to digest lactose, a sugar in milk that helps you absorb calcium from the intestine. If you are lactose intolerant, try taking an enzyme-replacement product such as Lactaid. These products replace the lactase you are missing and will digest the lactose for you. Another option is Lactaid milk. Available at most supermarkets, Lactaid milk is pretreated with the lactase enzyme.

Calcium supplements may be in order, too, particularly because three of every four Americans are believed to be deficient in calcium. The most bioavailable source of calcium as a supplement is calcium citrate. Calcium supplements are best taken with all of the other bone-building minerals such as magnesium, boron, and vitamin D.

The DRIs for calcium from food and supplements are as follows: women aged 19 to 50, 1,000 milligrams; women aged 51+, 1,200 milligrams; pregnant women, 1,000 milligrams; lactating women, 1,000 milligrams; men aged 19 to 50, 1,000 milligrams; and men aged 51+, 1,200 milligrams. The National Institutes of Health (NIH) recommends supplementation with calcium and vitamin D (which helps the body absorb calcium) by people not getting the DRIs, including women who develop the female athlete triad. If you have some calcium in your diet, don't take all 1,200 or 1,000 milligrams of calcium in a supplement. Too much calcium in the diet can cause kidney stones in some people.

For the prevention and treatment of osteoporosis in postmenopausal women, many physicians recommend 1,500 milligrams of calcium daily. Table 7.6 illustrates how to get a day's worth of calcium from food.

A word to women: If you have irregular menstruation, no menstrual cycle, or stop menstruating before a contest, you should see a good sports medicine physician or a gynecologist who is familiar with your sport. Loss of estrogen production at an early age can have a critical impact on your bone health. It's possible for osteoporosis to develop at a very early age.

Take care of your inside while you are taking care of your outside. Add some dairy to your diet, and you'll be standing straight and tall for many years to come.

## TABLE 7.6  A Day's Worth of Calcium

| Food | Amount | Calcium (mg) | Calories |
|------|--------|--------------|----------|
| Orange juice, calcium fortified | 1 cup (240 ml) | 300 | 112 |
| Nonfat milk | 1 cup (240 ml) | 301 | 86 |
| Tofu | 4 oz (120 g) | 120 | 88 |
| Low-fat yogurt, fruit | 8 oz (230 g) | 372 | 250 |
| Mozzarella cheese, part-skim | 1 oz (30 g) | 229 | 73 |
| Turnip greens cooked, chopped | 1 cup (72 g) | 250 | 60 |
| **Total** | | **1,572** | **669** |

## Iron

The major role of iron is to combine with protein to make hemoglobin, a special protein that gives red blood cells their color. Hemoglobin carries oxygen in the blood from the lungs to the tissues. Iron is also necessary for the formation of myoglobin, found only in muscle tissue. Myoglobin transports oxygen to muscle cells to be used in the chemical reaction that makes muscles contract.

As a strength trainer or bodybuilder, you are constantly tearing down and rebuilding muscle tissue. This process can create an additional need for iron, a mineral that is enormously essential to human health. What's more, there seems to be a common increase in iron losses from aerobic exercises or sports that involve pounding of the feet, such as jogging, aerobic dancing, and step aerobics. Also at risk for low iron are women who exercise more than three hours a week, have been pregnant within the past two years, or eat fewer than 2,200 calories a day.

Low iron can impair muscular performance. A shortfall of iron can lead to iron-deficiency anemia, the final stage of iron loss, characterized by a hemoglobin concentration below the normal level. Athletic training does tend to deplete iron stores for a number of reasons, including physical stress and muscle damage. Another reason for low iron and iron-deficiency anemia is an inadequate intake of iron. Studies of the diets of female athletes, who likely need to take in even more than the daily requirement (18 mg) to compensate for training-induced losses, indicate daily intakes of roughly 12 milligrams. Other possible reasons for low iron are losses that occur in the gastrointestinal tract, in sweat, and through menstruation.

Some people can have iron deficiency without anemia. This is characterized by normal hemoglobin but reduced levels of ferritin, a storage form of iron in the body. When iron is in short supply, your tissues become starved for oxygen. This can make you tire easily and recover more slowly. Several studies from Cornell University indicate that when untrained, iron-depleted women received an iron supplement during exercise training, they experienced greater increases in oxygen use and endurance performance. This goes to show how important iron is to performance. Taking iron supplements, however, will not enhance your performance if you have normal hemoglobin and iron status.

The best sources of dietary iron are liver and other organ meats, lean meat, and oysters. Iron is found in green leafy vegetables, too, although iron from plant sources is not as well absorbed as iron from animal protein.

Strength trainers and other active people tend to shy away from iron-rich meats because of their high fat content. But you can increase the iron in your diet without adding a lot of beef or animal fat. If you don't eat any meat at all, you must pay careful attention to make sure that you get the iron you need. Here are some suggestions:

- Eat fruits, vegetables, and grains that are high in iron. You won't get as much iron as from animal foods, but the plant foods are the lowest in fat. Green leafy vegetables such as kale and collards, dried fruits such as raisins and apricots, and iron-enriched and fortified breads and cereals are all good plant sources of iron.

- Enhance your body's absorption of iron by combining high iron-containing foods with a rich source of vitamin C, which improves iron absorption. For example, drink some orange juice with your iron-fortified cereal with raisins for breakfast. Or sprinkle some lemon juice on your kale or collards.

- Avoid eating very high-fiber foods at the same meal with foods high in iron. The fiber inhibits the absorption of iron and many other minerals. Avoid drinking tea and taking antacids with high-iron foods; they also inhibit the absorption of iron.

- Try to keep some meat in or add some meat to your diet. Lean red meat and the dark meat of chicken and turkey are highest in iron. Eating 3 to 4 ounces (90-120 g) of meat three times a week will give your iron levels a real boost. And if you combine your meat with a vegetable source of iron, you will absorb more of the iron from the vegetables.

- You might need an iron supplement. Eight milligrams for men and 18 milligrams for women 19 to 50 years old, or 100 percent of the DRI for iron, may be a big help. Don't pop huge doses of iron, though. The more iron you take at one time, the less your body will absorb. Also, excess iron can lead to hemochromatosis, a disorder that causes iron buildup in major organs and the eventual deterioration of liver function.

Because women are more prone to low iron than men are, the United States Olympic Committee (USOC) recommends that female athletes undergo blood testing periodically to check hemoglobin status. If you think you might be deficient in iron, talk to your physician or a registered dietitian who specializes in sport nutrition. Self-medicating with large doses of iron can cause big trouble and is potentially dangerous.

## Zinc

Zinc, one of the antioxidant minerals, is important for hundreds of body processes, including maintaining normal taste and smell, regulating growth, and promoting wound healing.

My research has revealed that female bodybuilders, in particular, don't get enough zinc in their diets. Zinc is an important mineral for people who work out. As you exercise, zinc helps clear lactic acid buildup in the blood. In addition, zinc supplementation (25 mg a day) has been shown to protect immunity during periods of intense training.

There is not much research on zinc supplementation and exercise performance. Interestingly, though, one study shows that if you're an endurance athlete who follows a diet that is rich in carbohydrate but low in protein and fat, you could be setting yourself up for a zinc deficiency, resulting in a loss of too much body weight, greater fatigue, and poor endurance.

Too much zinc might be a bad thing, however. It has been associated with lower levels of good cholesterol (HDL) and thus may increase your risk of cardiovascular disease. What's more, excess zinc over time may create mineral imbalances and produce undesirable changes in two substances involved in calcium metabolism: calcitonin, a hormone that boosts calcium in bones by drawing it from soft tissue, and osteocalcin, the key noncollagen protein needed to help harden bone.

By eating zinc-rich foods, you can get just the right amount, which is 8 milligrams a day for women and 11 milligrams a day for men. The best sources of zinc are meat, eggs, seafood (especially oysters), and whole grains. If you restrict your intake of meat, taking a multivitamin each day will help fill in the nutritional blanks.

### *Magnesium*

Magnesium, a mineral that is in charge of more than 400 metabolic reactions in the body, has been touted as an exercise aid. One study hints at a link between magnesium and muscle strength. Men in a test group were given 500 milligrams of magnesium a day, an increase over the DRI of 400 milligrams. Those in a control group took 250 milligrams a day, significantly less than the DRI. After both groups weight trained for eight weeks, their leg strength was measured. The supplemented men got stronger, whereas those in the control group stayed the same. But many researchers are not yet convinced that magnesium is a strength builder. They caution that the magnesium status of the subjects before the study was unknown. That's an important point, because supplementing with any nutrient in which you are deficient is likely to produce some positive changes in performance and health. Basically, the current train of scientific thought on magnesium supplementation is that it does not affect aerobic power or muscle strength.

Magnesium promotes calcium absorption and helps in the function of nerves and muscles, including heartbeat regulation. The DRI for magnesium for men aged 19 to 30 is 400 milligrams, and for men 31 and older it is 420 milligrams per day. The DRI for women aged 19 to 30 is 310 milligrams, and for women 31 and older it is 320 milligrams.

## Zinc–Magnesium Supplementation

Zinc–magnesium supplementation (ZMA) is widely marketed to strength athletes and bodybuilders as a muscle-building aid. Although one small study investigated the effects of a supplement containing zinc, magnesium, and vitamin $B_6$ on the muscle strength and functional power of college football players and suggested positive results, more current research proves otherwise.

In a study conducted at Baylor University, 42 strength-training men supplemented with ZMA or a placebo before going to sleep at night over an eight-week period. Researchers tested the subjects' muscular endurance, strength, anabolic and catabolic hormone status, and body composition at intervals. The results indicated that the supplementation during training did not enhance any of these variables. It appears that ZMA is not an effective muscle-building product.

---

The use of laxatives and diuretics can impair magnesium balance. If you use these products to make weight, be aware that you can compromise your health and that you risk nervous system complications from fluid and electrolyte imbalances.

The best dietary sources of magnesium are nuts, legumes, whole grains, dark green vegetables, and seafood. These foods should be plentiful in your diet. You can also supplement these foods with a daily multivitamin formulated with 100 percent of the DRI for magnesium.

## Boron

Boron is a trace mineral that has gained notoriety in recent years as a result of claims that it can build muscle mass by increasing testosterone in the body. The problem is that this theory is based on research with elderly women, not with athletes. I see no real point in supplementing with boron. You can get sufficient boron from fruits and vegetables.

## Vanadium

Vanadyl sulfate is a commercial derivative of vanadium, a trace mineral found in vegetables and fish. The body needs very little vanadium, and more than 90 percent of it is excreted in the urine. At high doses, vanadium is extremely toxic and may cause excessive fatigue. To the best of the knowledge of the medical community, no one has ever been diagnosed with a vanadium deficiency.

As a supplement, vanadyl sulfate is supposed to have a tissue-building effect by moving glucose and amino acids into the muscles faster and elevating insulin to promote growth, although the evidence for this has been found only in rats. Nevertheless, vanadyl sulfate is being aggressively marketed as a tissue-building supplement for strength trainers and athletes.

Does vanadyl sulfate work the magic manufacturers assert that it does? A group of researchers in New Zealand asked this question. In a 12-week study, 40 strength trainers (30 men and 10 women) took either a placebo or a daily dose of vanadyl sulfate in amounts matched to their weight (0.5 mg/kg of body weight). So that strength could be assessed, the strength trainers performed bench presses and leg extensions in 1- and 10-repetition maximum bouts during the course of the experiment.

The findings of the study were that vanadyl sulfate did not increase lean body mass. There were some modest improvements in strength-training performance, but these improvements were short-lived, tapering off after the first month of the study. About 20 percent of the strength trainers experienced extreme fatigue during and after training.

Some research hints that vanadyl sulfate supplementation might help treat type 2 diabetes, but the results are conflicting. In my opinion, there's no reason to supplement with vanadyl sulfate. You can get the benefits it promises with the nutritional methods discussed elsewhere in this book.

## Selenium

An antioxidant mineral, selenium works in partnership with vitamin E to fight damaging free radicals. Selenium is vital for a healthy immune system, boosting your defenses against bacteria and viruses, and it may reduce the risk of certain cancers, particularly in the prostate, colon, and lungs. As for performance, some studies have shown that selenium reduces lipid peroxidation after prolonged aerobic exercise, but this effect did not enhance athletic endurance in people who supplemented with selenium.

Selenium is found naturally in fish, meat, wheat germ, nuts (particularly brazil nuts), eggs, oatmeal, whole-wheat bread, and brown rice. Most people have to make sure they eat foods rich in selenium to get enough. You can supplement, but do so carefully. There is a narrow margin between the DRI of 55 micrograms and the UL of 400 micrograms.

## Food First

Always count on food first. Food is your body's best source of vitamins and minerals. Take the time to plan a healthy, well-balanced diet full of fruits, vegetables, grains, beans, lean meats, and nonfat dairy foods, and use the diet-planning guidelines in chapter 10. Along with dedicated training, a good diet with the correct balance of protein, the right kinds of carbohydrate, and the right kinds of fat is your best ticket to building a better body.

# 8

# Muscle-Building Products

You train hard. You're building body-hard muscle. Still, you want to know: Isn't there something else—besides intense workouts and healthy food—that can help you gain a little faster, something that will give you a muscle-building edge with less effort?

Definitely. You can do several things to pack on lean muscle. Unfortunately, not all of them are safe—or legal. Anabolic steroids, although approved for medical use and available by prescription only, are among the most abused drugs among athletes. *Anabolic* means "to build," and anabolic steroids tend to make the body grow in certain ways. They do have muscle-building effects, but they're also dangerous. Once practiced mainly by elite athletes, abuse of anabolic steroids has spread to recreational and teen athletes and is now a national health concern. The 2010 Monitoring the Future study funded by the National Institute on Drug Abuse showed that 0.5 percent of 8th-graders, 1.0 percent of 10th-graders, and 1.5 percent of 12th-graders had abused anabolic steroids at least once in the year prior to being surveyed. Table 8.1 lists some of the dangers associated with these drugs.

A trend related to anabolic steroid abuse is the use of androstenedione and androstenediol, prohormones or precursors to testosterone. Testosterone is the male hormone responsible for building muscle and revving up the sex drive. Legally considered a controlled substance in the same category as anabolic steroids, androstenedione is not without side effects, including acne, hair loss in genetically susceptible people, abnormal growth of breast tissue (gynecomastia), negative blood cholesterol profiles that can lead to the increased risk of heart disease, and potentially reduced testosterone output. Use of this family of compounds may also result in a positive drug test.

**TABLE 8.1　Health Dangers of Anabolic Steroids**

| | |
|---|---|
| Liver disease | Masculinization in women |
| High blood pressure | Muscle spasms |
| Increased LDL cholesterol | Headache |
| Decreased HDL cholesterol | Nervous tension |
| Fluid retention | Nausea |
| Suppressed immunity | Rash |
| Decreased testosterone | Irritability |
| Testicular atrophy | Mood swings |
| Acne | Heightened or suppressed sex drive |
| Gynecomastia | Aggressiveness |
| Lowered sperm count | Drug dependence |

In addition to using steroids and prohormones, athletes use other types of drugs, including stimulants, painkillers, diuretics, and drugs that mask the presence of certain drugs in the urine. Some athletes also use synthetic growth hormone (GH) because they believe it will increase strength and muscle mass. However, GH has many horrific side effects, including progressive overgrowth of body tissues, coronary heart disease, diabetes, and arthritis. GH is one of more than 100 drugs that have been banned by the International Olympic Committee (IOC). The full list of banned substances appears in table 8.2. Notice that not one of these substances is nutritional; they are drugs, not foods.

My advice is to forget health-destroying drugs. There are some natural aids you can use to enhance muscle building, give you an extra edge in training, and keep your body in healthy balance.

# Sport Supplements:
# Sorting Through the Confusion

On average, exercisers and athletes spend $3.2 billion on sport supplements—a sum that's growing every year. With so many supplements on the market, how do you know which will help you, which will hurt you, and which will just waste your money?

With many products, the real hazards and nutritional implications are not based on what the supplement does, but on what it doesn't do, and what other avenues of support it may impede. I call this the *laetrile effect*.

Laetrile, or amygdalin, is derived primarily from apricot pits and almonds. In the 1920s, a theory was formulated that laetrile could kill cancer cells. In the 1960s and 1970s, it became a popular cancer treatment promoted by nonmedical practitioners.

## TABLE 8.2 Drugs Banned by the IOC

**Stimulants**

Amineptine, amfepramone, amiphenazole, amphetamine, bambuterol, bromontan, carphedon, cathine, cocaine, cropropamide, crotethamide, ephedrine, ethamivan, etilamphetamine, etilefrine, fencamfamine, fenethylline, fenfluramine, formoterol, heptaminol, mefenorex, mephentermine, mesocarb, methamphetamine, methoxyphenamine, methylenedioxyamphetamine, methylephedrine, methylphenidate, nikethamide, norfenfluramine, parahydroxyamphetamine, pemoline, pentetrazol, phendimetrazine, phentermine, phenylephrine, phenylpropanolamine, pholedrine, pipradrol, prolintane, propylhexedrine, pseudoephedrine, reproterol, salbutamol, salmeterol, selegiline, strychnine, terbutaline

**Narcotics**

Buprenorphine, dextromoramide, diamorphine (heroin), hydrocodone, methadone, morphine, pentazocine, pethidine

**Anabolic agents**

Androstenediol, androstenedione, bambuterol, boldenone, clenbuterol, clostebol, danazol, dehydrochlormethyltestosterone, dehydroepiandrosterone (DHEA), dihydrotestosterone, drostanolone, fenoterol, fluoxymesterone, formebolone, formoterol, gestrinone, mesterolone, methandienone, methenolone, methandriol, methyltestosterone, mibolerone, nandrolone, 19-norandrostenediol, 19-norandrostenedione, norethandrolone, oxandrolone, oxymesterone, oxymetholone, reproterol, salbutamol, salmeterol, stanozolol, terbutaline, testosterone, trenbolone

**Diuretics**

Acetazolamide, bendroflumethiazide, bumetanide, canrenone, chlorthalidone, ethacrynic acid, furosemide, hydrochlorothiazide, indapamide, mannitol (by intravenous injection), mersalyl, spironolactone, triamterene

**Masking agents**

Bromontan, diuretics (see previous group), epitestosterone, probenecid

Peptide hormones, mimetics, and analogues

ACTH, erythropoietin (EPO), hCG,* nGH, insulin, IGF-1, LH,* clomiphene,* cyclofenil,* tamoxifen*

**Beta-blockers**

Acebutolol, alprenolol, atenolol, betaxolol, bisoprolol, bunolol, carteolol, celiprolol, esmolol, labetalol, levobunolol, metipranolol, metoprolol, nadolol, oxprenolol, pindolol, propranolol, sotalol, timolol

*Prohibited in males only.

Because it was not an approved medical treatment, patients seeking the cure had to travel to Mexico to acquire treatment. By 1982, medical science had proved that laetrile was not effective against cancer.

But in most cases, people who sought (and still seek) laetrile treatment did so by delaying standard medical treatment and at large financial expense, with no beneficial results but usually without harm from the treatment. However, by delaying or forgoing more proven treatment, these patients lost time, and their disease advanced. In some cases, the laetrile treatment was harmful and even deadly.

And so it is with many sport supplements. Looking for a shortcut, athletes and exercisers spend time and money on supplements that don't work while delaying the use of proven methods—good nutrition and intense training—to support their goals. Even worse, some supplements can be harmful and sometimes, though rarely, even deadly.

To help you sort through the confusion regarding sport supplements, I have developed a rating system for strength-training supplements and herbal supplements based on the concept of the laetrile effect:

**Meets marketing claims.** This supplement lives up to its marketing claims.

**Possibly meets marketing claims.** There is not yet enough research backing this supplement, although available data look promising.

**Does not meet marketing claims.** An abundance of negative data exists on this supplement.

**Potentially harmful.** This supplement does not meet marketing claims and is potentially harmful.

Now, here's a roundup of various sport supplements on the market, categorized according to this rating system. You can use table 8.4 at the end of the chapter to quickly refer to the ratings for all the supplements discussed in this chapter. Remember, this is not an exhaustive list of all supplements on the market. It is a focused list of supplements targeted for muscle building and developing strength and power.

# Meets Marketing Claims

The products in this category have numerous research studies that back up the marketing claims. In the right setting, these products work. When I say that the supplements meet their marketing claims, it doesn't mean that I recommend that you use them. It just tells you that what is claimed on the label is substantiated by research. You should choose to use or not use supplements based on your exercise goals, lifestyle, and attention to all the factors that support the enhancement of strength and power. Supplements will not help you if you don't have your diet, training, and rest dialed in.

## Caffeine

Caffeine, a drug found in coffee, tea, soda, and over-the-counter pharmaceutical preparations, can have a wide range of effects depending on your sensitivity to it. You might feel alert and wide awake, or you might get the jitters. Your heart might race, or you might race to the bathroom (caffeine in large amounts is a diuretic).

Caffeine lingers in the body, so even small amounts can accumulate over time. It has a half-life of four to six hours, meaning that it takes that long for the body to metabolize half the amount consumed. Because of its half-life, caffeine can become counterproductive. If you drink small amounts during the day, they add up, and you eventually reach a point at which your body has more caffeine than it can handle. By increasing anxiety or restlessness, caffeine reduces the body's ability to function. Other unwanted side effects are upset stomach, irritability, and diarrhea.

Caffeine also inhibits the absorption of thiamin (a vitamin important for carbohydrate metabolism) and several minerals, including calcium and iron. Women who consume caffeine regularly (4 or more cups [1 or more L] of coffee a day or 330 mg of caffeine) and have a low intake of calcium in their diet (fewer than 700 mg a day) may run a greater risk of developing osteoporosis, or brittle bone disease.

## How It Works

Most research on caffeine has focused on endurance sports. The main finding is that for many endurance athletes, caffeine may extend performance. There are three theories that offer possible explanations. The first was originally thought to be the most plausible theory and has to do with caffeine's ability to enhance fat use for energy. Caffeine stimulates the production of adrenaline, a hormone that accelerates the release of fatty acids into the bloodstream. At the beginning of exercise, the muscles start using these available fatty acids for energy while sparing some of your muscle glycogen. Some research has supported this theory.

The second theory goes like this: Caffeine may directly affect skeletal muscle by altering key enzymes or systems that regulate carbohydrate breakdown within the cells. However, the research on this theory has been conflicting and inconclusive.

The third theory may actually be at the root of why caffeine makes you perceive that you are doing less work than you really are during exercise. It states that caffeine, because of its direct effect on the central nervous system, might have the psychological effect of making athletes feel they are not working as hard, or it may somehow maximize the force of muscular contractions. We now know that caffeine can cross the blood–brain barrier and antagonize the effects of adenosine, the neurotransmitter that causes drowsiness by slowing down nerve cell activity. In the brain, caffeine looks like adenosine and can bind to adenosine receptors on brain cells. But caffeine doesn't have the same action as adenosine, so it doesn't slow down nerve cell activity. Instead, it stimulates brain chemicals to secrete epinephrine, the flight-or-fight hormone that makes you feel better while working out. Currently this is the prevailing theory most supported by the research.

## Caffeine Use in Power Sports

Does caffeine supplementation help with power sports? Yes, according to a mound of new research. A 2010 review report looked at 29 studies that tested caffeine's ability to enhance performance during power exercise, such as sprinting team sports and resistance training. Eleven of the 17 studies showed significant improvements in team sport exercise and power-based sports with caffeine ingestion, but the greatest improvements were shown in elite athletes who were not regular caffeine users.

Six of the 11 studies showed benefits of caffeine ingestion with resistance training.

The reason caffeine works in power sports probably has to do with its ability to trigger the release of epinephrine from the adrenal glands. This results in improved muscle contraction. When this happens, perceived exertion is reduced, letting you push more weight without making a conscious decision to work harder. Basically, it seems that caffeine can improve strength over time, which of course leads to greater muscle mass. Caffeine is a bona fide ergogenic aid: A large collection of studies shows that it can improve exercise performance by 22 percent. More good news: The amount of coffee it takes to enhance performance—about 16 ounces (480 ml), or 2 cups—does not have a dehydrating effect on the body.

## The Caffeine–Carbohydrate Duo

Some of the most breakthrough research on caffeine has to do with its interaction with carbohydrate. Basically, caffeine taken with carbohydrate boosts sport performance. Case in point: British scientists investigated the effects of the simultaneous consumption of carbohydrate and caffeine on athletic performance. Soccer players who drank a beverage with carbohydrate (6.4 percent) plus caffeine (160 mg) during a game simulation performed with higher intensity than they did when they drank with a carbohydrate drink alone or a placebo.

Another study, done with cyclists, found that, when taken with carbohydrate, caffeine increased fat use and decreased nonmuscle glycogen carbohydrate use over carbohydrate alone when participants were in negative energy balance; however, caffeine had no effect on the 20-kilometer cycling time trial performance. This study was published in the *Journal of Applied Physiology Nutrition and Metabolism* in 2008.

## Well-Trained Athletes Do Best

Studies also show that caffeine works best as a power booster if you're well conditioned. Proof of this comes from experiments with swimmers, whose sport is anaerobic as well as aerobic. Highly trained swimmers improved their swimming velocity significantly after consuming 250 milligrams of caffeine and then swimming at maximal speed. Untrained, occasional swimmers didn't fare as well. The same group of researchers had previously conducted experiments with untrained subjects who cycled against resistance after supplementing with caffeine. Again, caffeine didn't provide much of a performance boost in untrained people.

## The Final Word on Caffeine

The International Society of Sports Nutrition has taken the following position on caffeine and performance:

1. Caffeine is effective for enhancing sport performance in trained athletes when consumed in doses between approximately 3 to 6 milligrams per kilogram of body weight. Higher doses do not result in greater enhancements in performance.

2. Caffeine exerts a greater ergogenic effect when consumed in a dry state as compared to coffee.

3. Caffeine can enhance vigilance during bouts of extended exhaustive exercise.

4. Caffeine is ergogenic for sustained maximal endurance exercise, and has been shown to be highly effective for time trial performance.

5. Caffeine supplementation is beneficial for high-intensity exercise, including team sports such as soccer and rugby, both of which are categorized by intermittent activity within a period of prolonged duration.

6. Caffeine improves strength and power performance.

7. Caffeine can act as a diuretic, but athletes should not use it to trigger fluid losses.

One of the main reasons I like caffeine as a sport supplement is that it enhances certain aspects of mental performance, particularly vigilance, even if you're rested, and it has even more generalized effects if you're sleep deprived. By that, I mean that it improves cognitive (thinking) functions that are compromised by lack of sleep. Ultimately, this means that you can more easily push through those final reps, extra sets, or endurance laps or legs if you're feeling a little less fatigue.

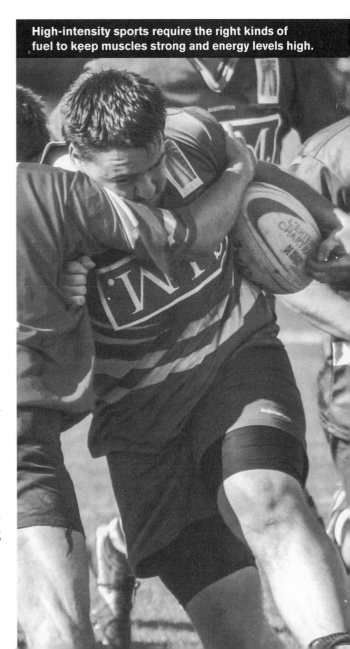

High-intensity sports require the right kinds of fuel to keep muscles strong and energy levels high.

Keep in mind, though, that caffeine may aggravate certain health problems, such as ulcers, heart disease, high blood pressure, and anemia, to name just a few. Stick to your doctor's advice. Above all, don't substitute caffeine for sound, commonsense nutritional practices for extending energy.

## Carbohydrate–Protein Sport Drinks

Unimaginable as it may seem, it is within your control to retool your body for more lean muscle and less fat—and do it naturally—all with a simple formulation. Here's how: Immediately after your workout, drink a liquid carbohydrate supplement that contains protein. This will jump-start the muscle-building process, plus boost your energy levels.

This simple formula is 12 ounces (360 ml) of carbohydrate and protein in liquid form taken immediately after your strength-training routine. This is the time your body is best able to use these nutrients for muscle firming and fat burning. The supplement I use with my clients is my Kleiner's Muscle-Building formulas, featured in chapter 17. For a long time, I've used these formulas with many of my bodybuilding clients, and soon after they begin drinking the formulas, we observed a major shift in their body composition from less fat to more muscle.

## How It Works

How does this formula help muscles get stronger and firmer? Exercise, of course, is the initial stimulus. You challenge your muscles by working out, and they respond with growth. But for muscle building to take place, muscles need protein and carbohydrate in combination to create the right hormonal climate for muscle growth.

What happens is this: Protein and carbohydrate trigger the release of insulin and GH in your body. Insulin is a powerful factor in building muscle. It helps ferry glucose and amino acids into cells, reassembles those amino acids into body tissue, and prevents muscle wasting and tissue loss. GH increases the rate of protein production by the body, spurring muscle-building activity, and it also promotes fat burning. Both hormones are directly involved in muscle growth. Your body is primed for growth thanks to this simple muscle-gain formula.

## Scientific Proof

Research into the effect of carbohydrate–protein supplements on athletes and exercisers supports what I've observed for years. Here are some examples:

- In one scientific study, 14 normal-weight men and women ate test meals containing various amounts of protein: none (a protein-free meal), 15.8 grams, 21.5 grams, 33.6 grams, and 49.9 grams. All subjects combined their protein intake with 58 grams of carbohydrate. Blood samples were taken at intervals after the meal. The protein-containing meals produced the greatest rise in insulin compared with the protein-free meal. This study points out that protein has an insulin-boosting effect.

- In another study, nine experienced male strength trainers were given water (which served as the control), a carbohydrate supplement, a protein supplement, or a carbohydrate–protein supplement. They took their designated supplement immediately after working out and again two hours later. Right after exercise and throughout the next eight hours, the researchers drew blood samples to determine the levels of various hormones in the blood, including insulin, testosterone, and GH.

    The most significant finding was that the carbohydrate–protein supplement triggered the greatest elevations in insulin and GH. The protein works hand in hand with postexercise carbohydrate to create a hormonal climate that's highly conducive to muscle growth.

- If you've started strength training later in life, consuming protein after your workout is very important. Researchers in Denmark instructed a group of men (aged 74 and older) to have a protein drink consisting of 10 grams of protein, 7 grams of carbohydrate, and 3 grams of fat either immediately after or two hours after each training session. The study lasted 12 weeks. By the end of the study, the best gains in muscular growth occurred when the subjects consumed liquid protein immediately after their workouts. The point here seems to be that the sooner you replenish with protein, the better results you can obtain.

## *More Energy*

If you supplement with a carbohydrate–protein beverage after your workout, you'll notice something else: higher energy levels. Not only does this nutrient combination stimulate hormone activity, but it also starts replenishing muscle glycogen, which means more muscle energy. The harder you work out, the greater your muscular gains will be.

When protein is added to the supplement mix, your body's glycogen-making process accelerates faster than if you just consumed carbohydrate alone. Some intriguing research proves this point. In one study, nine men cycled for two full hours during three different sessions to deplete their muscle glycogen stores. Immediately after each exercise bout and again two hours later, the men drank a straight carbohydrate supplement, a straight protein supplement, or a carbohydrate–protein supplement. By looking at actual biopsy specimens of the muscles, the researchers observed that the rate of muscle glycogen storage was significantly faster in men who consumed the carbohydrate–protein mixture.

Why such speed? It's well known that eating carbohydrate after prolonged endurance exercise helps restore muscle glycogen. When protein is consumed along with carbohydrate, there's a surge in insulin. Biochemically, insulin is like an acceleration pedal. It races the body's glycogen-making motor in two ways. First, it speeds up the movement of glucose and amino acids into cells, and second, it activates a special enzyme crucial to glycogen synthesis.

In another study, a group of athletes performed enough exercise to deplete their glycogen reserves. Afterward, part of the group consumed a carbohydrate–protein supplement; the other consumed a 6 percent glucose–electrolyte solution. Both groups exercised again. Endurance-wise, the carbohydrate–protein group outlasted the other group by 66 percent.

In a similar study, eight endurance-trained cyclists performed two 2-hour exercise bouts designed to deplete their glycogen stores. After exercise and again two hours later, they consumed either a carbohydrate–protein supplement or a carbohydrate-only formula. The carbohydrate–protein formula contained 53 grams of carbohydrate and 14 grams of protein, whereas the carbohydrate formula contained 20 grams of carbohydrate. The effects of the carbohydrate–protein supplement were quite remarkable: Glucose levels rose by 17 percent, and insulin levels increased by 92 percent. Furthermore, there was 128 percent greater storage of muscle glycogen when athletes took the carbohydrate–protein supplement compared with when they took the carbohydrate-only formula.

Scientific research indicates that for hard trainers, the optimal combination of protein and carbohydrate after exercise is one part protein to three parts carbohydrate, or approximately 50 to 60 grams of carbohydrate and 20 grams of protein. A question often arises as to whether you should eat your postexercise meal or drink it in the form of a carbohydrate–protein supplement. Let's turn to some scientific data for the answer. Researchers at Ithaca College in Ithaca, New York, tested whether a whole-foods meal, a supplemental drink of protein and carbohydrate, a carbohydrate-only beverage, or a placebo would have any effect on insulin, testosterone, or cortisol levels following resistance training. The study revealed that the supplemental drink of protein and carbohydrate had the most effect, but mostly in terms of increasing insulin levels. As noted before, insulin is essential for driving the manufacture of glycogen, so it looks as though your best meal after a workout is one that is in liquid form. That's why my clients love my smoothies! You can find a variety of smoothie recipes in chapter 17.

## Creatine

Creatine is one of the most important natural fuel-enhancing supplements discovered thus far for strength trainers. Unlike a lot of supplements, creatine has been extensively researched, with more than 500 studies conducted to date. Of these studies, 300 have focused on the performance-enhancing value of creatine, and about 70 percent of these studies report positive effects. These exciting experiments show that creatine produces significant performance improvements in sports that require high levels of strength and power, including strength training, rowing, and cycling sprints. Another big plus for creatine: Many studies have shown gains in body mass averaging 2 to 5 pounds (0.9 to 2.3 kg) during 4 to 12 weeks of training. Also, creatine improves overall performance, which means that you can train harder while supplementing with creatine. That translates into greater muscle gains. Thus, supplementing with creatine seems to be a safe and effective method to increase muscle mass.

Creatine received a major thumbs-up in a 2010 review article published in the *Journal of the International Society of Sports Nutrition*. The authors stated that creatine is the most effective nutritional supplement available to athletes to increase high-intensity exercise capacity and muscle mass during training.

Sound good? You bet. Who wouldn't prefer a bona fide natural supplement such as creatine over synthetic, dangerous compounds such as steroids? Creatine is the ticket to greater strength and improved muscularity.

### How It Works

Creatine is produced in the liver and kidneys at a rate of about 2 grams a day from arginine, glycine, and methionine, three nonessential amino acids. About 95 percent of the body's creatine travels by the blood to be stored in the muscles, heart, and other body cells. Inside muscle cells, it's turned into creatine phosphate (CP), a compound that serves as a tiny energy supply, enough for several seconds of action. CP thus works best over the short haul in activities such as strength training that require short, fast bursts of activity. CP also replenishes your cellular reserves of ATP, the molecular fuel that provides the power for muscular contractions. With more ATP around, your muscles can do more work.

There are now three major forms of creatine on the market (monohydrate, citrate, and pyruvate), and I'm sure you're wondering which form works the best. This issue has been widely studied. The bottom line of all the recent research is that all three are effective; however, creatine monohydrate works better at muscle building and performance than the other two forms do.

As a strength trainer, you load creatine into your muscles just as endurance athletes do with carbohydrate. Consequently, you can push harder and longer in your workouts because creatine boosts the pace of energy production in your muscle cells. Creatine supplementation doesn't build muscle directly. But it does have an indirect effect: You can work out more intensely, and this translates into muscle gains. Once in the muscles, creatine appears to induce swelling, which in turn may influence carbohydrate and protein metabolism.

## *The Latest Word on Creatine*

More than 500 articles have been written on the influence of creatine supplementation on strength, power, and athletic performance. A new area of creatine research, how creatine may influence medical conditions involving the nervous system, has greatly increased the number of publications addressing the possible benefits of creatine supplements. Here's the rundown of what the most current scientific literature says regarding creatine supplementation:

- By supplementing with creatine, lacto-ovo vegetarians (who typically have lower stores of creatine in their bodies) can increase their muscular stores of creatine to levels similar to those of people who eat meat and experience better synthesis of ATP.

- Supplementing with creatine has been shown to increase bone mineral content and bone density in older men who engage in strength training. This benefit may be related to enhanced muscle mass and strength due to taking the creatine. Men tend to lose both muscle mass and bone mass as they age, so this finding is quite promising in terms of quality of life as men age.

- Amateur swimmers who supplemented with creatine (5 mg) twice a day for seven days were able to sprint faster in the last 50 meters of a 400-meter swimming competition. This finding hints that creatine might give you a final surge of energy in the last leg of a race.

- During sleep deprivation, creatine levels decrease in the brain. Creatine supplementation, however, had a positive effect on sleep and mood in an experiment involving subjects who took 5 grams of creatine four times a day for seven days immediately before the experiment.

- More and more, creatine is being tested in medical settings to see whether it can enhance muscle recovery. Sometimes, the findings are promising; other times, they are not. In one study, researchers looked into the effect of strength training and creatine supplementation on patients with myasthenia gravis, a chronic autoimmune neuromuscular disease characterized by varying degrees of weakness of the skeletal (voluntary) muscles. They found that both interventions promoted gains in strength and in muscle mass. In another study, creatine supplementation was not found to help muscle strength when given before knee arthroplasty, nor did it help with recovery afterward.

## How Much?

Creatine supplements swell the ranks of creatine in your muscles, giving the working muscles another fuel source in addition to glycogen from carbohydrate. The question is, how much creatine do you need? You do get creatine from food—roughly 1 gram a day. But that's not enough to enhance strength-training performance.

Creatine usually comes in a powdered form. The latest scientific research shows that the most rapid method of increasing muscle creatine stores is to consume approximately 0.3 gram per kilogram of body weight per day of creatine for at least three days, followed by 3 to 5 grams of creatine per day thereafter to maintain elevated stores. Ingesting smaller amounts of creatine, 2 to 3 grams per day, will increase muscle creatine stores over a three- to four-week period.

Because creatine levels will be maintained in your muscles for about three weeks, another strategy is to cycle on and off creatine rather than using the loading maintenance phases. Start with a dose of 5 grams per day for about six weeks. It will take a little longer to reach saturation levels compared to the loading dose, but the results are virtually the same. Cycle off the creatine for about three weeks, and then go back on it again. Your muscle levels and training results will remain high during the off period. This strategy will lighten the strain on your wallet, while still giving you competitive results.

The question of when to supplement with creatine has been answered somewhat in research. A Canadian study conducted over a six-week period found that supplementing with creatine after working out can increase muscle size. This particular study focused on arm muscle, and the effect was more pronounced in men than in women. On the other hand, taking creatine before intense aerobic exercise improved energy production during exercise. More testing in terms of creatine timing is needed, but this study suggests some intriguing possibilities for when to take creatine.

Creatine is nontoxic, and studies have been unable to find any negative side effects to its use when dosage recommendations are followed. It does not interfere with normal body fluid shifts that occur when exercising or competing in the heat—good news to endurance athletes who often train or compete in hot weather. But if you take too much at once, you can experience an upset stomach. The only known side effect associated with creatine intakes of 1 to 10 grams per day is water weight gain. In addition, one report suggests that some people may experience muscle cramping and possibly muscle tearing when supplementing with creatine. However, these claims are unsubstantiated.

While loading with creatine, make sure to drink extra water. This may control cramping. And you're asking for trouble if you belt down daily dosages of 40 grams or more. Such high doses may cause liver and kidney damage, according to some reports. Thus, creatine is ill advised if you have preexisting kidney disease (e.g., renal dialysis or previous kidney transplant). In healthy people, however, creatine does not seem to adversely affect kidney function.

My stand has always been that you must have your nutrition, your training, and your rest dialed in before you add creatine to your program. Of course, always check with your physician before supplementing with creatine.

### Supercharge With Creatine and Carbohydrate

Here's an important fact about creatine supplementation: Creatine works best in combination with carbohydrate. This combination boosts the amount of creatine accumulated in muscles by as much as 60 percent!

That's the key finding of a recent study. Investigators divided 24 men (average age was 24) into experimental and control groups. The control group took 5 grams of creatine in sugar-free orange juice four times a day for five days. The experimental group took the same dose of creatine followed 30 minutes later by 17 ounces (510 ml) of a solution containing carbohydrate. Muscle biopsies after the five-day test period showed that both groups had elevated creatine levels, but with one dramatic difference—creatine levels in the experimental group were 60 percent higher than those in the control group. There were also higher concentrations of insulin in the muscles of the experimental group.

## Fractionated Starch: The New Wonder Carbohydrate

A new category of carbohydrate supplement is a patented amylopectin (starch) fraction that is the key ingredient in a new sport supplement product. It is made from a naturally occurring starch, but the very fast molecular fraction is selected out to create the unique product, and it has the research cred to support the claims. Unlike other types of carbohydrate added to drinks and powders, such as glucose, dextrose, and maltodextrin, this product's chief claim to fame is that it rapidly restocks muscle glycogen—about 70 percent faster than other forms of supplemental carbohydrate do. That means a faster uptake of carbohydrate after a workout, when your muscles are depleted of glycogen, and research has shown enhanced exercise performance. Currently only one brand, Vitargo, contains the fractionated starch ingredient because it is a unique, patented formula. Vitargo has these other research-proven benefits:

- Improves the uptake of creatine by muscles
- Helps enhance muscle growth after training by increasing insulin levels
- Makes a great postworkout choice for replenishing glycogen (muscle energy)
- Is sugar free
- Passes through the stomach 80 percent faster than other simple sugars and thus does not cause stomach upset or bloating

This product has been a game changer because it can target starch intake around exercise when it really works for you without inducing a feeling of fullness, and then pack the rest of your diet with nutrient-rich nonstarchy vegetables and fruits—an awesome lean and mean combination.

The implications of this study for strength trainers, athletes, and exercisers are enormous. Just think: By supplementing with creatine and carbohydrate at the same time, you're supercharging your body. With more creatine in your muscles, you have more power to strength train. The fact that the creatine–carbohydrate combination increases insulin is equally important. Insulin increases the uptake of glucose, which is ultimately stored as glycogen in the liver and muscles for fuel. The more glycogen you can stockpile, the more energy you'll have for exercise, including aerobics. The creatine–carbohydrate combination is a true energy booster for all types of exercise activity. Other studies have shown a similar benefit to combining creatine with protein and carbohydrate.

## Glucose–Electrolyte Solutions

Glucose–electrolyte solutions are beneficial for athletes competing in high-intensity sports lasting less than one hour or events that last an hour or longer. These solutions do two things: replace water and electrolytes lost through sweat, and supply a small amount of carbohydrate to the working muscles, decreasing the use of muscle and liver glycogen stores. During competition, athletes can thus run, bike, or swim longer because the supplemental carbohydrate has spared stored glycogen. Most drinks are about 6 to 8 percent carbohydrate. The carbohydrate may be glucose, a simple sugar; fructose, a fruit sugar; sucrose, ordinary table sugar (a blend of glucose and fructose); maltodextrin, a complex carbohydrate derived from corn; or a combination of these.

There's no evidence that electrolytes improve exercise performance for general workouts. For events lasting less than three hours, they're not required unless you have a mineral deficiency diagnosed by your physician or your daily sweat losses total more than 3 percent of your body weight, or 4.5 pounds (2 kg) in a 150-pound (68 kg) athlete. Endurance and ultraendurance athletes exercising more than three hours are among those who do need to replace electrolytes. Unless you count yourself in this elite class of athlete, if you are eating a diet rich in whole foods, you are getting enough of these minerals.

In addition to their ability to replenish fluids, electrolytes, and carbohydrate, glucose–electrolyte solutions may strengthen your immune system. This amazing news comes from Appalachian State University, where researchers put two groups of marathoners on some high-intensity treadmill exercise for two and a half hours. One group drank 25 ounces (750 ml) of a glucose–electrolyte solution (Gatorade) 30 minutes before exercise, 8 ounces (240 ml) every 15 minutes during exercise, and a final 25 ounces (750 ml) over a six-hour recovery period. The other group replenished fluids on the same schedule but with a noncarbohydrate placebo solution.

The researchers took blood samples from the marathoners and found that the glucose–electrolyte solution drinkers had lower levels of cortisol in their blood than the other exercisers did. Cortisol is a hormone that suppresses immune response. So apparently when the body is well fed, stress is reduced and cortisol levels remain at normal levels, helping to maintain more optimal immune function. Because this is just one study, obviously it offers no final and complete answers on the glucose–immunity connection. This research is intriguing, nonetheless.

In addition, other research has found that consuming a sport drink during aerobic exercise can enhance feelings of pleasure, meaning that you may not notice feelings of discomfort while working out. For people who don't like to exercise, sipping a sport drink may spark motivation simply because it makes them feel better.

Glucose–electrolyte solutions are designed primarily for endurance athletes. But they also have application for strength trainers in two important ways. First, if you train aerobically—particularly in the heat—these supplements prevent electrolyte and fluid depletion. Second, if you're training intensely for 45 minutes or more, extra fluid and fuel mean more energy.

A study conducted by Dr. Greg Haff at Appalachian State University examined the muscle glycogen levels and performance effect of supplementing with a glucose beverage or placebo just before and during resistance exercise. There was significantly less muscle glycogen degradation in the supplemented group versus the placebo group (15 percent versus 19 percent) after resistance exercise. Although this group of researchers has previously reported improvements in successive bouts of resistance exercise when subjects were supplemented with a glucose beverage, in this study no improvements in the single bout of resistance exercise were observed.

There has also been speculation on whether these drinks have any influence on oxidative damage in the aftermath of exercise. In strength trainers who were given a sport drink or a placebo, researchers could find no difference in oxidative stress. Sport drinks apparently don't help heal muscle damage following exercise. Adding protein to a sport drink in the form of amino acids has been shown to help with muscle recovery and muscle protein synthesis, however, particularly in novice strength trainers who drank a sport drink spiked with 6 additional grams of amino acids. The mixture significantly elevated insulin concentrations for an anabolic effect and decreased levels of the stress hormone cortisol, decreasing the stress effects of exercise on the body. Adding protein to these drinks has been shown to reduce the mental fatigue involved in exercise as well.

## What About Carbohydrate Gels?

Carbohydrate gels are highly concentrated sources of carbohydrate with a puddinglike consistency and are usually packaged in single-serve pouches. Designed for athletes and exercisers participating in endurance activity, these products are usually a mixture of simple carbohydrate with flavoring, and some are formulated with protein as well. These gels are quickly absorbed into the bloodstream and thus are a good source of immediate food energy, particularly during extended exercise. Research has found that carbohydrate gels that contain protein extend performance longer than plain carbohydrate gels and may be a better choice. When using these gels, make sure to take in sufficient water to process the carbohydrate and protein and to prevent dehydration.

The best time to swill one of these drinks is during an aerobic workout or during any period of exertion, especially if you're exercising or working in hot weather. Fluid loss is greater in the summer than at any other time of the year. You can lose more electrolytes, too, although the concentration of these minerals in sweat gets weaker the fitter you are. You also burn more glycogen working out in the heat—another good reason to quench your thirst with a glucose–electrolyte solution.

## Weight-Gain Powders

You've seen them: huge cans brightly labeled with alluring product descriptions such as "weight gainer," "solid mass," "lean mass enhancer," or "muscle provider." These products belong to a group of supplements known as weight-gain powders. Most contain various combinations of carbohydrate, protein, amino acids, vitamins, minerals, and other ingredients thought to enhance performance. The manufacturers of these products claim that their specific formulations will help you pack on muscle.

But do they? Actually, no one knows for sure whether there's really anything special about the formulas beyond what we already know: that when you train hard and give your body more energy in the right forms of protein and carbohydrate, your body increases mass. Because companies are not required to conduct research on their own products, studies on specific products are very rare. However, in 1996 a group of researchers at the University of Memphis put two weight-gain powders that are still on the market to the test. One was Gainers Fuel 1000, a high-calorie supplement that adds about 1,400 calories a day to the diet (290 g of carbohydrate, 60 g of protein, and 1 g of fat). Although the supplement contains many other ingredients, it's formulated with two minerals that have been hyped as muscle builders: chromium picolinate and boron.

Chromium picolinate is linked to muscle growth because it increases the action of insulin. But that's where the association ends. There's no valid scientific evidence that chromium directly promotes muscle building.

Boron has been touted as a supplement that promotes muscle growth by increasing the amount of testosterone circulating in the blood. But experiments have failed to verify this claim. In one recent study, 10 male bodybuilders took 2.5 milligrams of boron daily while 9 male bodybuilders took a placebo. Both groups performed their regular bodybuilding routines for seven weeks. Lean mass, strength, and testosterone levels increased in all 19 men to the same relative degree. Boron supplementation didn't make a bit of difference. It was the training, pure and simple, that did the trick.

Back to the 1996 study on weight-gain powder: The second supplement investigated was Phosphagain. It adds about 570 calories a day to the diet (64 g of carbohydrate, 67 g of protein, and 5 g of fat). As with most weight-gain powders, Phosphagain contains lots of other ingredients that are rumored to build muscle. Among the most notable are creatine (see the previous section), taurine, nucleotides, and l-glutamine. An amino acid found in muscles, taurine has been found in animal studies to enhance the effectiveness of insulin. Nucleotides are the building blocks of RNA and DNA; in Phosphagain, they are derived from the RNA in yeast. Nucleotides are fundamental to metabolism and integral to the cell division and replication involved in growth and development. As for l-glutamine, an amino acid, it theoretically regulates the water volume in cells and the protein-making process in muscles.

To check the effects of Gainers Fuel 1000 and Phosphagain on muscle growth, the University of Memphis researchers selected 28 strength-trained men around the age of 26. None was currently taking anabolic steroids, and none had a history of steroid use. The subjects had been training for an average of six years.

The researchers assigned them to one of three groups: a third of the men took a maltodextrin supplement three times a day (maltodextrin is a carbohydrate derived from corn); a third took two servings a day of Gainers Fuel 1000 according to the manufacturer's directions; and the remaining third took three servings a day of Phosphagain according to the manufacturer's directions. None knew which supplement they were taking. They all continued their normal workouts and diets during the course of the study. In addition, they were told not to take any other supplements two weeks before the study and during the study.

Here's a summary of what the researchers discovered:

- Both the maltodextrin supplement and Gainers Fuel 1000 promoted modest gains in muscle mass in combination with a strength-training program.

- In the group that supplemented with Gainers Fuel 1000, fat weight and percent body fat increased significantly.

- Phosphagain supplementation was more effective in promoting muscle gains than either maltodextrin or Gainers Fuel 1000 during strength training. In fact, muscle gains were significantly greater with Phosphagain, according to lead researcher Dr. Richard Kreider. The men who supplemented with Phosphagain did not gain any additional fat.

Before you draw your own conclusions, let me emphasize: It's still up in the air as to exactly which ingredients in Phosphagain were responsible for these results. More tests are needed on weight-gain powders in general as well as on the individual ingredients they contain to confirm these findings. But, carbohydrate with some protein (weight-gain powders contain both) taken at the proper times is an important supplement to a muscle-building diet. Importantly, the creatine in Phosphagain was highly likely to have been a factor in the results.

Weight-gain powders are helpful for increasing calories when you can't increase your calories from food alone. But keep in mind that these products are often quite high in calories (500 to 1,000 calories). Sure, those calories can help you gain weight, but that weight might wind up as fat. It is far easier to control your body composition by controlling your protein, carbohydrate, and fat ratios yourself.

# Possibly Meets Marketing Claims

The products in this category look promising based on early research, but there are not yet enough data for a definitive answer. In the end, they may or may not work. I suggest that you keep your eye on the magazines and research publications, because these are the supplements that will be in the news.

## Arginine

Arginine is an amino acid taken by athletes for a number of reasons. Supposedly, arginine activates the secretion of GH, which drives muscle growth, but no studies have demonstrated this benefit. Arginine is involved in the synthesis of creatine. However, that is not a good reason to supplement with arginine; just take creatine.

Arginine is also the chief ingredient in most nitric oxide (NO) products. NO works as a hemodilator that relaxes smooth muscle in the arteries. This helps reduce blood pressure and increase blood flow to the muscles, possibly delivering more nutrients and oxygen for enhanced muscle growth. So far, though, there is little evidence to support a muscle-building effect of arginine. Additional research is needed to better evaluate the role of arginine for strength trainers. Theoretically, it looks promising, but the data are clearly not there to support claims. Keep your eye on the research, but hold off on any product use.

Be careful with arginine supplementation—too much may damage the pancreas. At least one case study in the scientific literature indicates that arginine supplementation has been associated with pancreatitis, or inflammation of the pancreas.

## Beta-Alanine

Billed as the new performance-enhancing nutritional supplement that rocks, beta-alanine is a naturally occurring nonessential amino acid found in the muscle portion of animal protein, such as in beef, chicken, pork, fish, lamb, and others. It is a component of carnosine, a proteinlike compound that seems to be concentrated in actively contracting muscles. Beta-alanine appears to be a buffering agent, meaning that it prevents certain enzymatic reactions that increase lactic acid in working muscles and therefore dampens the "burn" in your muscles when you work out.

Scientists became interested in beta-alanine when they discovered a naturally occurring, unusually high level of carnosine in the muscles of a significant number of championship strength and power athletes. By controlling the natural rise in lactic acid that results from high-intensity exercise, these athletes could likely perform extra reps or perform a greater number of multiple sprints before muscle burn forced them to quit. To help those who are not naturally able to produce high levels of muscle carnosine, initial studies tried supplementing the diet with carnosine. It was found that carnosine is metabolized during digestion and does not raise muscle carnosine levels. So the researchers turned to supplementing with beta-alanine, an essential ingredient to carnosine production, and saw that it could raise muscle carnosine levels. The next step was to show that the more beta-alanine you have in your muscles, the better you can perform.

The research with beta-alanine has been methodical and primarily positive, although all studies are not in agreement. Supplementation with beta-alanine has been shown to increase muscle carnosine content and therefore total muscle buffer capacity, with the potential to elicit improvements in physical performance during high-intensity exercise. Studies of beta-alanine supplementation and exercise performance have demonstrated improvements in performance during multiple bouts of high-intensity exercise and in single bouts of exercise lasting more than 60 seconds. Similarly, beta-alanine supplementation has been shown to delay the onset of neuromuscular fatigue. Although beta-alanine does not improve maximal strength or aerobic capacity, some aspects of endurance performance, such as anaerobic threshold and time to exhaustion, can be enhanced.

Although most of the studies have used male subjects, two investigations from the University of Oklahoma studied women and resulted in different outcomes. In 2006, Dr. Jeff Stout and colleagues examined the effects of 28 days of beta-alanine supplementation on several parameters associated with intense exercise performance in 22 women. The subjects were supplemented with either beta-alanine or a placebo and performed an incremental exercise test on a cycle ergometer to exhaustion. The beta-alanine group significantly outperformed the placebo group in anaerobic, but not aerobic, metabolic and performance measurements.

In 2010, University of Oklahoma researchers again investigated the effect of beta-alanine supplementation, this time on 44 women performing high-intensity interval training (HIIT) for six weeks. The subjects were split into three test groups: beta-alanine, placebo, or control (no supplement at all). The training consisted of riding a cycle ergometer three times per week with five 2-minute work intervals separated by 1 minute of passive recovery at varying intensities of workload ranging from 90 to 110 percent of their maximum workload (recorded during an initial measure of peak aerobic capacity). All groups improved their cardiorespiratory fitness, but there was no difference in the measurements among the three groups. The scientists concluded that HIIT was "an effective and time-efficient method" to improve maximal oxygen uptake. No benefit from beta-alanine was shown.

So what's the bottom line? I can tell you that in my practice I have clients who wouldn't train without beta-alanine, and those who haven't seen any difference in their training or race results. Most likely, clients in this second set are not different from the original elite athlete subjects studied for their naturally high levels of muscle carnosine. Perhaps they have reached the stratosphere of athletic performance partly as a result of a natural ability to produce more muscle carnosine, so supplementation does not lead to any noticeable or statistically measurable effect. For those less capable of producing carnosine, supplementation may work seemingly like magic to decrease muscle burn and fatigue, thereby enhancing high-intensity training and conditioning, and performance.

My take on beta-alanine is that if you participate in high-intensity training, competition, or both, it's worth a try. Use it in the following way: The loading phase for beta-alanine appears to be 28 days (four weeks), although a recent five-week study showed no outcome difference between beta-alanine supplement and placebo groups. Dosages in research studies range from 3.2 to 6.4 grams per day, separated into four or more doses per day. Single dosage amounts greater than 800 milligrams can lead to a transient tingling and parasthesia in the extremities, which can be eliminated by using timed-release formulas and smaller doses. Beta-alanine is available in a number of supplement formulas, even mixed with creatine. Already, one study has shown that beta-alanine combined with creatine delayed the onset of muscular fatigue better than beta alanine or creatine alone.

## Beta-Hydroxy-Beta-Methylbutyrate

Found in grapefruit, catfish, and other foods, beta-hydroxy-beta-methylbutyrate (HMB) is a breakdown product of leucine, a branched-chain amino acid. The body produces it naturally from proteins containing leucine.

Studies show that HMB may be anticatabolic; that is, it inhibits the degradation of muscle and protein in the body, so you can possibly train harder on successive days. Preliminary research on HMB indicates that 1.5 to 3 grams a day can assist with increasing muscle mass, decreasing body fat, and boosting strength levels if you are just beginning a strength-training program. But there are few benefits for well-trained athletes, according to research.

## Branched-Chain Amino Acids (BCAAs)

The BCAAs are leucine, isoleucine, and valine. During endurance exercise, levels of these amino acids fall, which may contribute to fatigue during competition. Emerging but limited research suggests that supplementation with BCAAs may enhance performance, particularly if you compete in endurance events. One study found that marathoners who consumed a sport drink containing BCAAs increased their performance by as much as 4 percent. Not all studies have shown a positive effect, however.

Here are some guidelines based on what is currently known about BCAA supplementation: Dosages of 4 to 21 grams daily during training and 2 to 4 grams per hour with a 6 to 8 percent glucose–electrolyte solution before and during prolonged exercise have been shown to improve physiological and psychological responses to training. In other words, athletes felt better mentally and physically during exercise. Theoretically, BCAA supplementation during hard training may help reduce fatigue, too, as well as prevent protein degradation in your muscles. You can buy BCAAs in a bottle, but you can also find them in dairy products and in whey protein powder. Refer to chapter 2 for more information on BCAAs in food.

Future research opportunities point to BCAA supplementation for reduction of muscle soreness from resistance exercise. Keep your eyes open for publication of these studies.

## Carnitine

Found in red meat and other animal products, carnitine is a proteinlike substance once thought to be an important vitamin. Now scientists know carnitine is not an essential nutrient because the liver and kidneys can synthesize it without any help from food. Most people consume between 50 and 300 milligrams of this nutrient each day from food. Even if you don't eat that much carnitine, your body can produce its own from the amino acids lysine and methionine. About 98 percent of the body's carnitine is stored in the muscles.

The main job of carnitine in the body is to transport fatty acids into cells to be burned as energy. Because of this role, many theories have been floated regarding carnitine's potential benefits to exercisers. One theory is that carnitine boosts exercise performance by making more fat available to working muscles, thus sparing glycogen. Another theory is that, because of its role in cellular energy processes, carnitine reduces the buildup of waste products such as lactic acid in the muscles, thereby extending performance. Theories aside, what does scientific research show?

Numerous studies have evaluated the benefits of carnitine supplementation in both patient and athlete populations. With varying results, some studies indicate that carnitine (0.5 to 2 g a day) may increase fat oxidation and improve cardiovascular efficiency during exercise. New research suggests that supplemental carnitine can help you burn more of the fat found in muscle. It has also been shown to enhance carbohydrate metabolism. The ability to use more fat and stored carbohydrate from the muscle would certainly give you a tremendous competitive advantage for endurance activity.

New research is showing that carnitine is more effective as a sport supplement than previously believed. Researchers from the United Kingdom discovered that carnitine requires insulin for entry into muscle cells. (For carnitine to work, it has to get into muscles.) Sport nutritionists used to think that carnitine should be taken on an empty stomach, but now we know differently. Because carnitine needs insulin, it's best to take it with meals—particularly high-carbohydrate meals that digest quickly, because these meals elevate insulin in the body.

Research also shows that carnitine taken in partnership with choline reduces lipid peroxidation and conserves vitamin E and vitamin A in the body. Similarly, carnitine alone has been found to enhance the antioxidant capacity in rats during prolonged exercise, so it may have a protective effect on the immune system.

Based on what I've read in the research and observed in my own practice, I suggest that you take carnitine in the following manner: Take 2 grams of l-carnitine tartrate with 80 grams of carbohydrate while training and competing. Eighty grams of carbohydrate is the equivalent of the following:

- 10 grams more than 1 serving (2 scoops) of Vitargo S2 (the research showing the effectiveness of combining carnitine with carbohydrate used Vitargo S2 as the carbohydrate source)

- 48 ounces (1.44 L) of a 6 percent carbohydrate solution sport drink (e.g., Gatorade)

A word of caution: Some supplement preparations contain a mixture of L-carnitine and D-carnitine. The L-carnitine form appears to be safe; D-carnitine, on the other hand, can cause muscular weakness and excretion of myoglobin, the oxygen-transporting protein in the blood. If you supplement with carnitine, use products that contain L-carnitine only.

## Coenzyme Q10 (Ubiquinone)

Found in the mitochondria (energy factories) of cells, coenzyme Q10 (CoQ10), or ubiquinone, plays a central role in a series of chemical reactions that transport oxygen and produce energy. It also works as an antioxidant and thus may help destroy free radicals, particularly during aerobic exercise.

In addition, supplemental CoQ10 has been used successfully in patients with heart disease. As for its benefits for athletes and exercisers, the verdict is still out, although I've placed it in the "possibly useful" category because of its effectiveness in treating heart disease. For more information on CoQ10, refer to chapter 7.

A few studies have shown that CoQ10 may enhance aerobic performance in people who don't exercise. But in one study, trained triathletes took 100 milligrams of CoQ10, 500 milligrams of vitamin C, 100 milligrams of inosine, and 200 IU of vitamin E for four weeks, and no change in their endurance capacity was found.

It is important to add that CoQ10 in high doses may be harmful. In one study, supplementation with 120 milligrams daily for 20 days resulted in muscle tissue damage, possibly because of increased oxidation.

## Conjugated Linoleic Acid (CLA)

CLA is a family of fatty acids found in beef, dairy foods, and dietary supplements. Commercial preparations of CLA for supplements are made from safflower or sunflower oil. A mixture of CLA-like chemical structures, called isomers, is found naturally in foods as well as within the commercial CLA preparations. Two of these isomers, the cis-9, trans-11 isomer and the trans-10, cis-12 isomer, are the most biologically available. The t-10, c-12 CLA isomer appears to have the greatest antiobesity effect.

There has been a groundswell of research on this supplement. For example, in observing the action of CLA on isolated fat cells, researchers found that it encourages the breakdown of fat and stifles lipoprotein lipase, a fat-storage enzyme. In addition, CLA ferries dietary fat into cells where it is burned for energy or used to build muscle. Moreover, CLA investigators say that the supplement does not shrink fat cells (as dieting does), but rather, it keeps them from enlarging. Enlarged fat cells are the main reason we get pudgy.

Ever since CLA was shown to reduce body fat in animals, researchers have attempted to verify whether it does the same in humans. In one study, published in the *Journal of Nutrition*, CLA clearly reduced weight in a group of 60 overweight volunteers. They took either a placebo or CLA for 12 weeks; the CLA dosage ranged from 1.7 to 6.8 grams daily. By the end of the experimental period, those who supplemented with 3.4 grams of CLA daily had dissolved their body fat by 6 pounds (2.7 kg) on average. The researchers concluded that supplementing with 3.4 grams a day may be enough to pare down fat and manage weight.

One of the most intriguing areas of CLA research focuses on its apparent ability to trim abdominal fat, which is good news if you are trying to lose your belly bulge. To date, evidence for this waist-trimming effect has been observed only in men, but that doesn't necessarily rule out the same benefit for women. Let's look at the research.

In a Swedish study published in 2001 in the *International Journal of Obesity and Related Metabolic Disorders*, 25 men with abdominal obesity (aged 39 to 64) took either 4.2 grams of CLA or a placebo every day. At the end of the four-week experiment, those who took CLA had reduced their waists by 1.4 centimeters (0.5 in.), a reduction considered clinically significant by the researchers. The placebo group, by contrast, had insignificant reductions. The results of the study suggest that the effect of this safe and potentially helpful supplement on the reduction of abdominal fat is an avenue of research clearly worth further pursuit, particularly in women.

Even so, there is quite a bit of controversy about the effectiveness of CLA supplementation. Although animal studies have been very convincing in their results, showing benefits to body weight regulation, fat loss, and lean tissue maintenance, human studies have really had few positive results. Part of the confusion may lie in the mixture of isomers used, which resulted in diluting the most potent t-10, c-12 CLA isomer. Additionally, experimental animals showing positive results have been given CLA dosages based on weight that are 20 times greater than the dosages given to human subjects.

A recent human study has shown that CLA supplementation increased energy expenditure and fat burning and decreased body weight. The subjects in this study consumed 4 grams per day of a c-9,t-11 CLA and t-10, c-12CLA isomer mixture for six months. Another human study demonstrated increased lean body mass, which is associated with an increase in energy expenditure. These subjects were also given a CLA isomer mixture of 6.4 grams per day for 12 weeks.

We are getting closer to a firmer notion about the effectiveness of CLA, and of what works and what may not. An additional bonus may be that CLA supplementation may increase bone mineral density. In the meantime, I suggest you wait for more research on this supplement before running out to buy it by the boxload. However, including more CLA-rich foods in your diet may be a good idea. CLA is a naturally occurring dietary fatty acid found predominantly in whole milk, beef, eggs, and cheese. Significantly higher CLA levels are found in products from grass-fed animals. Because CLA is a fatty acid, low-fat or fat-free products are virtually CLA free.

## Glucosamine Sulfate and Chondroitin Sulfate

A supplement that combines glucosamine sulfate and chondroitin sulfate is being sold as an arthritis cure. Although research into this combination is ongoing, there is good evidence that this supplement does help relieve the pain and ease the movement of arthritis sufferers—perhaps as effectively as nonsteroidal anti-inflammatory drugs (NSAIDS) and without the long-term negative side effects.

One study of athletes with cartilage damage in their knees showed that 76 percent had complete resolution of symptoms and resumed full athletic training after 140 days of supplementation. However, there is no evidence demonstrating that glucosamine can repair damaged ligaments or tendons from sport-related injuries. More research is needed in this area, but supplementation with these compounds looks promising.

## Glutamine

Glutamine is the most abundant amino acid in your body. Most of it is stored in your muscles, although significant amounts are found in your brain, lungs, blood, and liver. It serves as a building block for protein, nucleotides (structural units of RNA and DNA), and other amino acids, and it is the principal fuel source for cells that make up the immune system.

Emerging evidence shows that glutamine may optimize recovery in at least four ways. Glutamine spares protein, stimulates the formation of glycogen, protects immunity, and enhances protein synthesis.

During intense exercise, the muscles release glutamine into the bloodstream. This can deplete muscle glutamine reserves by as much as 34 percent. Such a shortfall can be problematic, because a deficiency of glutamine promotes the breakdown and wasting of muscle tissue. But if sufficient glutamine is available, muscle loss can be prevented.

Glutamine also stimulates the synthesis of muscle glycogen. In a study involving subjects who cycled for 90 minutes, intravenous glutamine administered during a two-hour period after exercise doubled the concentration of glycogen in the muscles. It's not clear exactly how glutamine works in this regard, though. Scientists speculate either that glutamine itself can be converted into muscle glycogen or that it may inhibit the breakdown of glycogen.

In addition, glutamine is the chief fuel source for cells that make up the immune system. As noted, strenuous exercise depletes glutamine, and researchers believe that this shortage may be one of the reasons for the weakened immunity seen in hard-training athletes. Supplementing with glutamine may fend off infections that can sideline training.

Finally, glutamine assists with controlling the hydration levels of cells, or cell volumization. The maintenance of cell volume stimulates protein synthesis and decreases protein breakdown.

Glutamine thus may benefit anyone who wants to maximize performance, muscle repair, and immunity. The recommended dosage is between 5 and 15 grams a day.

## Glycerol

Glycerol is a syrupy substance that causes the body to store water and curtail urine output. It is an ingredient in some sport drinks and is available as a supplement you can add to water. A few studies indicate that glycerol supplementation can superhydrate your body. Research on whether glycerol supplementation actually enhances performance is equivocal, but one recent study in Australia showed enhanced fluid retention (600 ml) and improved endurance performance (5 percent) by cyclists in a hot environment when supplemented with glycerol.

The recommended dosage is 1 gram of glycerol per kilogram of body weight, with each gram diluted in 20 to 25 milliliters of fluid.

## Medium-Chain Triglyceride Oil

Processed mainly from coconut oil, medium-chain triglyceride oil (MCT oil) is a type of synthetically derived dietary fat that was first formulated in the 1950s by the pharmaceutical industry for patients who had trouble digesting regular fat. Still used in medical settings today, MCT oil is also a popular fitness supplement, marketed as a fat burner, muscle builder, and energy source.

At the molecular level, MCT oil is structured quite differently from conventional types of fat such as butter, margarine, and vegetable oil. Conventional fat is made up of long carbon chains, with 16 or more carbon atoms strung together, and are thus is known as long-chain triglycerides (LCTs). Body fat is also an LCT. MCT oil, on the other hand, has a much shorter carbon chain of only 6 to 12 carbon atoms, which is why it is described as a medium-chain triglyceride.

As a result of this molecular difference, MCTs are digested, transported, and metabolized much more quickly than fatty acids from regular oil or fat and thus have some interesting properties. To begin with, MCTs are burned in the body like carbohydrate. Unlike conventional fat, MCTs are not stored as body fat but are shuttled directly into the cells to be burned for energy. MCT oil is burned so quickly that its calories are turned into body heat during thermogenesis, which boosts the metabolic rate. The higher your metabolism is, the more calories your body burns.

Does that mean that if you take MCT oil you can rev up your metabolism and therefore burn more fat? Researchers at the University of Rochester looked into this possibility. In an experiment involving seven healthy men, they tested whether a meal of MCTs would increase the metabolic rate more than a meal of LCTs. The men ate test meals containing 48 grams of MCT oil or 45 grams of corn oil given in random order on separate days. In the study, metabolic rate increased 12 percent over six hours after the men ate the MCT meals but increased only 4 percent after they ate the LCT meals. What's more, concentrations of triglycerides in plasma (the liquid portion of blood) were elevated 68 percent after the LCT meal but did not change after the MCT meal. These findings led the researchers to speculate that replacing LCTs with MCTs over a long period of time might promote weight loss.

Other researchers aren't so sure. In a study at Calgary University in Alberta, Canada, healthy adults were placed on a low-carbohydrate diet supplemented with MCT oil. The researchers found that the diet had no real effect on elevating the metabolism. The calories burned over a 24-hour period were less than 1 percent of total caloric intake. However, there was a decrease in muscle protein burned for energy. Although MCT might not be a fat burner per se, it may help preserve lean mass by inhibiting its breakdown.

In most studies on MCT oil and fat burning, volunteers ingest huge amounts of the fat—usually 30 grams or more—to bring on metabolic-boosting results. Such amounts are not tolerable for most people, because too much MCT oil produces intestinal discomfort and diarrhea. In my opinion, taking such huge doses of MCT oil to spur fat burning just isn't practical.

There's another problem with using MCT oil to try to burn fat. The recommended way to take MCT oil is with carbohydrate, a practice that prevents ketosis. In ketosis, by-products of fat metabolism called *ketones* build up if carbohydrate isn't available to assist in the final stages of fat breakdown. But when MCTs are taken with carbohydrate, there is no effect on fat burning whatsoever. Here's why: Carbohydrate triggers the release of insulin, which inhibits the mobilization of fat for energy. Thus, there's simply no benefit to the use of MCT oil as a fat burner. You have to do it the old-fashioned way, by exercising and watching your diet.

Because MCT oil is processed in the body much like carbohydrate, it may help boost endurance. Case in point: At the University of Capetown Medical School in South Africa, researchers mixed 86 grams of MCT oil (nearly 3 tbsp) with 2 liters of 10 percent glucose drink to see what effect it would have on the performance of six endurance-trained cyclists. The cyclists were fed a drink consisting of glucose alone, glucose plus MCT oil, or MCT oil alone. In the laboratory, they pedaled at moderate intensity for about two hours and then completed a higher-intensity time trial. They performed this cycling bout on three separate occasions so that each cyclist used each type of drink once. The cyclists sipped the drink every 10 minutes. Performance improved the most when the cyclists supplemented with the MCT–glucose mixture. The researchers did some further biochemical tests on the cyclists and confirmed that the combination spared glycogen while making fat more accessible for fuel. Thus, when combined with carbohydrate, MCT oil may improve aerobic endurance performance by sparing muscle glycogen.

Another claim attached to MCT oil is that it helps you put on muscle; however, there are no controlled studies to prove this. Using some MCT oil to sneak in extra calories for harder workouts makes some sense, though. Go easy at first by taking 0.5 to 1 tablespoon (7 to 15 ml) a day. Its fast absorption can cause cramping and diarrhea if you take too much. Before experimenting with MCT oil, get your doctor's okay.

## N-Acetylcysteine (NAC)

NAC is an altered form of cysteine, an amino acid that helps the body synthesize glutathione (an antioxidant involved in boosting immunity). This supplement is used in the treatment of respiratory disorders, including acute and chronic bronchitis. What's more, it may help treat cardiovascular disease and might be useful in treating diabetes and some cancers.

In the exercise arena, NAC has been tested mostly with endurance athletes. In one study, eight men took either NAC or a placebo while cycling for 45 minutes at a very high intensity meant to simulate a race. NAC improved performance by 26 percent, probably as a result of its ability to enhance oxygen-carrying molecules and decrease oxidation in the muscle. It's too early to tell whether NAC will be a true performance-enhancing supplement, but it is worth watching.

# Phosphatidylserine (PS)

Phosphatidylserine (PS) is a fat-soluble nutrient that is most concentrated in the brain, where it supports many crucial nerve cell functions, including mood and brain health. It is available as a supplement (extracted from soybeans), and it has been well studied. Here's what some of the research shows:

- Taking 300 milligrams daily of PS for a month helped young adults better cope with stress (from taking a mental arithmetic test).

- Male soccer players who supplemented with 850 milligrams of PS for 10 days increased their running time to exhaustion. This benefit probably has to do more with the ability of PS to reduce anxiety and improve mood than anything else, because the nutrient had no real effect on preventing muscle damage, oxidative stress, or lipid peroxidation. A study with cyclists looked at similar parameters and also found that PS has a positive effect on performance. Again, this may have occurred because of the ability of PS to improve mood. If your mood is good, you're naturally going to feel like exercising because you have better mental energy.

If you wish to supplement with PS, I suggest 750 milligrams daily. I believe that supplementation with PS may have some benefit in any brain health program.

# Protein Supplements

Protein supplements are a convenient way to consume high-quality, fat-free, lactose-free protein after workouts or between meals. A variety of these supplements are on the market. Each has unique benefits to exercisers, strength trainers, and other athletes.

Table 8.3 guides you through the differences in processing. Here's a rundown of the different protein sources.

## TABLE 8.3 Supplemental Protein: What's the Difference?

| Forms of protein | Characteristics |
| --- | --- |
| Hydrolysates | Hydrolysates are proteins that have been partially broken down. This makes them taste more bitter, but taste has fortunately improved with newer products. Hydrolysates are extremely well absorbed and virtually free of any potential allergens. |
| Isolates | Isolates have the highest protein concentration (90-95%) and contain very little (if any) fat, lactose, and minerals. These have been removed to "isolate" the protein. |
| Concentrates | Concentrates have a protein concentration ranging from 25 to 89%. Concentrates are less processed than the other forms of protein and contain some lactose, fat, and minerals. |

### Bovine Colostrum

A clear premilk fluid and life's first food for every newborn mammal, colostrum is loaded with growth factors, amino acids, and bioactive protein that help the newborn develop in its first week of life. Several brands are on the market, including one called Intact. Studies have been conducted on this low-heat processed colostrum for its role in athletic performance, showing promising results for strength and power improvements in repetitive bouts of exercise.

Colostrum is similar to whey protein in both protein efficiency ratio (PER) (3.0) and protein digestibility score (PDCAAS) (1.0). What's more, it is low in fat and free of lactose. Because of its naturally high content of insulin-like growth factors, colostrum is banned by the National Collegiate Athletic Association (NCAA) and the USOC. If you are not affected by these organizations, you might try colostrum for its easy digestibility if you are looking for any possible strength-building edge.

### Egg Protein

The protein obtained from egg whites (ovalbumin) is considered the reference standard against which to compare types of protein. Egg protein was traditionally the protein of choice for supplements but is rather expensive. The PER of egg protein is 2.8; the PDCAAS is 1.0. If you like variety in your protein supplements, this one has value.

### Soy Protein

Despite being low in the amino acid methionine, soy is an excellent source of quality protein. Soy protein concentrate (70 percent protein) and isolate (90 percent protein) are particularly good protein sources for vegetarians. Soy protein isolate also contains isoflavone glucosides, which have a number of potential health benefits. The PER of soy protein is 1.8 to 2.3; the PDCAAS is 1.0. The downside of soy protein is that it is not as effective at muscle building as whey protein. On the other hand, if you are a vegetarian or you don't consume milk proteins, soy protein is an excellent alternative for boosting protein intake, especially immediately after exercise.

### Whey Protein

Whey is a component of milk that is separated off to make cheese and other dairy products. It is high in B-complex vitamins, selenium, and calcium. In addition, whey appears to boost the levels of the antioxidant glutathione in the body.

## Protein Supplements and Weight Loss

In addition to being used in muscle-building diets, protein supplements are frequently used in weight-loss diets. Increasing dietary protein has been shown to be a successful weight-loss strategy, and protein supplements are an easy way to increase protein without increasing carbohydrate and fat.

Could whey protein possibly ward off oxidative stress? Yes, says at least one study. Twenty athletes (10 men and 10 women) took a whey protein supplement (20 g a day) for three months. A control group supplemented with a placebo. Researchers assessed the athletes' power and work capacity during bouts of cycling. Both aspects of physical performance increased significantly in the whey-supplemented group, whereas there was no change in the placebo group. The researchers concluded that prolonged supplementation with a product designed to shore up antioxidant defenses resulted in improved performance.

Along with colostrum, whey protein represents the highest-quality protein available in supplements. It is digested rapidly, allowing for fast uptake of amino acids. Also available are whey protein hydrolysate, ion exchange whey protein isolate, and cross-flow microfiltration whey protein isolate. These differ slightly in their amino acid profiles, fat content, lactose content, and ability to preserve glutamine. It is unclear whether these small differences would have any impact on exercise performance. Using the isolated form of whey is a good idea if you want to reduce the amount of carbohydrate you consume. However, you will get less calcium and other minerals from this form of whey.

A 2011 study published in the *Journal of Nutrition* found that whey protein works better than soy protein for weight loss. In this clinical trial covering 23 weeks, the body weight and fat mass of the group consuming the whey protein were lower by 1.8 kilograms (4 lb) and 2.3 kilograms (5 lb), respectively, than those same measures in the group consuming carbohydrate. Whey protein also trimmed belly fat more significantly than soy protein did.

One reason whey protein is so effective for weight loss is that it is high in leucine, an amino acid that regulates muscle mass, but also helps you reduce body fat during weight loss. Research shows that 2.5 grams is the ideal dose of leucine for fat loss, that whey protein contains 10 percent leucine, and that other proteins contain slightly less. So a dose of 25 grams of whey protein will contain the ideal dose of leucine.

## Quercetin

As a result of the successful marketing of quercetin-based supplement by the company FRS, this nutrient has become very popular for cyclists, triathletes, and anyone who cross-trains. Quercetin is an antioxidant found naturally in fruits and vegetables such as red apples, grapes, and berries.

A major review study concluded that there is a very small but statistically significant benefit of quercetin for endurance athletes. The reason it is beneficial is that it may increase $\dot{V}O_2$max (how much oxygen you can process) by 3 percent. The greater your $\dot{V}O_2$max is, the stronger your performance will be and the less fatigue you will feel. In reality, this is a trivial difference that may only matter at the most elite levels of competition. I've concluded that much more research needs to be done before quercetin can be considered a supplement that works.

# Ribose

Found in every cell of your body, ribose is a simple sugar that forms the carbohydrate backbone of DNA and RNA, the genetic materials that control cellular growth and reproduction, thus governing all life. Ribose is also involved in the production of ATP, the main energy-producing molecule of all living cells, and is one of its structural components. Cells need ATP to function properly.

Normally, your body can produce and recycle all the ATP it needs, especially when there is an abundant supply of oxygen. But under certain circumstances—namely, ischemia (lack of blood flow to tissues) and strenuous exercise—ATP cannot be regenerated fast enough, and energy-producing compounds called *adenine nucleotides* may be lost from cells. This can impair muscle function and tax strength, because cells need adenine nucleotides to produce sufficient amounts of ATP.

In animal research, ribose supplementation increased the rate of nucleotide synthesis in the resting and exercising muscles of rats by three to four times. Other animal studies have found that ribose can restore nucleotides to near normal levels within 12 to 24 hours of intense exercise.

Some medical studies indicate that ribose supplementation (10 to 60 g a day) can increase ATP availability in certain patients and protect against ischemia in others. But what about athletes and exercisers? Does ribose, now marketed as a sport supplement, have any benefit? Two abstracts of research presented at the 2000 ACSM meeting have convinced me to move ribose to the possibly meets marketing claims category. Both studies indicate that ribose taken before, during, and after hard exercise quite possibly helps energize muscles and enhance power.

In one small study, six subjects consumed 2 to 10 grams of ribose. As a result, their blood glucose levels were maintained over 120 minutes, whereas subjects who took a placebo experienced no such benefit. This study hints that ribose may make more energy (blood glucose) available to working muscles.

The results of the second study were a little more convincing because it was an actual performance test. This study investigated whether short-term ribose supplementation improved anaerobic performance in eight young men compared with a taste-matched placebo. Subjects performed a series of six 10-second cycle sprints separated by 60-second rest periods.

There were two familiarization rides before the series of six and then four depletion rides and two posttest rides. Four 8-gram doses were given over a period of 36 hours, with a final dose given 120 minutes before posttesting. In four of six sprints, values for peak power were improved by 2.2 to 7 percent, and overall power improved by 2 to 10 percent. The researchers are now hoping to confirm these results in a larger study.

Supplemental ribose is available in sport drinks, energy bars, tablets, and powders. The usual recommended dosage is 3 to 5 grams daily as maintenance dose and 5 to 10 grams daily for hard-training athletes.

As a way to restore muscular energy, ribose looks promising. So stay tuned: There is much more to learn about this intriguing new supplement and what it holds for athletes and exercisers.

## Taurine

One of the most abundant amino acids in the body, taurine is found in the central nervous system and skeletal muscle and is very concentrated in the brain and heart. It is manufactured from the amino acids methionine and cysteine, with help from vitamin B6. Animal protein is a good source; taurine is not found in vegetable protein.

Taurine appears to act on neurotransmitters in the brain. There have been reports on the benefits of taurine supplementation in treating epilepsy to control motor tics such as facial twitches. The effectiveness of taurine in treating epilepsy is limited, however, because it does not easily cross the blood–brain barrier.

Taurine is also an effective cellular protector against exercise-induced DNA damage. It appears to reduce muscle damage caused by exercise, thereby accelerating recovery between workouts. Other research indicates that supplemental taurine may improve exercise performance by increasing the muscles' force of contraction (strength). In addition, taurine may exert an insulin-like effect. Research hints that it might improve insulin resistance and help the body better use glucose. It also appears to reduce triglycerides and blood levels of harmful cholesterol.

With high-intensity exercise, blood levels of taurine increase, possibly as a result of its release from muscle fibers. Because of its association with neurotransmitters in the brain, taurine has recently been advocated as a supplement to enhance attention, cognitive performance, and feelings of well-being. One study investigated these possibilities with a supplement containing caffeine, taurine, and glucuronolactone (a natural detoxifier derived from carbohydrate metabolism) and found that these ingredients had positive effects on human mental performance and mood. But because a combination of ingredients was tested, there's no way of knowing how much of the effect was the result of taurine alone.

Research into taurine in athletes is very limited, and many more studies need to be done to verify its benefits. However, because of the possible effectiveness of supplemental taurine in other populations, it is a supplement to watch.

# Does Not Meet Marketing Claims

The products in this category either have no scientific data or they have negative data, poor studies, or only animal studies to support their claims. You might still keep your eye on any research publications, but I wouldn't waste my money or my time on them.

## Inosine

Inosine is a natural chemical that improves oxygen use, possibly by forcing additional production of ATP. However, research does not support claims that supplemental inosine increases physical power. If it really created more ATP, it would give you more energy. But again, no research supports this claim.

## Pyruvic Acid

Pyruvate, or more specifically, pyruvic acid, is made naturally in the body during carbohydrate metabolism and is involved in energy-producing reactions that occur at the cellular level. Pyruvate is also found in many foods in tiny amounts. The dietary supplements sold as pyruvate are derived from pyruvic acid, which is bonded to a mineral salt, usually calcium, sodium, or potassium. Little data support the claims that the dosages currently marketed to promote fat loss (0.5 to 2 g a day) affect fat loss or improve exercise performance. Nor is there enough research to support the effectiveness of newer supplements that pair pyruvate with creatine.

## Tryptophan

Tryptophan is an amino acid supplement used by athletes to increase strength and muscle mass, although it does neither. People have used tryptophan to relieve insomnia, depression, anxiety, and premenstrual tension. In 1989, thousands of Americans developed a crippling illness called eosinophilia-myalgia syndrome after taking tainted tryptophan made by a Japanese chemical company. As a result, tryptophan was yanked from the market. There are some new tryptophan products on the market, but I don't see any reason to use them. If you'd like to give your brain a serotonin boost by consuming more tryptophan, try turkey and milk instead.

## Zinc and Magnesium

Zinc and magnesium are mineral elements required in adequate amounts to maintain health and physiological function, and they promote increased energy expenditure and work performance. Zinc and magnesium are being formulated together as a supplement and marketed as a strength-building formula. But to date no formally published studies have proved that this combination even works.

# Potentially Harmful

Products in this category have been shown to cause harm and are not worth the risk. All medications come with a ratio of risks to benefits. Just because these products are potentially harmful doesn't necessarily mean that they don't work. What it does mean is that the risks outweigh any potential benefits.

## Amino Acids

Amino acid supplements are heavily marketed to bodybuilders and other strength-training athletes with claims that they build muscle as a safe alternative to steroid drugs. But these supplements are bought not only by bodybuilders but also by average exercisers lured by promises that amino acids, the building blocks of protein, build lean mass and burn fat. Although data support the claim that essential amino acids taken after exercise will lead to increased muscle growth and strength,

6 grams of essential amino acids are required. This is a very costly endeavor and is not without risks. The Federation of American Societies for Experimental Biology (FASEB) recently conducted an exhaustive search of available data on amino acids and concluded that insufficient information exists to establish a safe intake level for any amino acids in dietary supplements, and that their safety should not be assumed. Eighteen to 20 grams of whey protein will safely give you approximately 6 grams of essential amino acids.

## Androstenedione

Androstenedione is a hormone that occurs naturally in the body and is a direct precursor to testosterone. Androstenedione is found in some plants, notably pollen, and in the gonads of mammals. Athletes take it to increase blood levels of testosterone for a strength- and muscle-building effect. Supposedly, it is safer than taking anabolic steroids. However, there has not been much reliable research to prove the marketing claims made by supplement companies that androstenedione really works. And because it is a controlled and banned substance, drug-tested athletes beware!

## Bee Pollen

Bee pollen supplements sold are actually a loose powder of bee saliva, plant nectar, and pollen compressed into tablets of 400 to 500 milligrams or poured into capsules. Bee pollen also comes in pellets to be sprinkled on foods. It is rich in amino acids, with a protein content that averages 20 percent but ranges from 10 to 36 percent. Ten to 15 percent is simple sugars. There are traces of fat and minerals in bee pollen. Bee pollen has been marketed as an athletic supplement for improving physical performance. Some European studies have found benefits, but American studies have not. Can bee pollen hurt you? Possibly. It does contain pollen, so you could suffer an allergic reaction if you're prone to allergies, or worse, death from anaphylactic shock.

## Dehydroepiandrosterone

Dehydroepiandrosterone, more commonly known as DHEA, is a steroid that's naturally secreted by the adrenal glands. Promoted as an antiaging product, DHEA is probably the most talked about, most hyped supplement on the shelves. Near-magical properties have been attributed to DHEA, ranging from increased sex drive to enhanced immunity to weight loss to higher energy levels. Bodybuilders, strength trainers, and other athletes take it with the hope that it will build muscle and burn fat. But there's no real evidence to support this effect; in fact, research shows that supplementation with DHEA does not increase strength. As with all anabolic steroids, DHEA has side effects, including excessive hair growth and other virilizing effects in women and breast enlargement in men. A major concern with DHEA is that there have been no long-term human experiments with it.

## Dimethylglycine

Dimethylglycine (DMG, or vitamin B15) is a dietary supplement rather than a vitamin and supposedly increases aerobic power and endurance. However, there are no studies to substantiate these claims. What most people don't realize is that supplements containing DMG may cause chromosome damage in cells.

## Gamma Butyrolactone

Gamma butyrolactone (GBL) is commercially available as an industrial solvent and is used as an ingredient in cleaners, solvents, paint removers, and engine degreasers. It is also sold as a natural supplement over the Internet and in some health food stores and gymnasiums, and it is marketed as a natural, nontoxic dietary supplement. Manufacturers of GBL claim that it builds muscle, improves physical performance, and acts as an aphrodisiac.

Although labeled as a dietary supplement, GBL and products containing it are illegal drugs marketed under various trade names, including Renewtrient, Revivarant, Blue Nitro, GH Revitalizer, Gamma G, and Remforce. The FDA has issued a recall on products containing GBL because of at least 55 adverse events, including one death. Read ingredient labels on supplements to make sure you avoid this substance.

## Plant Sterols

Plant sterols are naturally occurring steroids extracted from plants that are promoted to exercisers, strength trainers, and athletes. They include gamma oryzanol, found in rice bran oil; Smilax, an herbal extract that is advertised as a natural form of testosterone; beta-sitosterol, a lipid extract; and ferulic acid, another type of lipid extract. The research that has been done so far with these supplements indicates that they have no effect on body composition in people who exercise. Some people may be sensitive to these substances, which can cause allergies and possibly anaphylactic shock.

# Diet Is Still Key

Building fit, firm muscle isn't as easy as just exercising and supplementing; there's a lot more to it than that. You can't neglect a good diet. Learn how to develop your Power Eating plan in chapters 10 and 11, and refer to the sample strength-training diets in chapters 12 through 16. Above all, eat enough quality calories each day to fuel your body for exercise and activity.

## TABLE 8.4　Rating of the Supplements

| Supplement | Meets marketing claims | Possibly meets marketing claims | Does not meet marketing claims | Potentially harmful |
|---|---|---|---|---|
| Caffeine | ✔ | | | |
| Carbohydrate–protein sport drinks | ✔ | | | |
| Creatine | ✔ | | | |
| Glucose–electrolyte solutions | ✔ | | | |
| Weight-gain powders | ✔ | | | |
| Arginine | | ✔ | | |
| Beta-alanine | | ✔ | | |
| Beta-hydroxy-beta-methylbutyrate (HMB) | | ✔ | | |
| Branched-chain amino acids (BCAAs) | | ✔ | | |
| Carnitine | | ✔ | | |
| Coenzyme Q10 (CoQ10) | | ✔ | | |
| Conjugated linoleic acid (CLA) | | ✔ | | |
| Glucosamine/chondroitin sulfate | | ✔ | | |
| Glutamine | | ✔ | | |
| Glycerol | | ✔ | | |
| MCT oil | | ✔ | | |
| N-acetyl cysteine (NAC) | | ✔ | | |
| Phosphatidylserine (PS) | | ✔ | | |
| Protein supplements | | ✔ | | |
| Quercetin | | ✔ | | |
| Ribose | | ✔ | | |
| Taurine | | ✔ | | |
| Inosine | | | ✔ | |
| Pyruvate | | | ✔ | |
| Tryptophan | | | ✔ | |
| Zinc–magnesium | | | ✔ | |
| Amino acids | | | | ✔ |
| Androstenedione | | | | ✔ |
| Bee pollen | | | | ✔ |
| Dehydroepiandrosterone (DHEA) | | | | ✔ |
| Dimethylglycine (DMG; vitamin $B_{15}$) | | | | ✔ |
| Gamma butyrolactone (GBL) | | | | ✔ |
| Plant sterols | | | | ✔ |

# 9

# Botanicals for Performance

Herbs are the most popular self-prescribed medication. They now come in capsules, tablets, liquids, and powders. Of the $20 billion spent on dietary supplements in the United States, more than $5 billion is spent on herbal supplements alone. Those sales figures increase by 3 to 5 percent each year. Herbs are heavily promoted as bodybuilding supplements with little evidence that they work (although we have more data now than ever before) Also, herbs can even do harm.

An herb is a plant or part of a plant valued for its medicinal qualities, its aroma, or its taste. Herbs and herbal remedies have been around for centuries. Even Neanderthal people used plants for healing purposes. About 30 percent of all modern drugs are derived from herbs. Cooking with herbs and botanicals is a very powerful way to influence your mind–body health. I encourage you to enhance the healing properties of your foods by adding more herbs and botanicals to your diet. In this chapter, however, I'll be focusing more on supplements. The information in this chapter can help guide you through the often-confusing maze of which herbs can be helpful and which may be harmful.

## Natural, but Not Always Safe

It's a common but dangerous notion to think that because herbs are natural, they are safe. What separates plant-derived drugs from herbal supplements is careful scientific study. Makers of herbal supplements in the United States are not required to submit their products to the FDA, so there is no regulation of product quality or safety. Without the enforcement of standards, there is only a meager chance that the contents and potency described on labels are accurate. Some eye-opening proof of this was found in a study conducted at the UCLA Center for Human Nutrition. Researchers analyzed commercial formulations of saw palmetto, kava kava, echinacea, ginseng, and Saint-John's wort. They purchased six bottles each of two lots of supplements from nine manufacturers and analyzed their contents. There were differences in what was actually in the product versus what was stated on the labels, particularly with echinacea and ginseng. Even the product labels varied in the information provided. Dosage recommendations and information about the herbs often varied.

This study reflects an important problem with herbal products. When products that are not standardized are tested for effectiveness, conclusive evidence on what works and what doesn't is hard to come by, no matter how well the study is designed. What you are taking may not be the same in any way as the extract that was tested.

Many herbal supplements are contaminated, too, although this is usually not the case with well-known mainstream store brands. For this reason, try to purchase herbal supplements from reputable manufacturers. Also, make sure the product lists all ingredients on the label and that it is certified by a good laboratory. Given all the time you spend making sure your food is clean and the exercise you do is at peak levels, why unintentionally mess up your health and performance with a dubious supplement?

Herbs are classified as food supplements by the FDA. Labeling them as medicines would require stringent testing to prove their safety and effectiveness. This costs millions of dollars per herb, an investment few manufacturers are willing to make.

Fortunately for consumers, supplements can no longer be labeled with unsubstantiated claims. The latest government regulations require that the supplement industry abide by the same labeling laws that govern packaged foods. This means that any supplement bearing a health claim must support the claim with scientific evidence that meets government approval. Any product marketed as a way to cure, modify, treat, or prevent disease is regulated as a drug by the FDA.

What you see on supplement labels now are structure and function claims. This means that manufacturers are allowed to make claims about the impact of dietary supplements on the structure or function of the body, but these claims must be truthful. An example of such a claim is, "Vitamin C is involved in immune function."

It's not uncommon to have an allergic reaction to drugs, even those that have been tested and manufactured with strict safeguards. Therefore, it is even more likely that untested herbs, which are consumed in large amounts, may also produce allergic reactions. These reactions can sometimes be fatal. Herbs can interact with prescribed medications, too. If you're taking any medications, you should consult your physician, pharmacist, or dietitian before using any herbal supplement.

In addition, if you're scheduled for surgery and are taking herbal supplements, let your physician know well in advance of your operation. Certain herbs, particularly *Ginkgo biloba*, garlic, ginger, and ginseng, interfere with normal blood clotting and can lead to excessive blood loss during surgery. Mood-boosting herbs such as Saint-John's wort and kava kava dangerously heighten the sedative effects of anesthesia.

Pregnant and nursing mothers should avoid all herbal preparations. If you are pregnant or nursing, ask your physician or dietitian about specific herbal teas, because even these can cause harmful reactions in a developing baby or nursing infant. Don't give herbal supplements or remedies to children, either. There is virtually no medical information about the safety of herbs for children. Your best intentions could result in serious harm.

Because there's no universal quality-control regulation of the industry, the danger of chemical contamination of herbal supplements is real. Were the plants sprayed with any chemicals before harvesting or processing? Other toxic contaminants or banned or illegal substances may enter the product during processing as well. For instance, a study testing herbal products for prohibited anabolic androgen steroids and GH found that 15 percent contained prohormones (variants of hormones) that were not declared on the label. Most of these substances were manufactured in the United States but were sold in European countries. Products that are purchased by mail order from other countries are even more questionable than those purchased in the United States. The following is a rundown of well-known herbs, either sold alone or as an ingredient in fitness supplements. I have classified these herbs similarly to the way I classified sport supplements in chapter 8. According to current sport science research, some meet their marketing claims, and others are possibly useful. Table 9.2, located at the end of the chapter, provides a quick reference for the effectiveness of the many performance herbs on the market.

## Meets Marketing Claims

Much of the research on herbal supplements has been conducted outside the United States, but experts agree that the products listed here have been well tested for efficacy. Even so, herbs can act as powerful drugs. Approach them with the same respect as you would any prescription medication.

### Buchu

Culled from a shrub native to South Africa, the leaves of this herb are usually made into a tea and other supplement forms. Buchu is a mild diuretic, and in that regard it may help rid your body of excess water weight. It is also an antiseptic that fights germs in the urinary tract.

Buchu is generally considered safe, although herbalists recommend taking no more than 2 grams two or three times a day.

### Fo-Ti

Ancient Chinese herbalists swore that this member of the buckwheat family is one of the best longevity promoters ever grown. According to herbalists, fo-ti exhibits different properties depending on the size and age of its root. A fist-sized 50-year-old plant, for example, keeps your hair from turning gray. A 100-year-old root the size of a bowl preserves your cheerfulness. At 150 years old and as large as a sink, fo-ti makes your teeth fall out so that new ones can grow in. And a 200-year-old plant restores youth and vitality. Or so the folk tales go.

Fo-ti has a reputation as a good cardiovascular herb. Supposedly, it lowers cholesterol, protects blood vessels, and increases blood flow to the heart. Fo-ti does act as a natural laxative, however, and in this regard it's probably a safe herb.

## Guarana

Guarana is a red berry from a plant grown in the Amazon valley. It contains seven times the caffeine as coffee beans and is widely sold in health food stores as a supplement to increase energy. It is also found in energy drinks and energy waters. The supplement is made from the seeds of the berry.

Guarana is used in a number of natural weight-loss supplements. It is believed to increase thermogenesis (body heat) and thus stimulate the metabolism. In large doses, guarana may also cause the body to lose water because the caffeine it contains is a diuretic. As for a possible performance benefit, guarana has been shown to increase blood glucose in animals. Whether that holds true for humans, however, remains to be seen. A note of caution: If you're sensitive to caffeine, it's best to leave guarana alone.

## Maté

Another caffeinated herb is maté. Touted as a natural upper, it has a caffeine content of 2 percent. Maté is found in some natural weight-loss supplements because it is believed to help control appetite. Like guarana, it is found in energy drinks and energy waters. It also has a mild diuretic effect and thus may produce temporary water weight loss. Medical experts say the herb is relatively safe when taken in small quantities for short periods of time.

Please keep in mind that both guarana and maté contain caffeine. I've had clients come to me thrilled that they are off caffeine, only to find out that they've been drinking energy waters containing one of these herbs! They haven't quit caffeine at all; they went from caffeine in their coffee to caffeine in their herbal water. Read labels to watch for these herbs. You do have to be well informed about herbs that naturally contain caffeine; the label will not list caffeine unless caffeine itself is an additive ingredient.

# Possibly Meets Marketing Claims

Research is still not clear on whether the claims made about the herbs in this category are true—maybe they are; maybe they aren't. If you try these herbs, remember that you are being the guinea pig. It may be preferable to wait and see how the research pans out before trying them yourself.

## Beetroot Juice

If you watched the 2012 London Olympics, you may have heard something about beetroot juice as a possibly effective endurance supplement. Beetroot juice appears to help prolong time to exhaustion by reducing oxygen intake and making exercise less tiring.

Studies with beetroot juice show that athletes who took this botanical needed less oxygen and had lower blood pressure than those who did not take it. Other benefits found in research included better performance and heart function while exercising.

Nitrates are compounds found naturally in various foods, including beetroots, green leafy vegetables, cured meats, and tea. Nitrates are converted in the body to various other compounds, including sodium nitrite, and part of this process involves bacteria found in the mouth and digestive tract.

Dietary nitrates used to be forbidden for fear of increased cancer risk from the converted nitrites, but new science tells us that they aren't necessarily bad for our health, and can even jack up blood flow and energy during exercise. Nitrates are likely the active natural compound in beetroot juice. They are also found abundantly in celery, spinach, and collard greens.

The conclusion that nitrates cause cancer has been shown to be the result of research flaws, and these conclusions were retracted. Unfortunately, the media spent significantly more time covering the fear of nitrates than they have the retraction. Today, the National Academy of Sciences, the American Cancer Society, and the National Research Council all agree that there's no cancer risk from consuming sodium nitrite. Although lowering your total sodium content is a positive outcome of this effort, you will notice that most "nitrate-free" cured products contain celery juice or other natural source of nitrates to serve as important antibacterial preservatives. Without them, the cured meat would have virtually no shelf-life.

Among the many studies done on beetroot juice is an experiment conducted with cyclists at the University of Exeter. Researchers found that beetroot juice boosts energy by making muscles more fuel efficient. The study focused on male cyclists aged 19 to 38 training on exercise bikes. Drinking half a liter of beetroot juice a day for a week enabled them to cycle 16 percent longer before getting tired out. Other research has shown the same benefits with walking, running, and resistance training.

How exactly does beetroot juice work? Basically, it doubles the amount of nitrate in the blood and reduces the rate at which muscles use their source of energy, ATP.

See chapter 17 for my banana beet orange antioxidant smoothie that includes beets in its ingredient list. this does not give the efficacious dose of beetroot juice, it certainly adds to your total nitrate intake for the day.

Using beetroot juice supplements may be the easiest way to ingest adequate amounts of dietary nitrate, but a side effect of this strategy may be red urine and stools. There are other great sources of nitrates (see table 9.1). The beneficial amount of dietary nitrate consumed in most studies ranges from 300 to 500 milligrams.

## Cayenne

Cayenne pepper, that spice you use to make foods taste hot, may be a bona fide fat burner. It contains a compound called capsaicin, which has been shown in studies to enhance energy expenditure and increase fat burning. Chapter 5 discusses the

### TABLE 9.1    Dietary Nitrate in Foods

| 250 mg/100 g: celery, cress, chervil, lettuce, red beetroot, spinach, arugula | |
|---|---|
| 100-250 mg/100 g: celeriac, Chinese cabbage, endive, fennel, kohlrabi, leeks, parsley | |
| **Amount of nitrate in normal serving:** | |
| 1 cup raw spinach | 900 mg nitrate |
| 1/2 cup cooked collard greens | 200 mg nitrate |
| 1 cup raw leaf lettuce | 100 mg nitrate |
| 1/2 cup vegetable juice | 40 mg nitrate |

Source: E. Coleman, 2012, "Reap the benefits of beetroot juice—evidence suggests it improves heart health and athletic performance," *Today's Dietitian* 14(2): 48.

best fat-burning foods and includes capsaicin from hot peppers. Supplementing with a new nonspicy formulation is an exciting new option for this fat burner.

A lot of athletes have trouble using this supplement, however. It tends to create a burning sensation in the stomach. Fortunately, a less-hot form of capsaicin, the capsinoid dihydrocapsiate, has been developed from sweet peppers. Available data suggest that it's best to take 3 milligrams daily to obtain the fat-burning benefit without the burning sensation in the stomach.

## Echinacea

Echinacea is a member of the sunflower family. There are three species used medicinally—*purpurea*, *angustifolia*, and *pallida*. The German Commission E, Germany's equivalent to the U.S. FDA, has approved *Echinacea purpurea* as supportive therapy for colds and chronic infections of the respiratory tract. The Commission's monograph, a publication describing scores of herbs and their therapeutic applications, notes that echinacea preparations increase the number of white blood cells in the body. White blood cells destroy invading organisms, including cold viruses.

A stringent scientific review study of echinacea conducted in 2006 analyzed 16 trials of the herb. It concluded that some evidence has found that the aerial parts of *Echinacea purpurea* are effective for the early treatment of colds in adults, but that these results are not fully consistent.

Weakened immunity is often seen in athletes and highly active people— which is why many sport scientists recommend supplementing with echinacea. However, I am not one of them. One reason is that if you suffer from hay fever, taking echinacea puts you at risk for a severe reaction, even anaphylactic shock, a life-threatening allergic reaction. Allergies in general appear to be on the rise, so I believe that taking an herb such as this is not worth the risk.

Don't supplement with echinacea if you have an autoimmune disease such as lupus or a progressive illness such as multiple sclerosis, because the herb may overstimulate your immune system and do further damage. Also, don't take echinacea orally for longer than eight weeks.

# Ginseng

Used for thousands of years in the Far East as a tonic to strengthen and restore health, ginseng has more recently been touted as a performance-boosting herb for exercisers and athletes. For background, ginseng comes from the root of a medicinal plant in the ginseng family (*Araliaceae*). There are various types of ginseng, including those in the *Panax* classification and a botanical cousin called Siberian ginseng, also known as eleuthero or its Chinese name, Ciwujia, for short.

*Panax* ginseng and eleuthero are approved medicines in Germany. In fact, the German Commission E states in its monographs that these ginsengs can be used "as a tonic for invigoration and fortification in times of fatigue and debility, for declining capacity for work and concentration, also during convalescence" (Blumenthal, 174).

In the United States, the FDA considers ginseng a food. According to one nutritional analysis, 100 grams of *Panax* ginseng root contain 338 calories; 70 grams of carbohydrate; appreciable amounts of vitamins A, $B_1$ (thiamin), $B_2$ (riboflavin), $B_{12}$, C, and E; as well as the minerals niacin, calcium, iron, and phosphorus.

The main active constituents of the *Panax* species are plant steroids called ginsenosides. Eleuthero's active constituents are plant steroids known as eleutherosides, which differ in chemical structure from ginsenosides but have similar properties. The mechanisms of action of these chemical components are complex, but scientists theorize that they increase the size of the mitochondrion (the energy factory of the cell), stimulate the production of adrenal hormones, and enhance the transmission of brain chemicals called neurotransmitters, among other functions.

In herbal medicine, all ginsengs are considered to be "adaptogens." Coined by a Soviet scientist in 1947, the term refers to a class of agents that build resistance to physical stress, enhance performance, extend endurance, and stimulate the body's recovery power after exercise.

Summarizing much of the research that's been done, Dr. Luke Bucci in a review paper noted that *Panax* ginseng supplements may enhance physical and mental performance if taken long enough and in sufficient enough doses. Further, he stated that ginseng is more effective in untrained or subjects older than 40 years. There are no acute or immediate effects from ginseng supplementation, either. It is a supplement that acts over at least an eight-week period of time.

In other research, when doses are at least 2 grams of the standardized extract for longer than eight weeks, significant improvements in physical or psychomotor performance are almost always seen. Siberian ginseng, different from *Panax* ginseng, has not shown any influence on physical performance. Further studies and better studies are needed on both Siberian ginseng and *Panax* ginseng.

Clearly, there is conflicting research on ginseng. How do we make sense of the data? The most valid explanation is the wide variability among commercial ginseng products. An analysis of 24 roots and products (including softgels, tablets, dry-filled capsules, and teas) showed great variations in the concentrations of ginsenosides. Another study revealed that ginseng products vary in content even across lots of the same brand, and that some products contain no ginsenosides at all. In addition, the chemical composition of commercial ginseng products varies according to the age of the root, its cultivation, the part of the root used, and manufacturing methods.

When it comes to ginseng, knowing what you're buying can be difficult. And taking ginseng is a questionable practice. There are known side effects of large doses and long-term use: high blood pressure, nervousness, insomnia, low blood pressure, sedation, painful breasts, breast nodules, and vaginal bleeding. In addition, ginseng reacts with many drugs. Ginseng is contraindicated for use with stimulants, including excessive use of caffeine. Talk to your physician and pharmacist about potential interactions with any medications you're taking.

## Green Tea

Derived from the leaves and leaf buds of an evergreen plant native to Asia, green tea is of interest to fitness-minded people because it may help encourage weight loss. Certain natural chemicals called catechins are abundant in green tea; animal and human studies show that these chemicals appear to increase fat burning and stimulate thermogenesis, the calorie-burning process that occurs as a result of digesting and metabolizing food. Green tea is also an excellent anti-inflammatory.

A study by Japanese researchers in 2001 reported that tea catechins (600 mg/day) taken with the diet for 12 weeks in men promoted weight loss, a decrease in body mass index (BMI), and a decrease in waist circumference compared to subjects consuming a placebo with a small amount of catechins.

Green tea used in conjunction with caffeine has also been widely studied. In 2011, researchers published a review of the mechanisms contributing to the antiobesity effects of green tea and reported their findings in the *Journal of Nutritional Biochemistry*. They stated that the predominant hypothesis is that the green tea catechins influence the sympathetic nervous system, increasing energy expenditure and promoting fat oxidation. Caffeine also influences sympathetic nervous system activity, acting synergistically to increase the antiobesity effects. The researchers speculate that other potential mechanisms are involved, too, including appetite suppressing, an increase in fat-burning enzymes, and less absorption of calories.

Does green tea help boost exercise performance? Studies looking into this have found no effect. I believe more research is needed in this area.

Even the amount that you need to consume for weight loss isn't yet clear. A 1999 study in Maryland used 6 1/4 cups (1.5 L) of tea per day for four days. The more recent Japanese study on men (mentioned earlier) found successful results from 2 1/2 cups (600 ml) every day for 12 weeks. If you are caffeine sensitive, you might want to start with the lower dose, and definitely don't drink the tea in the evening before bed.

Whether or not green tea pans out as a true antiobesity agent, it's worth drinking for other reasons. Research has found that the natural chemicals in green tea may protect against periodontal disease, some cancers, and heart disease.

Unless you're sensitive to caffeine, green tea or extracts containing it are very safe and probably beneficial to health.

# Does Not Meet Marketing Claims

The following products don't have enough research to back up their marketing claims. I wouldn't waste my money on them. At another time in history, this category would have been called "snake oil."

## Burdock

Burdock is a relative of the dandelion and is often called a blood purifier, a diuretic, a treatment for skin diseases such as acne and psoriasis, and a diaphoretic (sweat producer). None of these claims has been verified scientifically, and no solid evidence exists that burdock has any useful therapeutic effects. In addition, there have been reports of poisonings caused by burdock tea contaminated with belladonna, a harmful herb.

## Canaigre

Canaigre is deceptively promoted as a less expensive American alternative to real ginseng, but in no way is it related to ginseng, either botanically or chemically. Native to the southwestern United States and Mexico, canaigre has been recommended by herbal enthusiasts for a variety of problems ranging from lack of energy to leprosy. The trouble is, canaigre is potentially cancer causing because of its high content of tannin.

## Citrus Aurantium

Citrus aurantium (also known as bitter orange or synephrine) is the botanical name of the Chinese fruit zhishi. An alkaloid called synephrine is extracted from this fruit and used as an ingredient in numerous fitness supplements. Synephrine is a chemical cousin to ephedrine (an alkaloid found in the herb ephedra) but has few of ephedrine's adverse side effects. Synephrine is thought to suppress the appetite, increase the metabolic rate, and help burn fat by stimulating the action of fat-burning enzymes inside cells. To date, though, there are no published studies on synephrine as a fat burner.

## Coleus Forskohlii

Coleus forskohlii is a member of the mint family and has been used extensively for many applications in Indian (ayurvedic) medicine. Its active ingredient, diterpene forskolin, activates adenylate cyclase, an enzyme that increases cyclic adenosine monophosphate (cAMP) in cells. The synthesis of cAMP influences many biological systems, including the breakdown of stored fat in animal and human fat cells. This enzyme also regulates the body's thermic response to food, increases the metabolic rate, and activates fat burning.

The theory behind using this herb is that if you can stimulate fatty acid metabolism, then you can lose body fat while saving lean muscle tissue. Even so, research on coleus forskohlii does not substantiate this effect, and the herb does not appear to promote weight loss.

## Cordyceps

Cordyceps is a mushroom native to mountainous regions of China and Tibet, and it is unusual in that it grows on caterpillar larvae. Cordyceps is available as a performance supplement, believed to open breathing passages to let more oxygen circulate. With more oxygen available to cells, endurance increases. Research fails to substantiate this effect, however. Although cordyceps is described as safe and gentle, little information exists on its safety.

## Damiana

Damiana comes from the leaves of a Mexican shrub. Around the turn of the century, it was touted as a powerful aphrodisiac. Closer scientific scrutiny of damiana revealed that it has no aphrodisiac properties or beneficial physiological action whatsoever.

## Gotu Kola

Gotu kola, a member of the parsley family, is a common weed usually found growing in drainage ditches in Asia and orchards in Hawaii. A known effect of this herb is that it fights water retention by helping the body eliminate excess fluid. It is also a central nervous system stimulant and believed to be a lipotropic, or fat-burning, herb. Gotu kola is also a constituent of numerous cellulite-fighting supplements. However, the *Physician's Desk Reference (PDR) for Herbal Medicines* does not cite research supporting any of these claims for gotu kola.

Because of its stimulating effect, you should avoid gotu kola if you have any chronic medical conditions. Side effects include insomnia and nervousness.

## Hoodia

Hoodia (*Hoodia gordonii*) is a spiny succulent that grows in the Kalahari Desert on the border of South Africa and Namibia. For thousands of years, it has been used by the Xhomani Bushmen, a people indigenous to the region, to stave off pain, hunger, and thirst during long-distance travel over the vast desert. In the 1960s, South African researches began studying the plant after the Xhomani revealed the plant's secrets to the South African army. Since then, hoodia has been studied for its various properties, including its ability to reduce weight by suppressing appetite. Only recently has it been introduced as a natural dietary supplement for weight control. But there haven't really been any human studies on hoodia, so we just don't know if the claims are valid.

## Saw Palmetto

Saw palmetto is one of several plants approved in Germany to help men with benign prostatic hypertrophy (BPH), an enlargement of the prostate gland. Purportedly, saw palmetto increases urinary flow, cuts the frequency of urination, and makes it easier to pass urine. It is used by more than 2 million men in the United States to treat BPH. But does it work? Well-designed research shows that the herb does not improve symptoms of BPH, nor does it help improve prostatitis, or chronic pelvic syndrome, which causes pain in the groin with or without urinary symptoms such as an urgency or frequency in the need to urinate.

## Tribulus Terrestris

Tribulus terrestris, also known as puncture weed, is a popular strength-training herb. This herb is believed to be a natural steroid that increases testosterone, enhances muscle mass, and boosts strength. Unfortunately, it does none of these, according to recent research.

# Potentially Harmful

The products in this category have been shown to cause harm and are not worth the risk. Although some of them may offer a few benefits, the risks are not worth the benefits.

## Ephedra

Ephedra is the world's oldest known cultivated plant. Also known as ma huang, Chinese ephedra, or Mormon tea, it is a short-acting stimulant and effective weight-loss aid and may be found in some cold remedies. Ephedra in dietary supplements was banned by the FDA several years ago because of safety concerns, including its harmful effect on the cardiovascular system. In April 2005, however, a federal judge struck down the ban, saying that the FDA was regulating ephedra as a drug and not as a food. The ruling allows supplement companies to bring back ephedra, but most haven't because of the bad press. In fact, many supplement makers now proudly market their products as ephedra free.

Ephedra has a lot of side effects, including nervousness, agitation, and rapid heartbeat. It can make the heart race and blood pressure soar, and it can be lethal in people with heart conditions, high blood pressure, or diabetes.

## Pau d'Arco

Pau d'arco, as an herbal agent, is found as a tea or in cosmetic preparations. The name refers to the bark of various species of trees. Pau d'arco is often billed as a cancer cure. Indeed, the bark contains a tiny amount of lapachol, an agent shown in research to have anticancer properties, but pau d'arco is potentially toxic and not to be fooled with.

Sassafras, usually found as a tea, is a well-known herb that may sound like a cure-all. It has been promoted as a stimulant; a muscle relaxant; a sweat producer; a blood purifier; and a treatment for rheumatism, skin diseases, and typhus. However, none of these benefits has been supported or even documented by medical science. Furthermore, sassafras contains an oil called safrole, which is carcinogenic.

## Yohimbe

Yohimbe is an herb derived from the bark of an evergreen grown in West Africa. It is best known for its aphrodisiac properties, because it stimulates erection. An extract of the herb, yohimbine, is available as a prescription drug for treating erectile dysfunction.

# Anti-Inflammatory Botanicals

A big part of Power Eating is including anti-inflammatory foods in your diet. One way to do this is to use botanicals that fight inflammation. Here are my top picks for anti-inflammatory botanicals.

## Mood-Boosting Botanicals

Several botanicals influence mood. They are typically not as potent as drugs and take longer to show an effect. Although side effects may also not be as potent as the negative side effects from drugs, because they do exist, dosages should always be according to label directions. Here's a rundown of these mood boosters:

- Passion flower—helps with calming, anxiety reduction, and better sleep.
- Chamomile—helps with calming, anxiety reduction, and better sleep.
- *Ginkgo biloba*—improves blood flow to the brain for clearer thinking.
- Kava kava—elevates mood and well-being, induces relaxation, and may lower anxiety. (I don't recommend it, though, because there are serious and dangerous side effects, including liver damage.)
- Saint-John's wort—relieves mild depression. (Caution: This herb can interfere with other drugs and should be used only under the care of a physician.)

## Ginger

This popular herb helps relieve symptoms of mild muscle pain and works like nonsteroidal anti-inflammatory drugs but without the negative side effects on your digestive tract. The recommended dose is between 2 and 7 grams daily. Ginger is also helpful for mild nausea; I recommend it to my clients who get nervous prior to competing in an event or race. Ginger comes in capsules and lozenges.

## Turmeric

This spice is used widely in Indian cooking. It contains a potent anti-inflammatory and antioxidant called curcumin. Curcumin works through several well-established pathways. As an antioxidant, it boosts levels of glutathione, one of the body's chief antioxidants. It also blocks the formation of prostaglandin E2, a compound that promotes inflammation within the body. You can reap the benefits of curcumin by spicing your foods with turmeric.

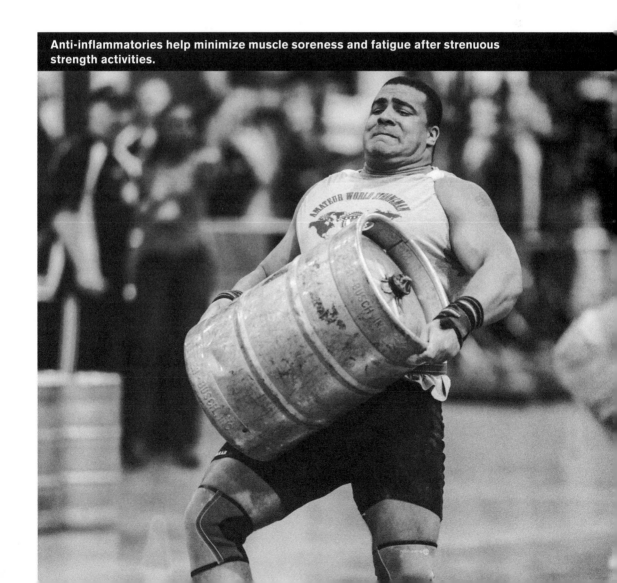

Anti-inflammatories help minimize muscle soreness and fatigue after strenuous strength activities.

## Flavonols

These phytochemicals are strong antioxidants and anti-inflammatories. They include quercetin, kaempferol, and myricetin, as well as the citrus bioflavonoids that include naringenin, hesperetin, and others. Green tea also contains flavonols. These beneficial compounds are easy to obtain from food. Foods rich in quercetin include capers, the green leafy vegetable lovage, apples, and chamomile tea. Kaempferol is found in tea, broccoli, cabbage, kale, beans, endives, leeks, tomatoes, strawberries and grapes, and in botanical supplements including *Ginkgo biloba* and propolis. Myricetin is found in grapes, berries, onions, tea, and walnuts. Flavonols are found most abundantly in citrus fruits, dark chocolate, and all types of teas.

## Botanicals That Beat the Bloat

Are you a physique competitor or someone who wants to look ripped? If so, there are botanicals that can help. For perspective, bloat is typically the result of too much salt in your diet, not enough fluid, or yo-yo dieting. Thus, the first thing to do is cut back on the salt in your diet or simply use herbs and spices to season your food. Then, make sure to drink enough water every day to help your kidneys excrete fluids.

Foods and botanicals that prevent bloat and balance fluid in your body are those high in electrolytes. Here are examples:

### Fruits and Vegetables
Asparagus
Celery
Cranberry juice
Cucumber
Dandelion
Eggplant
Fennel

### Herbs and Teas
Alfalfa tea
Black tea
Cardamom
Chamomile tea
Coriander
Dandelion or green tea
Parsley

Word of caution: Be careful not to overconsume these foods and herbs. You don't want to dehydrate yourself unnecessarily.

## Sport Nutrition Fact Versus Fiction: Are Functional Foods the New Training Staple?

If you've ever bitten into a sport bar, swilled a glass of calcium-fortified orange juice, or slurped a soup beefed up with herbs such as Saint-John's wort or echinacea, you've feasted on a functional food.

Technically, the term *functional food* refers to a food product that enhances performance or is beneficial to health. In its position paper on functional foods, the Academy of Nutrition and Dietetics defines these products as "any modified food or food ingredient that may provide a health benefit beyond the traditional nutrients it contains" (American Dietetic Association, 735-746).

Products that fit this definition include the following:

- **Foods in which sugar, fat, sodium, or cholesterol have been reduced or eliminated.** Fat-free cheese, reduced-sugar jam, or low-sodium soup are all examples. Functional foods such as these are beneficial to people on restricted diets and may be helpful in preventing or controlling obesity, cardiovascular disease, diabetes, and high blood pressure.

- **Foods in which naturally occurring ingredients have been increased.** Breakfast cereal and pasta that have been enriched with additional fiber or vitamins are good examples. Foods modified in this way can play an important role in preventing disease.

- **Foods enhanced with nutrients not normally present.** Folic acid–enriched bread and soups or soft drinks spruced up with therapeutic herbs are good examples. Enriched foods help people take in higher levels of health-protective nutrients and can be important in maintaining general wellness.

- **Probiotic yogurt and other dairy products to which special healthy bacteria have been added as a part of the fermentation process.** These foods are believed to enhance the growth of healthy flora in the intestines, which improve digestion and prevent disease.

- **Sport foods targeting the nutrient and energy needs of athletes and exercisers.** These include sport drinks with added electrolytes; protein powders formulated with creatine, amino acids, and other nutrients; and sport bars packed with vitamins, minerals, or herbs. Functional foods such as these are designed to provide energy, enhance muscle growth, and replenish nutrients lost during exercise.

Should you incorporate these foods into your diet if you're not already doing so? The answer is yes, particularly if convenience is important and you're trying to enhance muscular health, strength, and growth. Sport foods, in particular, can help you achieve those goals. However, think of functional foods as supplements to your diet rather than as substitutes for real food. Ultimately, the best way to fuel your body is always to eat a varied, nutrient-rich diet of lean protein and dairy products, fruits, whole grains, vegetables, and the right kinds of fat.

Other important and potent anti-inflammatory and antioxidant botanicals with good supporting evidence include grape seed extract, elderberry, pomegranate, nettles, devil's claw, frankincense, flaxseed, milk thistle, and white willow bark.

## Precautions

If you're still curious and want to try an herbal supplement, do so with care by following a few precautions:

- Choose good-quality supplements by reputable manufacturers.
- Keep in mind that cost is not always a reliable gauge of quality.
- Do not exceed recommended dosages.
- Get advice from a trained health care professional.
- In general, supplement with simpler rather than more complicated formulas.
- Liquid forms may be easier during active treatment (easier to swallow and more easily absorbed).
- Consider taste and ease of swallowing in choosing the form of a supplement.
- Disclose any use of botanicals and herbal supplements to your health care team.

## TABLE 9.2 Rating Herbal Supplements

| Supplement | Meets marketing claims | Possibly meets marketing claims | Does not meet marketing claims | Potentially harmful |
|---|---|---|---|---|
| Buchu | ✔ | | | |
| Fo-ti | ✔ | | | |
| Guarana | ✔ | | | |
| Maté | ✔ | | | |
| Beetroot juice | | ✔ | | |
| Cayenne | | ✔ | | |
| Echinacea | | ✔ | | |
| Ginseng | | ✔ | | |
| Green tea | | ✔ | | |
| Burdock | | | ✔ | |
| Canaigre | | | ✔ | |
| Citrus aurantium | | | ✔ | |
| Coleus forskohlii | | | ✔ | |
| Cordyceps | | | ✔ | |
| Damiana | | | ✔ | |
| Gotu kola | | | ✔ | |
| Hoodia | | | ✔ | |
| Saw palmetto | | | ✔ | |
| Tribulus terrestris | | | ✔ | |
| Ephedra (ma huang) | | | | ✔ |
| Pau d'arco | | | | ✔ |
| Sassafras | | | | ✔ |
| Yohimbe | | | | ✔ |

# Plans and Menus

This part of the book is where you put your knowledge to work. You have the foundation, the information, and hopefully, the inspiration. Now let's put it all into practice, designing your own personalized Power Eating plan. To begin, determine your goals: do you want to maintain weight, build muscle, lose weight, or cut fat? Are you in your off-season trying to gain, or approaching a championship and planning for a peak? Are you new to strength training, or have you been training for years? Chapter 10 will walk you through the steps I take when I design a client's customized nutrition plan. With the information here, you can figure your calories and map out your protein, carbohydrate, and fat needs based on your personal goals, just as I would if you came to my office. Chapter 10 also provides the information you need to customize all of the menu plans presented later in this part. Chapter 11 gives you the ultimate competitive nutrition strategies for preparing your body to peak for competition. I've kept no top-level professional secrets from these pages—it's all here.

Each of the five diet strategies (maintaining weight, building muscle, cross-training, losing weight, and cutting fat) in chapters 12 through 16 offers a menu plan designed especially for novice strength trainers, or those who work out three or four times per week, and one for highly muscled strength trainers who work out five or more times per week. The menu plans are also divided into plans geared for women and those geared for men. The plans begin with the mathematical models I designed to create the menus. By plugging in your weight, you can create your own personalized diet plan. The menus in this section are examples based on the needs of a 180-pound (82 kg) man and a 130-pound (59 kg) woman. If your weight is different, just plug it into the formulas and you can create a personalized plan.

The menus are similar in food choices so you can easily move from one strategy to the next as your training goals change. Some menus place exercise in the morning and others place it in the late afternoon so you can see how to customize a menu to your training schedule. Always make sure to have a preworkout snack and a postworkout snack or meal. Menu planning takes some time and effort, but the results are worth it!

Once you've designed your diet, have some fun with the recipes in chapter 17. This chapter includes the special power drinks I created for the clients and teams I've worked with over the years. These drinks can be used in place of liquid supplements. Add liquid or powdered supplements to them for an extra boost. My family and I particularly enjoy the smoothies, and we make them daily. They're a great way to sneak in extra protein, fruit, and vegetable servings. Don't miss power breakfasts, either—they will give your day a tasty and energy-charged start. And I am very proud to include recipes designed by Shar Sault, two-time consecutive winner of the drug-tested World Figure Title of Ms. Natural Olympia. Shar is an awesome role model and a dear friend.

Most of all, train hard and Power Eat!

# 10

# Developing a Power Eating Plan

There are different schools of thought regarding the ideal way to help people change their dietary behaviors. One school has a less defined approach, giving guidelines and strategies for menu selection, but no specific menu plans. I have found that this method works best with people who don't have highly specific goals or those who are doing just about everything right but need a tweak here and there. For most people this approach leaves too much room for error and results in their never quite accomplishing their performance and physique goals. People with very idealized goals need a targeted plan so that they make strategic choices. That is why I offer specific plans that outline exactly how to eat to achieve your goals. You undertake rigorous training and need a diet to support that training.

The Power Eating plan begins with determining the proper calorie level and then the right distribution of protein, fat, and carbohydrate to meet your goal. Menu development is based on a food group plan that I have tweaked just a bit based on state-of-the-art nutrition science. Food groups force you to have variety in your diet and at the same time allow you to personalize your program through food choices and exchanges among groups. Use the sample diets as a starting point, and then add or subtract servings to meet your protein, carbohydrate, and fat needs.

I provide a lot of examples of fat servings to give you the freedom to personalize your plan. Lower-fat and nonfat milk and very lean and lean protein sources are the primary choices in the meal plans. The one exception is a whole egg, which is a medium-fat protein. There is also space in your diet for healthier fat from sources such as vegetable oils, olive oils, nuts, and seeds in place of animal fat that is higher in saturated fat. Consider any low-fat or fat-free protein supplements as very lean protein servings.

To use more medium-fat protein sources such as soy products, as well as the occasional high-fat protein source, just exchange one very lean protein serving plus one fat serving for one medium-fat protein serving. Exchange one lean protein serving plus one fat serving for one high-fat protein serving. Refer to the Nutrients per Food Group Serving chart to become proficient at food group exchanges. Remember that you can easily determine your fat grams once you have calculated your total calories and your protein and carbohydrate needs. All the leftover calories are fat calories. Divide fat calories by 9 to get your total fat grams per day.

You will also be able to add in teaspoons of sugar mostly as sport drinks and learn how to use these to your advantage. These high-glycemic foods can assist you in muscle recovery and work best around exercise.

A note on alcohol: Alcohol is metabolized more similarly to fat than any of the other macronutrients. Too much alcohol on a regular basis will slow your training, halt your fat loss, and even impair your health and safety. Thus, alcohol is not part of the Power Eating plan.

## Creating Your Diet Plan

Once you have calculated your daily nutrient and calorie needs, use the Nutrients per Food Group Serving table that follows to design your diet. This table shows the amount of nutrients in one serving from each food group. Make sure that you include choices from all of the food groups to ensure a well-balanced diet. Add liquid supplements to meet additional carbohydrate, protein, and calorie needs. Refer to the serving size charts in the next section to learn about serving sizes for each food group.

### Nutrients per Food Group Serving

| Food groups | Carbohydrate (g) | Protein (g) | Fat (g) | Calories |
|---|---|---|---|---|
| Bread and starch | 15 | 3 | 1 or less | 72-81 |
| Fruit | 15 | - | - | 60 |
| Nonfat milk | 12 | 8 | 0-1 | 80-89 |
| Low fat milk | 12 | 8 | 3 | 107 |
| Added sugar (1 tsp, 4 g) | 4 | - | - | 16 |
| Vegetables | 5 | 2 | - | 25 |
| Very lean protein | - | 7 | 0-1 | 35 |
| Lean protein | - | 7 | 3 | 55 |
| Medium protein | - | 7 | 5 | 75 |
| Fat protein | - | - | 5 | 45 |

Adapted from American Diabetes Association and American Dietetic Association, 1995, *Exchange lists for meal planning* (Alexandria, VA: American Diabetes Association).

# Knowing Your Portions

A portion is the amount of food used to determine the numbers of servings for each food group. It is not always the amount of food that you would think of as a serving, however. For example, one portion of cooked pasta is just 1/2 cup (70 g). But if you have pasta for dinner, you would likely eat at least 1 cup (140 g). One cup of pasta equals two servings from the bread and starch group.

Learning the portion sizes for servings is the foundation of success. It is the method by which calorie control is built into the Power Eating plan. If you are eating portions that are too large or too small, the plan will not work. The following charts list serving sizes for each food group. In the beginning, you should refer to this chart frequently, as well as weigh and measure foods to get a handle on portion sizes. After a few weeks, you will be able to do it on your own.

## Milk and Yogurt Group
*A portion equals 90 to 110 calories.*

| Food | Size of one portion |
|------|---------------------|
| Nonfat or low-fat milk | 1 cup (240 ml) |
| Evaporated nonfat milk | 1 cup (240 ml) |
| Nonfat dry milk powder | 1/3 cup (22 g) |
| Plain nonfat yogurt | 1 cup (230 g) |
| Nonfat or low-fat soy or rice milk, fortified with calcium and vitamins A and D | 1 cup (240 ml) |

## Vegetable Group
*Each portion contains 25 calories.*

| Food | Size of one portion |
|------|---------------------|
| Most cooked vegetables | 1/2 cup (81 g) |
| Most raw vegetables | 1 cup (30-100 g) |
| Raw lettuce | 2 cups (56 g) |
| Sprouts | 1 cup (30 g) |
| Vegetable juice | 6 oz (180 ml) |
| Vegetable soup | 1 cup (240 ml) |
| Tomato sauce | 1/2 cup (120 ml) |
| Salsa (made without oil) | 3 tbsp (45 g) |

# Fruit Group
*A portion contains 60 calories.*

| Food | Size of one portion |
| --- | --- |
| Most fruits, whole | 1 medium |
| Most fruits, chopped or canned in own juice | 1/2 cup (120 g) |
| Melon, diced | 1 cup (156 g) |
| Berries, cherries, grapes (whole) | 3/4 cup (80 g) |
| Fruit juice | 1/2 cup (120 ml) |
| Banana | 1 small |
| Grapefruit, mango | 1/2 |
| Plums | 2 each |
| Apricots | 4 each |
| Strawberries (whole) | 1 1/4 cup (180 g) |
| Kiwi | 1 each |
| Prunes, dried | 3 each |
| Figs | 2 each |
| Raisins | 2 tbsp (28 g) |
| Juice–cranberry, grape, fruit blends (100% juice) | 1/3 cup (80 ml) |
| Cranberry juice cocktail (reduced calorie) | 1 cup (240 ml) |

# Bread and Starch Group
*Each portion has 60 to 100 calories.*

| Food | Size of one portion |
| --- | --- |
| Bread | 1 slice |
| Pita | 1 small (1 oz) |
| Bagel, English muffin, bun | 1/2 small (1 oz) |
| Roll | 1 small |
| Cooked rice, cooked pasta | 1/2 cup (97 g) |
| Tortilla | 6 in. round (15 cm) |
| Crackers, large | 2, or 3-4 small |
| Croutons | 1/3 cup (13 g) |
| Pretzels, baked chips | 1 oz (30 g) |
| Rice cakes | 2 each |
| Cooked cereal | 1/2 cup (119 g) |
| Cold cereal, unsweetened | 1/2-1 cup (15-30 g) |
| Granola | 1/2 cup (30 g) |
| Corn, green peas, mashed potato | 1/2 cup (105 g) |
| Corn on the cob | 1 medium |
| White or sweet potato baked with skin | 1 small |

# Protein

*Each protein portion contains about 35 to 75 calories. Very lean servings contain 35 calories and 0 to 1 grams of fat; lean, 55 calories and 3 grams of fat; and medium-fat, 75 calories and 5 grams of fat.*

| Food | Size of one portion |
|---|---|
| **Very lean** | |
| White meat skinless poultry | 1 oz (30 g) |
| White fish | 1 oz (30 g) |
| Fresh or canned tuna in water | 1 oz (30 g) |
| All shellfish | 1 oz (30 g) |
| Beans, peas, and lentils* | 1/2 cup (100 g) |
| Cheeses and processed sandwich meat with 1 g of fat | 1 oz (30 g) |
| Egg whites | 2 each |
| **Lean** | |
| Select or choice grades of lean beef, pork, lamb, or veal trimmed to 0 fat | 1 oz ( 30 g) |
| Dark-meat skinless poultry or white-meat chicken with skin | 1 oz ( 30 g) |
| Oysters, salmon, catfish, sardines, tuna canned in oil | 1 oz (30 g) |
| Cheese and deli sandwich meat with 3 g of fat | 1 oz (30 g) |
| Parmesan cheese | 1 oz (30 g) |
| **Medium-fat** | |
| Most styles of beef, pork, lamb, veal—trimmed of fat, dark-meat poultry with skin | 1 oz (30 g) |
| Ground turkey or chicken | 1 oz (30 g) |
| Cheese with 5 g of fat | 1 oz (30 g) |
| Cottage cheese, 4.5% fat | 1/4 cup (56 g) |
| Whole egg | 1 each |
| Tempeh | 4 oz or 1/2 cup (120 g) |
| Tofu | 4 oz or 1/2 cup (120 g) |

*One portion counts as one very lean protein and one starch.

# Fats and Oils

*Each portion contains 45 calories.*

| Food | Size of one portion |
|---|---|
| Butter margarine | 1 tsp (5 g) |
| Cream cheese, cream, sour cream | 1 tbsp (15 g) |
| Cream cheese, whipped cream, sour cream (low fat or nonfat) | 1 tbsp (15 g) |
| Salad dressing (full fat) | 1 tbsp (15 g) |
| Salad dressing (low fat or nonfat) | 1 tbsp (15 g) |
| Avocado | 1/8 medium (2 tbsp, 30 g) |
| Olives, black | 8 large |
| Nuts | 6-10 |
| Seeds | 1 tbsp (9 g) |
| Peanut butter and other nut butters | 1/2 tbsp (8 g) |

# Added Sugar

*There is no way that I could give you an exhaustive list of all the added sugar in foods. No food manufacturer puts that information on the label. But you can figure it out yourself, just as I do, by following these basic guidelines. Every 1 teaspoon, or serving, of sugar contains 4 grams of carbohydrate and 16 calories (no protein or fat).*

## Cereals and grains

Grains do not contain any sugar. By looking at the Nutrition Facts label on the side of a box of cereal such as Shredded Wheat, you'll see 0 grams of sugar in a serving. Therefore, the manufacturer adds any sugar contained in a cereal. Most sweetened cereals contain 8 grams of sugar per serving, which is the equivalent of 2 teaspoons of added sugar, and many contain much more. The exception is cereals with added fruit. Some of the sugar in these cereals comes from the fruit. Look at the ingredient label. If any kind of sugar is listed ahead of the fruit, you know that the greatest proportion of the added sugar is not from the fruit. The same concept goes for breads, crackers, and other grain products. Any sugar on the label is added in processing.

## Yogurt and milk

One cup (8 oz, or 240 ml) of milk contains 12 grams of natural milk sugar, or lactose. If you look at the Nutrition Facts label on a carton of milk, you will see that one serving (1 cup) contains 12 grams of sugar. Any amount of sugar above that is added, as in chocolate milk and other flavored milks.

Yogurt cartons are generally 6 oz (180 g). A carton of plain yogurt will contain about 12 grams of natural milk sugar. Anything above that is added sugar. Most yogurts are sweetened with at least 4 teaspoons of added sugar, and many use 6 teaspoons or more.

## Fruit and fruit juices

A medium-sized piece of fruit contains about 15 grams of carbohydrate. Some of that is fiber, often 2 to 3 grams, and the rest is natural fruit sugar. When purchasing canned or frozen fruits and fruit juices, you must read the ingredients label to check for added sugar. Any amount of sugar above 15 grams for 1/2 cup (120 g) of canned or frozen fruit or 1/2 cup (120 ml) of fruit juice is added to the product.

## Vegetables, vegetable juices, and soups

A medium-sized vegetable contains 5 grams of carbohydrate and no sugar. Any sugar listed on the Nutrition Facts label is added to the product.

## Beverages

Obviously, water has no amount of natural sugar. So if you're looking at the Nutrition Facts label on the side of a can of soft drink, all the sugar is added, and it usually amounts to about 10 teaspoons (50 g) per 12-ounce (360 ml) can. Typical sport drinks contain about 12 grams of sugar per cup, equivalent to 3 teaspoons (15 g) of added sugar per serving. This same principle can be applied to most bottled beverages that do not contain any milk or fruit juice. When it comes to fruit juice concentrates added as sweeteners to beverages and foods, the juice is highly refined in the processing and is little more than sugar syrup. Ingredients such as white grape juice concentrate are virtually the same as added sugar.

# Personalizing the Plan

To achieve the greatest strength and muscle gain, follow these guidelines when designing your diet:

## 1. Assess Calorie Needs Based on Body Weight

As your weight changes, you must recalculate energy and nutrients. Chapters 12 through 16 outline the calorie needs for each phase of the plan to help you do this.

### Training to Maintain Muscle

Men who train five or more times per week need 42 calories per kilogram of body weight a day (3,444 calories a day for a 180 lb [82 kg] man). Women who train five or more times per week may be able to increase muscle at 44 to 50 calories per kilogram of body weight a day (2,950 calories for a 130 lb [59 kg] woman) and maintain at about 38 to 40 calories per kilogram of body weight a day (2,360 calories). The larger and more muscular a woman is, the more calories she can handle for maintenance.

Smaller women may need fewer than 38 calories per kilogram of body weight per day to maintain weight. There is a lot of trial and error with women, because all the research has been done on men and because levels of activity vary widely.

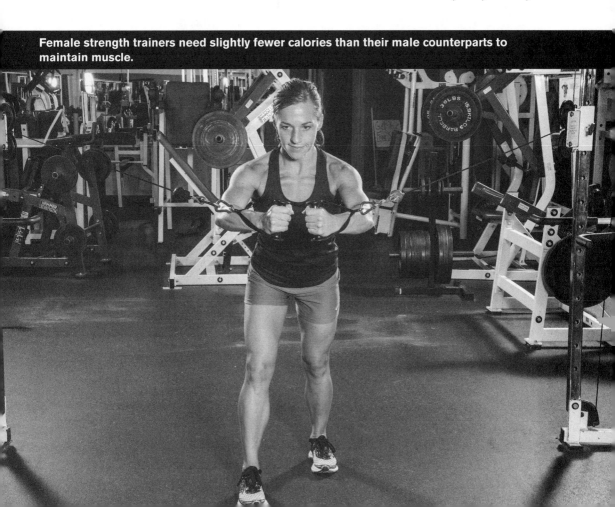

Female strength trainers need slightly fewer calories than their male counterparts to maintain muscle.

For the rest of the phases, women should generally choose the lower end of the calorie ranges. This diet is great for bodybuilders, powerlifters, and weightlifters, as well as for recreational strength trainers. Novice trainers should follow the novice guidelines.

### Building

This plan requires 44 to 52 or more calories per kilogram of body weight a day, depending on the intensity of training (4,264 or more calories for a 180 lb [82 kg] man; 2,596 to 2,950 calories for a 130 lb [59 kg] woman). Start low and add calories as needed. As stated earlier, women will likely be able to build at 44 calories per kilogram of body weight a day. Smaller women should try slightly fewer calories when beginning a building program and work up from there. This diet is good for all competitive and recreational strength trainers. Novice trainers should follow the novice guidelines.

### Losing Fat

To lose fat and begin to sculpt (10 to 12 weeks of precontest dieting), you'll need 35 to 38 calories per kilogram of body weight a day (3,116 calories for a 180 lb [82 kg] man; 2,065 calories for a 130 lb [59 kg] woman). Because it's more difficult for women to lose fat than it is for men, women should choose the lower calorie range and increase aerobic exercise in order to burn 300 to 400 calories a day. Again, smaller women may need fewer calories. This recommendation is primarily for bodybuilders. Novice trainers should follow the novice guidelines.

### Cutting

This plan requires 29 calories per kilogram of body weight a day (7 to 14 days maximum) for women (1,711 calories for a 130 lb [59 kg] woman) and 32 calories per kilogram of body weight a day for men (2,624 calories for a 180 lb [82 kg] man). If you are a smaller woman who has been losing fat at a lower calorie level, decrease recommended calories here as well. Use this approach only when absolutely necessary. This diet is only for bodybuilders or others trying to make a weight class—not for powerlifters or Olympic weightlifters.

### Powerlifters and Weightlifters Trying to Make a Weight Class

After dieting to build muscle, go back to the maintenance diet for two weeks before your meet and use your goal weight for the calculations. This will allow for loss of body fat without loss of muscle, strength, or power. This strategy is also a good basic diet for overweight strength trainers who want to lose body fat.

## 2. Calculate Your Protein Needs

Protein needs change with both energy intake and training goals. Although the menu plans in chapters 12 through 16 provide grams per pound of body weight, you can easily convert your weight from pounds to kilograms by dividing your weight by 2.2. Make sure to cover your protein needs during all four diet strategies. If you are a vegan, add 10 percent more protein to all of the plans.

| | |
|---|---|
| Maintenance | 1.4 grams per kilogram of body weight a day |
| Building | Women: 2.0-2.2 grams per kilogram of body weight a day |
| | Men: 2.5 grams per kilogram of body weight a day |
| Losing fat | 2.2 grams per kilogram of body weight a day |
| Cutting | 2.3 grams per kilogram of body weight a day; 2.5 grams per kilogram of body weight a day for those eating a mostly vegetarian or vegan diet |

## 3. Calculate Your Carbohydrate Needs

Calculate your carbohydrate needs as 5 to 7 grams per kilogram of body weight a day. Strength trainers need closer to 5 to 6 grams per kilogram of body weight a day for maintenance and 6.5 to 7 grams per kilogram of body weight a day for building. Cross-trainers who do an intense ultra type of sport such as an Ironman event need closer to 8 to 10 grams per kilogram of body weight a day. Novice athletes need less carbohydrate at all levels of training, but the amount will increase as they increase their training intensity.

During fat-loss and cutting phases, women and men need different amounts of carbohydrate. Here is the amount of carbohydrate needed per kilogram of body weight per day.

| | |
|---|---|
| Losing fat | Women: 2.5 to 3.5 grams per kilogram |
| | Men: 3 to 4 grams per kilogram |
| Cutting | Women: 1.8 to 2.9 grams per kilogram |
| | Men: 2.3 to 3 grams per kilogram |

## 4. Calculate Your Fat Needs

The rest of your calories will be 25 to 30 percent of the total. Fat sources should be predominantly monounsaturated and polyunsaturated, including omega-3 fat, with much less saturated fat.

To find the number of fat grams you need in your plan, first determine the calories of protein and carbohydrate that you have calculated for yourself (1 g protein = 4 calories; 1 g carbohydrate = 4 calories). Then subtract those calories from the total number of calories needed for your weight and training phase, and you have the number of fat calories you need. Fat contains 9 calories per gram, so if you divide the fat calories by 9, you have your grams of fat.

Here's an example of a maintenance diet for a novice 180-pound (82 kg) man:

| | |
|---|---|
| Calories: | 33 calories per kilogram |
| | $33 \times 82$ kg = 2,706 calories |

| | |
|---|---|
| Protein: | 1.4 grams per kilogram |
| | $1.4 \times 82$ kg = 115 g protein |
| Carbohydrate: | 4.5 grams per kilogram |
| | $4.5 \times 82$ kg = 369 g carbohydrate |
| Fat: | The leftover calories, or about 1 g per kilogram |

Calculate the calories in the protein and carbohydrate grams:

$$115 \text{ g protein} \times 4 \text{ calories/g} = 460 \text{ protein calories}$$
$$369 \text{ g carbohydrate} \times 4 \text{ calories/g} = 1{,}476 \text{ carbohydrate calories}$$
$$460 + 1{,}476 = 1{,}936 \text{ protein and carbohydrate calories}$$

Then, calculate the fat calories and grams.

$$2{,}706 \text{ total calories} - 1{,}936 \text{ protein and carbohydrate calories} = 770 \text{ fat calories}$$
$$770 \text{ fat calories} / 9 \text{ calories} = 86 \text{ g of fat}$$

So, the diet consists of 2,706 calories, 115 grams of protein, 369 grams of carbohydrate, and 86 grams of fat. Then, by using the chart of the nutritional content of food groups, you can write your own diet. Use the menus that I have written as your guide. An easy solution is to add or subtract portions from the menus that I have already written for you. For instance, if you need to subtract carbohydrate grams, remove some servings of sugar; if you need to subtract fat grams, remove some servings of fat, and so on.

## POWER PROFILE: A Winning Formula

A championship high school football team in Pennsylvania was accused by the local newspaper of taking creatine—even performance-enhancing drugs—because the players had gotten so big. But when confronted with these accusations, the coach replied, "All we are using is Dr. Susan Kleiner's Power Eating diet. That is our winning formula."

This high school won five district football championships and four state championships through 2000. In 2004 they were the Suburban One League American Conference Champs. They just won their fourth championship in a row. Since 1998, I have been working with the strength coach on nutrition strategies for the players. The players have more energy, endurance, muscle, and power during training, practices, and games. The team is always ranked in the top 20 in the nation or among those to watch nationwide.

# Adjusting the Plan for Competitive Bodybuilders and Physique Athletes

If you're preparing for a contest, begin the fat-loss phase 10 to 12 weeks before your contest. Decrease calories and increase your aerobic exercise. However, if you simply up the intensity and duration of your aerobic exercise, you'll lose some muscle, along with fat. The solution is to do high-intensity interval training (HIIT). It enables you to get extremely defined, without burning up precious muscle mass. HIIT involves performing intervals of high-intensity exercise at a rate near 90 percent of your maximum heart rate (MHR) interspersed with intervals of slower-paced activity. It is fine to do some aerobic work, but ramp up your HIIT training.

If you're not looking as ripped as you would like, follow the cutting program for one or two weeks prior to your contest. Consume 29 to 32 calories per kilogram of body weight a day for this phase. This will allow for a final loss of 3 to 4 pounds (1.4 to 1.8 kg), as long as you keep up your HIIT. Make sure to increase your protein intake to 2.3 grams per kilogram of body weight a day.

## Sticking to Your Plan

For these strategies to work, you have to stick to your Power Eating plan. Design your diet with foods that you like. Use the sample diets in chapters 12 through 16 to help you design your personal plan. If you don't like the foods you're supposed to eat, you won't stick to the plan. If you're using liquid supplements, try different brands and flavors to find ones you like.

Pay attention to your body and plan to eat when you're hungry. You might want to pick specific times of the day to eat rather than depending on the pace of each day. But also be aware of whether you are hungry or thirsty; sometimes we confuse thirst with hunger. Keep food and drink on hand wherever you go. The most successful strength trainers always have a backpack full of food and drink that goes with them everywhere. This way, they can stick to their timed eating patterns, and if they get hungry, they're not dependent on vending machines or other snack foods that are high in fat and sodium.

### POWER PROFILE: Plan, Don't Panic

Here's a familiar story: Melody B., a 35-year-old female executive, was a yo-yo dieter who could never keep her lost weight off, despite a regular program of strength training and aerobic exercise. At 5 feet, 6 inches (168 cm) and 150 pounds (68 kg), Melody had tried every fad diet, product, and diet drug there was, all to no avail. She was muscular, but her body-fat percentage was too high.

In just six weeks on the Power Eating diet, Melody lost 1 percent of her body fat and one whole dress size. After this experience, she became so excited about fitness and nutrition that she started her own health and fitness promotion company. After going on the diet, Melody had this to say: "Susan saved my life. Before, I couldn't go on any longer thinking about food all the time. Now I just know what to do and I do it, because it feels good."

When you're trying to lose fat, you might find it difficult to eat at restaurants, and it might be especially difficult to travel. If you must do either, try to find restaurants that specialize in healthy fare. They should be able to easily adjust their menu to meet your personal needs. Don't forget to ask what's in the recipe. A menu description may be misleading. You can even ask for foods that aren't on the menu—restaurants may be able to accommodate your request.

Remember to always recalculate your requirements based on your present weight. If you have gained weight during a building or bulking phase and now want to lose weight, use your new weight rather than that of the prebulking phase.

No one can do this for you. You know that to get big and strong, you have to work your body hard. You also have to fuel your body to grow, and this is the best way. Plan your diet and stick to it. You'll be thrilled with how you feel, how you look, and how you perform.

## Sport Nutrition Fact Versus Fiction: Fast-Food Nutrition

If yours is an on-the-go lifestyle, I've included many fast and delicious recipes that you can prepare in under 10 minutes and take with you on the road. Alternatively, it's fine to eat at fast-food restaurants on occasion. The key is to make the right choices—those that are low in fat and high in nutrition. Fortunately, fast-food restaurants today cater to the healthier preferences of consumers. So if you're really serious about your training, get serious about your eating, too (see appendix B for a guide to restaurant eating and healthy fast food).

When you get caught without the food you need, here are some fast-food tips to keep you on track.

- Always order the regular-sized (vs. large) sandwiches, because they are lower in unhealthy fat and calories.
- Instead of ordering a bigger sandwich, order a salad and low-fat milk.
- Stay away from fried foods.
- Don't eat the high-fat tortilla shells from taco salads.
- Request that sour cream and secret sauces be left off your order.
- Top your baked potato with chili instead of fatty cheese sauce.
- Whatever you order, order just one!

# Power Eating Grocery Shopping List

Meal planning also includes grocery planning. I advise going to the grocery store with a list of Power Eating foods you'll need, week by week. Sticking to your list will help you stay on track. What follows is an example of a good shopping list.

## Lean Proteins

- [ ] Turkey
- [ ] Chicken
- [ ] Salmon
- [ ] Tuna
- [ ] Other fish
- [ ] Lean beef, lamb, pork

---

- [ ] Omega-3 eggs
- [ ] Mixed beans
- [ ] Veggie sausage links

## Dairy

- [ ] Fat-free or low-fat milk
- [ ] Fat-free or low-fat plain yogurt
- [ ] Low-fat sour cream
- [ ] Low-fat cheeses

## Fruits and Vegetables

- [ ] Mixed berries
- [ ] Citrus fruit
- [ ] Other fruits (apples, bananas, mangos)

---

- [ ] Raw spinach
- [ ] Carrots
- [ ] Broccoli, cauliflower, cabbage
- [ ] Tomatoes
- [ ] Lettuce, kale
- [ ] Whole mushrooms
- [ ] Cucumbers
- [ ] Lemons
- [ ] Green beans
- [ ] Onions
- [ ] Fresh garlic
- [ ] Red and green peppers
- [ ] Other veggies (okra, sweet potatoes)

---
---

## Nuts and Seeds

- [ ] Peanut or other nut butters
- [ ] Mixed raw nuts (almonds, pecans)
- [ ] Whole or ground flaxseed

## Grains

- [ ] Whole-grain bread
- [ ] Steel-cut oats
- [ ] Oat bran
- [ ] Wheat bran
- [ ] Quinoa grain
- [ ] Whole-wheat tortillas
- [ ] Brown rice
- [ ] Taco shells
- [ ] Other grains

## Fats and Oils

- [ ] Extra-virgin olive oil
- [ ] Cooking spray (canola or olive)
- [ ] Butter, coconut oil, or spread

## Other

- [ ] Sea salt
- [ ] Black pepper
- [ ] Garlic powder
- [ ] Cinnamon
- [ ] Cumin
- [ ] Turmeric
- [ ] Paprika
- [ ] Fajita seasoning
- [ ] Stevia or Truvia
- [ ] Lemon juice
- [ ] Fat-free salad dressing
- [ ] Non-Dutched, non-alkali cocoa powder
- [ ] Salsa
- [ ] Mustard
- [ ] Balsamic vinegar
- [ ] Raspberry vinegar

# 11

# Planning a Peak

Perhaps you've decided to fine-tune your physique to look more trim, fit, and muscular. Maybe you desire to take your strength training up a notch—to competitive bodybuilding, powerlifting, or weightlifting. Or perhaps you're already a competitive strength trainer who's searching for that extra edge. No matter what your ambition, proper nutrition is the key.

You may not realize it, but the same nutritional techniques that work for bodybuilders and other athletes can also be applied to recreational exercisers and strength trainers. That's because the goals are generally the same: increasing muscularity (degree of muscular bulk), etching in definition (absence of body fat), and training for symmetry (shape and size of muscles in proportion to each other).

Whether you're trying to get in shape for swimsuit season, preparing for a bodybuilding competition, cross-training to support another sport, or building strength for your sport, you strive to reduce body fat without sacrificing muscle mass so as to reveal as much muscular definition as possible. Or perhaps one of your chief goals is building strength and muscle mass, either for looks and health or because you're a competitive powerlifter and weightlifter. In these cases, your goal is to lift as much weight as possible when you train and compete.

If you're a competitor, you'll be required to make weight to qualify for a specific weight class. You must focus on gaining and preserving muscular weight and losing body fat to achieve your contest weight. Diet therefore plays a critical role in precontest preparation for all competitive strength trainers who want to achieve peak shape.

Until recently, most strength athletes partitioned their diets into two distinct phases: a bulking phase, in which the competitor eats huge amounts of food without much regard to sound nutrition practices or to the type of calories taken in from food, and a cutting phase, in which drastic measures such as starvation dieting and drugs are used to lose weight rapidly in the weeks before a contest. Even if you're not a competitor, you've probably done something similar: bulking up in the winter; then crash dieting to get in shape for summer.

Unless sound nutritional practices are followed, the cutting phase, much like a crash diet, can be unhealthy, rigid, monotonous, and damaging to performance. And bulking up tends to pile on fat weight, which is that much harder to lose when it comes time to get in shape or prepare for competition.

Today, though, more strength athletes choose to stay in competition shape year-round. That way, it's easier to lose body fat because there's less to lose, and the process of cutting is much safer and more successful. And we all want to look our best all the time. You never know when you might have a photo shoot opportunity!

This chapter outlines a step-by-step diet strategy called tapering that lets you lose maximum body fat, retain hard-earned muscle, and perform at your best. This strategy works for exercisers, bodybuilders, and strength athletes—anyone who wants to become lean and muscular. The end of the chapter covers key issues for bodybuilders, powerlifters, and weightlifters.

# Step 1: Plan Your Start Date

The length of time you spend dieting depends on how out of shape you are to begin with. If you've let yourself get too fat by bulking up, then you'll really have to stretch your dieting out by several months.

A caution for bodybuilding competitors: Don't start your dieting too close to your contest. You'll be too tempted to resort to crash dieting, which can result in loss of muscle, decreased strength and power, low energy, moodiness and irritability, and low immunity. Losing lots of fat in a short period of time is virtually impossible for most people, anyway. Physiologically, no one can lose more than 4 pounds (1.8 kg) of pure fat a week even by total fasting. Instead, take a gradual approach to dieting.

Start your diet or contest preparation about 10 to 12 weeks before your competition. During this period, make slight adjustments to your calorie and nutrient intake, as well as to your aerobic exercise level. In addition, supplement with creatine and drink one of my muscle-building formulas (see chapter 17).

# Step 2: Determine a Safe Reduction in Calories

Getting cut is essential for achieving physique perfection, as well as for achieving competitive success in a sport such as bodybuilding. One way to begin this process is by slightly reducing your caloric intake. I use this strategy with any of my athlete clients who need to reduce body fat to enhance performance. By consuming fewer calories, you can gradually reduce body fat. However, you don't want to cut calories too much. A drastic reduction in calories will slow down your resting metabolic rate (RMR) for two reasons. The first has to do with the thermic effect of food (TEF), which is the increase in RMR after you eat a meal as food is digested and metabolized. Eating more calories increases the thermic effect of food and, along with it, your RMR. Likewise, cutting calories decreases the TEF as well as your RMR. Without enough calories to drive your metabolic processes, your body has a harder time burning calories to lose body fat.

Second, long periods of calorie deprivation—that is, diets under 1,200 calories a day—lower your RMR as a result of the starvation adaptation response. This response simply means that your metabolism has slowed down to accommodate your lower caloric intake. Your body is stockpiling dietary fat and calories rather than burning them for energy. You can actually gain body fat on a diet of fewer than 1,200 calories a day.

The starvation adaptation response has been observed frequently in undernour-ished endurance athletes. In a study of triathletes, researchers found that these athletes weren't consuming enough calories to fuel themselves for training and competition. When calories were increased, the athletes' weight stayed the same. This occurred because their RMRs returned to normal with the introduction of ample calories. To keep your metabolism running in high gear, you have to eat enough calories to match your energy requirements.

When you drastically cut calories, you also slash your fat intake too much. That's a problem because you starve your brain of the fat it requires for nourishment. Consequently, your brain sends messages to your body to hang on to fat rather than burn it. In men, the low fat intake also diminishes the production of anabolic hormones. So there's no good reason to slash your fat intake.

While dieting, reduce your calories by up to 300 each day if you are a woman and 400 each day if you are a man. This is the ideal metabolic window for fat burn-ing and will not adversely affect your RMR. (See chapter 5 for a discussion of this metabolic window.) At the same time, increase your aerobic exercise to burn up to 300 to 400 calories a day. This type of caloric manipulation will help you burn fat efficiently. You'll lose more fat in the initial weeks, and then you'll need to increase your exercise and probably lower your calories as you continue to shed body weight. I've designed the Power Eating fat-loss (chapter 15) and cutting (chapter 16) plans with exactly these scientific concepts in mind.

You might wonder, "Why can't I just crash diet for a few weeks to get in shape?" After all, I'm training hard with weights. Shouldn't strength training protect me from losing muscle?

As logical as this argument sounds, scientific research proves otherwise. Case in point: In one study, overweight women were divided into two groups: a group that only dieted and a group that dieted and strength trained. The diet provided only 800 calories a day, and the study lasted four weeks. The results revealed that both groups lost the same amount of weight (11 lb, or 5 kg). Even the composi-tion of the lost weight was the same. All the women lost 8 pounds (3.6 kg) of fat and 3 pounds (1.4 kg) of muscle. The bottom line is that strength training does not preserve muscle under these low-calorie dieting conditions, but it does when caloric restriction isn't so severe.

The implications are clear: In just four short weeks, you can lose precious muscle if you crash diet. Watch how low you go in decreasing your caloric intake. Research with bodybuilders confirms that you can lose muscle in just seven days on calories as low as 18 per kilogram (8.2 per pound) of body weight a day.

## Step 3: Increase Aerobic Exercise

To sculpt a fit physique, increase the intensity and duration of your aerobic exercise. Aerobic exercise stimulates the activity of a fat-burning enzyme called *hormone-sensitive lipase*, which breaks down stored fat and moves it into circulation to be burned for energy. Aerobic exercise also increases $\dot{V}O_2$max—the capability to process oxygen and transport it to body tissues. Fat is burned most efficiently when sufficient oxygen is available.

If you put a lot of effort into your aerobic exercise, you may not have to reduce your calories. That's the conclusion of a recent study from West Virginia University. Women of normal weight were able to decrease their body fat within three months simply by exercising aerobically four days a week for about 45 minutes each time at a heart rate between 80 and 90 percent of their maximum. They didn't have to cut calories, yet still lost plenty of body fat. But they trained hard!

Here's some more good news: The better trained you are aerobically—and the leaner you are—the better your body can burn fat for energy. By increasing $\dot{V}O_2$max and thus the oxygen available to tissues, aerobic exercise enhances the ability of your muscles to combust fat as fuel. At the cellular level, the breakdown of fat speeds up, and it's released faster from storage sites in fat and muscle tissue.

In addition, focus on HIIT, which alternates short bursts (one to two minutes) of high-intensity exercise with short bursts (one to two minutes) at a lower intensity. Research has shown this form of exercise to keep your metabolic rate elevated for many hours following your workout and is thus an effective fat-burning strategy. Plus, it maximizes your time in the gym and gives you a great whole-body workout.

Women's bodies can burn a lot of fat with regular aerobic exercise, including HIIT, which will result in their staying very lean. Men, however, burn more carbohydrate through aerobic exercise than they do fat. Too much aerobic exercise can be detrimental to a man's ability to burn fat; in fact, it may cause muscle loss. I recommend that men focus on HIIT three or four times a week at most to protect their muscle.

There's no doubt about it: Aerobic exercise, particularly when done in addition to HIIT, is a miracle worker when it comes to fat burning. Stay aerobically fit year-round and you'll have no trouble shedding those last few pounds of pudge.

## Step 4: Eat More Protein

To shed body fat, you should be eating at least 2.2 grams of protein per kilogram of body weight a day. This level will help you maintain muscle mass. Increasing your protein intake during a time of calorie reduction helps protect against muscle loss; the extra protein can be used as a backup energy source in case your body needs it.

## Step 5: Plan Your Diet to Go From Heavy to Light

Eat your largest meal first thing in the morning. You guessed it: I'm talking about breakfast. Strength trainers and other health-conscious people need to take breakfast as seriously as they take their other meals and snacks.

Breakfast literally "breaks the fast" to get nutrients to your famished bodies. Plus, it can actually boost your metabolism. By contrast, there is also proof that skipping breakfast actually lowers your metabolic rate. The thermic effect of food—how many calories are used to digest your food—is higher in the morning and tapers off slightly throughout the day.

What makes a good breakfast? Clean carbohydrate such as that found in whole-grain cereal or bread and fresh fruit and some lean protein, maybe a little fat, make an excellent first meal of the day. Carbohydrate, in particular, helps with appetite control and boosts fat burning all day long. You don't have to be limited to break-fast foods, either. Enjoy some whole-grain bread and light cheese, or some chicken or fish, if you wish.

## Step 6: Time Your Meals and Exercise

When you are well fueled throughout the day, you can train harder and burn more calories. Before, during, and directly after exercise, put your high-glycemic, fast carbohydrates to work for you. Depending on your goal, sometimes it is best to consume them during and after exercise. That's when your body can best burn them for the energy you need to build solid muscle. The rest of the day, focus on slow carbohydrate sources such as vegetables and beans.

After your workout, be sure to take in protein, carbohydrate, and fat to replenish your glycogen stores and create a hormonal environment in your body that is conducive to building muscle.

As you time your meals, be careful about overrestricting food. This can backfire and make you lose control by bingeing. It's better to allow yourself foods you consider "treats" than try to shun them altogether. Research supports the concept of controlled "cheating" to help you stay the course. I encourage my clients to enjoy a few of their favorite foods every so often, but to try to eat them when they can best burn them off—say, at breakfast or after a workout. That way, these foods become "recovery rewards." This optimistic attitude toward treats will keep you on track to meet your goals.

## Step 7: Don't Neglect Carbohydrate

As far as the rest of your diet is concerned, don't cut too much carbohydrate, or you're going to be really sluggish and out of sorts. A lack of carbohydrate will adversely affect your energy levels and mood. It's critical to have some carbohydrate in your diet throughout the tapering phase. The best choices are slow carbohydrates such as veggies, whole grains, beans, and low-fat dairy.

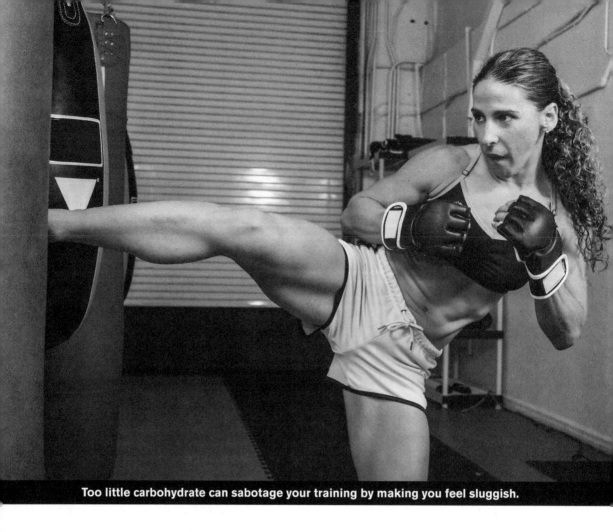

Too little carbohydrate can sabotage your training by making you feel sluggish.

I do, however, recommend cutting back on added sugars—sweets, nondiet sodas, and table sugar in your coffee or tea. As I've mentioned previously, added sugars are beneficial only around exercise when they're efficiently burned off for energy.

With the recommended increase in your protein intake, for the peaking diet your total calories might look something like this: protein, 30 to 35 percent; carbohydrate, 40 percent; and fat, 25 to 30 percent. As long as you don't cut calories too drastically, you'll still have enough carbohydrate to support your training requirements. You can even have a minimal amount of added sugar (if you really can't live without it) and still meet the 40 percent carbohydrate requirement, although I prefer that you use your carbohydrate calories to eat nutritionally dense foods such as milk, vegetables, and fruits.

Some very low-carbohydrate diets can hinder your training. Case in point: A study published in the Journal of the International Society of Sports Nutrition pointed out that the Atkins diet decreased exercise capacity in nine exercisers. Yes, they lost weight; however, they had a significant drop in their blood glucose levels, and this caused them to fatigue very early on during their workouts. This type of diet and others like it are neither appropriate nor necessary for active people.

## Solving the Problem of Added Sugars in Performance and Recovery

When fueling for exercise and recovery, high-glycemic index (fast) carbohydrates are king. That means some combination of added sugar or sugarlike ingredients. These range from sucrose, glucose, and fructose to maltodextrin and isomaltulose.

Ideally, if you are doing long-duration exercise, you should front-load your fuel with these types of sugars. But here is a red flag warning: Too much added sugar can cause stomach and GI discomfort—not a helpful feeling if you're competing in a marathon or triathlon and want to finish strong.

I don't give a shoutout to a specific brand unless it stands alone in terms of quality and research evidence. This is one of those times. A promising new solution to the sugar issue is a patented amylopectin (starch) fraction used in the starch-based product Vitargo S2. Backed by a number of peer-reviewed research studies from the same laboratory that did work on carbohydrate loading, creatine, and beta-alanine, as well as from other labs, this unique starch fraction empties from the stomach and is delivered to the muscle cells nearly twice as fast as any other carbohydrate available. This is true even when compared to the fastest carbohydrate typically used in top sport drinks, maltodextrin. A published performance study showed enhanced work output and endurance performance during a cycling time trial in subjects supplemented with Vitargo S2 versus those taking a 98 percent maltodextrin and 2 percent sugar carbohydrate supplement or water.

Based on this research, I have begun to suggest Vitargo S2 to my clients. It is not only very well tolerated as a sport supplement, but also has enabled me to create even healthier diet plans. Because it is so rapidly emptied from the stomach, athletes can load carbohydrate before exercise better than they could before. They can therefore take in the majority of their dietary starch before, during, and after exercise to best support performance and recovery. Because they can minimize if not eliminate added sugar, they have lots of room for an abundance of vegetables all day long. They don't have to have so many added sugar and starch servings just to get in the levels of carbohydrate that they needed to previously, especially in building and cross-training diets.

If you want to try what I now do frequently in my practice, substitute grams of starch carbohydrate from Vitargo S2 for grams of added sugar in sport drinks. You'll be able to pack in much more, in fact, and perhaps minimize some of the starch servings in your diet the rest of the day as well. For fat and weight loss, this offers the edge you need. But be aware that this product works best to support intense exercise. It even says so on the label!

# Step 8: Focus on High-Performance Fat

When your goal is to build lean muscle mass (the building diet), there is plenty of room in your plan for the right types of dietary fat. However, when you are trying to peak in a fat-loss or cutting diet, there isn't any room for the wrong kinds of fat. Fat is critical to your success and should be eaten in the right proportions with protein and the right types of carbohydrate.

The key is to focus on healthy monounsaturated fat, including fat from vegetable oils, olives, nuts, and avocados. Continue to obtain your omega-3 fat from fatty fish and a little flaxseed meal. And make sure to supplement with omega-3 (DHA and EPA) supplements.

Always avoid saturated and trans fat from processed snack foods, commercially baked goods, and fried foods, because they will sabotage your progress.

# Step 9: Space Your Meals

Your body will better use its calories for energy, rather than deposit them as fat, if you eat several small meals throughout the day. Most bodybuilders and other strength athletes eat five, six, or more meals a day. Spacing meals in this manner keeps you fueled throughout the day. Plus, the more times you eat, the higher your metabolism stays, thanks to the thermic effect of food. In other words, every time you eat, your metabolism accelerates. Eating multiple meals throughout the day is a good dietary practice regardless of whether you're dieting for competition.

# Step 10: Include Anti-Inflammatory Foods

Exercise can increase free radical production and inflammation in the body. However, you can mitigate these processes by choosing anti-inflammatory foods and immune-boosting foods, all of which are loaded with antioxidants. The key is to choose bright, colorful vegetables and fruits (I'm not talking about Fruit Loops or Trix cereals, either!), from green spinach to sweet oranges. You can also get many of these healing nutrients from dairy products, eggs, and fish. Fish is especially high in omega-3 fatty acids, which have very effective anti-inflammatory properties.

Here is a list of healing foods to consider:

| | | |
|---|---|---|
| Citrus fruits | Broccoli | Tomatoes |
| Carrots | Pineapple | Apples |
| Oranges | Bananas | Star fruits |
| Papayas | Mangos | Kiwi fruits |
| Blood oranges | Passion fruits | Prickly pears |
| Strawberries | Cherries | Cranberries |
| Raspberries | Blueberries | Red grapes |
| Black currants | Green tea | |

At the same time, stay away from or limit "pro-inflammatory foods." These are foods that activate inflammation in your body. The biggest offender here is added sugar; by shunning processed foods and sweets, you automatically reduce harmful inflammation in your body. Pro-inflammatory foods include omega-6 fat sources, such as safflower oil, sunflower oil, soybean oil, and corn oil.

## Step 11: Supplement Prudently

There are some real nutritional horror stories among people who crash diet or diet stringently for contests. They tend to suffer deficiencies in calcium, magnesium, zinc, vitamin D, and other nutrients. Generally, these deficiencies occur because dieters and bodybuilders eliminate dairy foods and red meat while dieting. I commonly hear about contest dieters eating only chicken breast and canned tuna, period. However, you don't need to shy away from any healthy foods. You can include red meat in your diet as long as it's lean and cooked appropriately. You can also include nonfat dairy foods, an important source of body-strengthening minerals and fat-burning whey protein. Neither of these foods will make you gain fat, as long as you eat them in moderation.

Because calories are cut during diets, supplement with an antioxidant vitamin and mineral formula that contains at least 100 percent of the DRI for all essential nutrients. This type of supplement will help cover your nutritional bases. See chapters 7, 8, and 9 for additional supplement recommendations.

## Step 12: Watch Water Intake

Fitness-conscious people live in dread of water retention, medically known as edema. Water retention can keep you from looking lean even after you've pared down to physique perfection. Water swells up in certain areas, and you look like you have body fat even though it's only water weight.

How can you prevent water retention? Ironically, the best defense is to drink plenty of water throughout your tapering period. This means drinking at least 8 cups (2 L) of water or more daily. With ample fluid, your body automatically flushes itself of extra water. Not drinking enough water can make your body cling to as much fluid as it can, and you'll end up bloated. Dehydration can sap your energy, and you won't be able to work out as intensely.

Besides drinking plenty of water, follow these strategies to prevent water retention.

- **Be cautious with your sodium intake.** Sodium has gained a bad reputation, but it's an essential element in our diets. Our bodies have a minimum requirement of 500 milligrams a day. The body tightly regulates its electrolyte levels, including sodium. Decreasing sodium levels really doesn't have much of an effect; your body holds on to the amount of sodium it needs, even if you reduce your intake. It's essential to consume the minimum requirement to maintain fluid balance and electrolyte balance. Otherwise, nerve and muscle function will be impaired, and exercise performance will definitely diminish. Some bodybuilders have passed out just before their competitions because of dehydration and possible electrolyte imbalance.

If you're sodium sensitive—that is, sodium causes you to retain water—you probably should reduce your intake slightly. Don't go to extremes, though. Simply avoid high-sodium foods such as snack foods, canned foods, salted foods, pickled foods, cured foods, and lunch meats. Certainly don't add any extra salt to your food. But eliminating natural, whole foods because of their sodium content is usually unnecessary. Concentrate your food choices on whole grains, fresh fruits and vegetables, nonfat dairy foods, and unprocessed meats.

- **Eat naturally diuretic vegetables.** Some foods naturally help the body eliminate water, including asparagus, cucumbers, and watercress. You might try eating these while dieting, especially if water retention is a concern. Add a serving or two of these foods to your diet every day. Avoid pharmacological forms of diuretics at all cost. Diuretic drugs flush sodium and other electrolytes from your body, causing life-threatening imbalances.

- **Continue aerobic exercise.** Aerobic exercise improves the resiliency and tone of blood vessels. Unless blood vessels are resilient, water can seep from them and collect in the tissues, and water retention is the result. A regular program of aerobics helps prevent this.

## For Powerlifters and Weightlifters Only

As a powerlifter or weightlifter, you probably don't care much about getting ripped. Rather, you want to be as strong and as powerful as possible in your weight class. Here's what you should do to get strong for training and competition:

- **Load your muscles with energy sources.** Carbohydrate and creatine are your best bets. Stay on a carbohydrate-dense diet, supplemented with creatine. Take your creatine with carbohydrate, as recommended in chapter 8, to supercharge your muscles with energy. Numerous studies on creatine have shown that this supplement is a sure thing for boosting strength and power.

  You don't need to carbohydrate load. There's no scientific evidence that this method has any performance-enhancing benefit for strength athletes. Simply maintain a high-carbohydrate diet throughout your training and competition preparation. Going into competition well fueled is critical.

- **Manipulate your aerobics and carbohydrate intake.** Increase your aerobics and slightly lower your carbohydrate intake if you need to make weight. This will help you lose fat to qualify for your weight class. You may need to decrease your calories slightly, and you can do this by cutting carbohydrate. However, try to go no lower than 40 percent of your total calories. That way, you can reduce weight but maintain strength.

  Give yourself plenty of time to make weight—at least 10 to 12 weeks. If your contest is fast approaching, you can cut your calories down to 30 per kilogram of body weight a day. That will result in a loss of 3 to 4 pounds (1.4 to 1.8 kg) a week. But keep in mind that you may lose some muscle mass, too.

If you do cut to 30 calories per kilogram of body weight a day, stay on this regimen for no longer than seven days. Prolonged restrictive dieting slows your RMR—and your ability to burn fat.

- **Avoid dangerous practices for making weight.** Before a meet, it's fairly common for some lifters to exercise in rubberized suits or sit in steam or sauna baths for extended periods—all without drinking much water. This practice can lead to dehydration so severe that it can harm the kidneys and heart. Dehydrated lifters also usually do poorly in competition.

 Fasting isn't a good idea, either, even for a day or two. You'll lose water rapidly, and with it, you'll gain the health problems caused by dehydration. Glycogen depletion sets in, too, making it virtually impossible to perform well on competition day.

## Sport Nutrition Fact Versus Fiction: Night Eating—An Anabolic Secret

Eating at night used to be considered a no-no if you wanted to stay lean and muscular. This is a myth that I want to bust wide open. It probably exists because people mistakenly believe that when you're in bed and inactive, you don't burn off all the calories and fat from that meal you've eaten. The reality, however, is not that simple. On the contrary, it turns out that eating at night is another way to gain muscle mass, according to recent studies. Here's why: Your body actually stays in an anabolic condition throughout the night. The reason is that, at night, testosterone (a muscle-building hormone) is naturally elevated. Thus, the right late-night snack can maximize the effects of elevated testosterone. Food also blunts cortisol (a fat-producing hormone) and boosts the availability of muscular building blocks such as branched-chain amino acids and glutamine.

The trick is to create the right anabolic late-night snack. It should feature carbohydrate with a low-to-moderate glycemic index so it doesn't cause much insulin release, which could increase fat accumulation. Avoid fat, sugar, and processed sweets, too. Your snack should also focus on lean protein, such as whey, yogurt, or nuts. I recommend having a small whey protein shake made with low-fat milk, whey protein powder, and berries (fructose is low glycemic). Just remember: Eating at night is a win-win for building muscle—while you sleep!

# 12

# Maintaining Physique Menu Plans

The Power Eating maintaining physique diet outlined in this chapter is for exercisers; bodybuilders; and novice and recreational strength trainers, powerlifters, and weightlifters. Often during training you are not trying to gain or lose weight. Sometimes, it's a timing issue; you're just too busy to spend time in the gym. Sometimes, it is a planned part of your training schedule, such as after the competitive season. Whatever the reason, this menu plan will keep you right where you want to be.

Please note: For all listings of added sugar in each of these diet plans, you can choose to substitute starch. Please see the section Solving the Problem of Added Sugars in Performance and Recovery in chapter 11 before making the substitution.

## Power Eating Maintaining Physique Diet

| Workouts per week | Woman | | Man | |
|---|---|---|---|---|
| | Three or four (novice) | Five or more (experienced) | Three or four (novice) | Five or more (experienced) |
| Calories/kg | 29-33 | 38-40 | 33 | 42 |
| Calories/lb | 13-15 | 17-18 | 15 | 19 |
| **Protein** | | | | |
| g/kg | 1.4 | 1.4 | 1.4 | 1.4 |
| g/lb | 0.64 | 0.64 | 0.64 | 0.64 |
| **Carbohydrate** | | | | |
| g/kg | 3.5 | 5.5 | 4.5 | 6.0 |
| g/lb | 1.75 | 2.3 | 2.0 | 2.7 |
| **Fat\*** | | | | |
| g/kg | ~0.85-1.0 | ~1.0-1.3 | ~1.0 | ~1.4 |
| g/lb | ~0.39-0.45 | ~0.45-0.59 | ~0.45 | ~0.64 |

\*Total fat varies based on total calories. To find your fat grams, determine your total calories, protein grams, and carbohydrate grams. Add your protein and carbohydrate calories (1 g protein = 4 calories, 1 g carbohydrate = 4 calories), subtract this total from the total calories, and divide by 9 (1 g fat = 9 calories). See chapter 10 for more information.

# 130-POUND (59 KG) NOVICE WOMAN
## (three or four workouts per week)

1,690 calories (29 calories/kg); 83 grams protein; 228 grams carbohydrate; 50 grams fat

| Food groups | Number of servings |
|---|---|
| Bread/starch | 4 |
| Fruit | 5 |
| Nonfat milk | 3 |
| Teaspoons of added sugar | 3 |
| Vegetable | 8 |
| Protein: | |
|   Very lean | 4 |
|   Lean | 3 |
|   Medium-fat | 1 |
| Fat | 6 |

| Food group servings | Menu |
|---|---|
| **Breakfast** | |
| 1 bread/starch | 1 cup (25 g) Kashi Whole Grains Puffs cereal |
| 1 milk | 1 cup (240 ml) fat-free milk |
| 2 fruit | 1/2 cup (120 ml) orange juice<br>3/4 cup (110 g) blueberries for cereal |
| 2 vegetable | 1 cup sautéed vegetables to scramble with egg |
| 1 medium-fat protein | 1 whole egg, scrambled in nonstick skillet |
| 2 fat | 1 tbsp ground flaxseed sprinkled on cereal<br>1 tsp oil for skillet |
| | Water |
| **Snack** | |
| 1 fruit | 8 dried apricots halves |
| 1 vegetable | 1 cup (128 g) mini carrots |
| 1 fat | 6 almonds |
| | Green tea (or other tea) |

| Food group servings | Menu |
| --- | --- |
| **Lunch** | |
| 2 bread/starch | 2 slices whole-grain (ideally sprouted grain) bread |
| 2 vegetable | Fill sandwich with vegetable choices<br>Veggie sticks |
| 2 very lean protein | 2 oz (60 g) turkey |
| 1 fat | 1/8 avocado |
| | Water |
| **Preworkout snack** | |
| 1 milk | 1 cup (230 g) plain yogurt |
| 1 fruit | 1 small banana |
| | Water |
| **Workout** | |
| | Water |
| **Postworkout smoothie** | |
| 1 fruit | 1 1/4 cups (180 g) whole strawberries |
| 1 milk | 1 cup (240 ml) nonfat milk |
| 3 tsp added sugar | 3 tsp honey |
| 2 very lean protein | 14 g isolate whey protein |
| **Dinner** | |
| 1 bread/starch | 1/2 baked sweet potato |
| 3 vegetable | 1 cup (180 g) steamed asparagus<br>2 cups (56 g) mixed green salad |
| 3 lean protein | 3 oz (90 g) wild salmon, grilled |
| 2 fat | 1 tsp olive oil for salmon<br>1 tsp butter or Heart Smart margarine for potato<br>2 tbsp reduced-fat salad dressing |
| | Green tea (or other tea) |

# 130-POUND (59 KG) EXPERIENCED WOMAN
## (five or more workouts per week)

2,340 calories (40 calories/kg); 83 grams protein; 325 grams carbohydrate; 79 grams fat

| Food groups | Number of servings |
|---|---|
| Bread/starch | 7 |
| Fruit | 7 |
| Nonfat milk | 3 |
| Teaspoons of added sugar | 8 |
| Vegetable | 10 |
| Protein: | |
|   Very lean | 4 |
|   Lean | 3 |
|   Medium-fat | 1 |
| Fat | 11 |

| Food group servings | Menu |
|---|---|
| **Breakfast** | |
| 2 bread/starch | 2 slices whole-grain (ideally sprouted grain) bread |
| 1 milk | 1 cup (240 ml) fat-free milk |
| 3 fruit | 1 cup (240 ml) orange juice<br>3 tbsp no-sugar-added apple butter for bread |
| 1 medium-fat protein | 1 whole egg, scrambled |
| 2 fat | 1/8 avocado, sliced and cooked with eggs<br>1 tsp Heart Smart Omega margarine for cooking eggs |
| | Water |
| **Snack** | |
| 1 fruit | 8 dried apricot halves |
| 3 fat | 18 almonds |
| | Green tea (or other tea) |

| Food group servings | Menu |
|---|---|
| **Lunch** | |
| 3 bread/starch | 6 in. (15 cm) Subway sandwich (choose from "6 grams of fat or less" list) |
| 2 vegetable | Fill sandwich with vegetable choices |
| 2 very lean protein | Included in sandwich |
| 2 fat | 2 tsp olive oil or 2 tbsp salad dressing |
| | Water |
| **Preworkout snack** | |
| 1 milk | 1 cup (230 g) plain yogurt |
| 1 fruit | 3/4 cup (110 g) blueberries |
| 3 tsp added sugar | 3 tsp honey |
| 1 vegetable | Red pepper spears |
| | Water |
| **Workout** | |
| | Water |
| **Postworkout smoothie** | |
| 1 fruit | 1 1/4 cups (180 g) whole frozen strawberries |
| 1 milk | 1 cup (240 ml) nonfat milk |
| 4 tsp added sugar | 4 tsp sugar |
| 2 very lean protein | 14 g isolate whey protein |
| **Dinner** | |
| 2 bread/starch | 1 baked sweet potato |
| 1 fruit | 3 oz (about 15) red grapes |
| 4 vegetable | 1 cup (180 g) steamed asparagus<br>4 cups (112 g) mixed green salad |
| 3 lean protein | 3 oz (90 g) wild salmon, grilled |
| 4 fat | 1 tsp olive oil for salmon<br>1 tsp butter or Heart Smart margarine for potato<br>4 tbsp reduced-fat salad dressing |
| | Green tea (or other tea) |

# 180-POUND (82 KG) NOVICE MAN

## (three or four workouts per week)

2,700 calories; 115 grams protein; 360 grams carbohydrate; 89 grams fat

| Food groups | Number of servings |
|---|---|
| Bread/starch | 8 |
| Fruit | 7 |
| Nonfat milk | 3 |
| Teaspoons of added sugar | 16 |
| Vegetable | 9 |
| Protein: | |
| Very lean | 6 |
| Lean | 4 |
| Medium-fat | 1 |
| Fat | 11 |

| Food group servings | Menu |
|---|---|
| **Preworkout snack** | |
| 1 milk | 1 cup (230 g) plain yogurt |
| 1 fruit | 3/4 cup (110 g) blueberries |
| 3 tsp added sugar | 3 tsp honey |
| | Water |
| **Workout** | |
| 8 tsp added sugar | 16 oz (480 ml) sport drink |
| | Water |
| **Breakfast** | |
| 1 bread/starch | 1 slice whole-grain bread |
| 1 milk | 1 cup (240 ml) fat-free milk |
| 2 vegetable | 1 cup sautéed veggies in margarine, add eggs |
| 2 fruit | 1 cup (240 ml) orange juice |
| 3 tsp added sugar | 1 tbsp 100% fruit spread for bread |
| 1 medium-fat protein | 1 whole egg, scrambled in nonstick skillet |

| Food group servings | Menu |
|---|---|
| **Breakfast,** *continued* | |
| 2 very lean protein | 4 egg whites, cooked with whole egg |
| 2 fat | 1/8 avocado, sliced and cooked with eggs<br>1 tsp Heart Smart Omega margarine for cooking eggs |
| | Water |
| **Snack** | |
| 2 vegetable | 2 cups (125 g) carrot and celery sticks (or others) |
| 3 fat | 1.5 tbsp natural peanut butter |
| **Lunch** | |
| 5 bread/starch | 12 in. (30 cm) Subway sandwich (choose from "6 grams of fat or less" list) |
| 2 vegetable | Fill sandwich with vegetable choices |
| 1 fruit | Banana |
| 4 very lean protein | Included in sandwich |
| 2 fat | 2 tsp olive oil or 2 tbsp salad dressing |
| **Snack** | |
| 2 fruit | 16 dried apricot halves |
| 1 milk | 1 tall nonfat latté |
| 1 tsp added sugar | 1 tsp sugar |
| 2 fat | 12 almonds |
| **Dinner** | |
| 2 bread/starch | 1 baked sweet potato |
| 1 fruit | 3 oz (about 15) red grapes |
| 1 tsp added sugar | 1 tsp sugar or honey for tea |
| 3 vegetable | 1/2 cup (90 g) steamed asparagus<br>4 cups (112 g) mixed green salad |
| 4 lean protein | 4 oz (120 g) wild salmon, grilled |
| 2 fat | 1 tsp olive oil for salmon<br>2 tbsp reduced-fat salad dressing |
| | Green tea (or other tea) |

# 180-POUND (82 KG) EXPERIENCED MAN

## (five or more workouts per week)

3,420 calories; 115 grams protein; 486 grams carbohydrate; 113 grams fat

| Food groups | Number of servings |
|---|---|
| Bread/starch | 10 |
| Fruit | 9 |
| Nonfat milk | 3 |
| Teaspoons of added sugar | 27 |
| Vegetable | 11 |
| Protein: | |
| Very lean | 6 |
| Lean | 4 |
| Medium-fat | 1 |
| Fat | 18 |

| Food group servings | Menu |
|---|---|
| **Preworkout snack** | |
| 1 milk | 1 cup (230 g) plain yogurt |
| 1 fruit | 3/4 cup (110 g) blueberries |
| 3 tsp added sugar | 3 tsp honey |
| | Water |
| **Workout** | |
| 16 tsp added sugar | 32 oz (950 ml) sport drink |
| | Water |
| **Breakfast** | |
| 2 bread/starch | 2 slices whole-grain bread |
| 1 milk | 1 cup (240 ml) fat-free milk |
| 3 vegetable | 1 1/2 cups sautéed veggies, add eggs |
| 3 fruit | 1 cup (240 ml) orange juice<br>1 cup (170 g) melon cubes |
| 6 tsp added sugar | 2 tbsp 100% fruit spread for bread |
| 2 tsp added sugar | 2 tsp sugar (for tea or coffee) |

| Food group servings | Menu |
|---|---|
| **Breakfast,** *continued* | |
| 1 medium-fat protein | 1 whole egg, scrambled in nonstick skillet |
| 2 very lean protein | 4 egg whites, cooked with whole egg |
| 5 fat | 1/4 avocado, sliced and cooked with eggs<br>3 tsp Heart Smart Omega margarine for cooking veggies and eggs |
| | Tea or coffee |
| | Water |
| **Snack** | |
| 2 bread/starch | 8 whole-wheat crackers |
| 2 vegetable | 2 cups (125 g) carrot and celery sticks (or others) |
| 6 fat | 3 tbsp natural peanut butter |
| **Lunch** | |
| 5 bread/starch | 12 in. (30 cm) Subway sandwich (choose from "6 grams of fat or less" list) |
| 2 vegetable | Fill sandwich with vegetable choices |
| 1 fruit | Banana |
| 4 very lean protein | Included in sandwich |
| 2 fat | 2 tsp olive oil or 2 tbsp salad dressing |
| **Snack** | |
| 2 fruit | 16 dried apricot halves |
| 1 milk | 1 tall nonfat latté |
| 2 fat | 12 almonds |
| **Dinner** | |
| 1 bread/starch | 1/2 baked sweet potato |
| 2 fruit | 6 oz (about 30) red grapes |
| 4 vegetable | 1 cup (180 g) steamed asparagus<br>4 cups (112 g) mixed green salad |
| 4 lean protein | 4 oz (120 g) wild salmon, grilled |
| 3 fat | 1 tsp olive oil for salmon<br>4 tbsp reduced-fat salad dressing<br>Green tea (or other tea) |

# 13

# Building Muscle Menu Plans

My Power Eating diet for building muscle is for novice or experienced exercisers, bodybuilders, powerlifters, weightlifters, and other serious strength trainers who are interested in building quality muscle. The larger you are and the greater your muscle mass is, the more calories it will take for you to build muscle. If you are not seeing gains at these levels, increase your calories by 300 to 400 per day by primarily increasing carbohydrate (75 percent of the calorie increase) and secondarily increasing fat (25 percent of the increase). If you are cross-training with intense aerobic exercise, increase your carbohydrate intake by another 1 to 2 grams per kilogram of body weight per day.

### Power Eating Building Muscle Diet

| Workouts per week | Woman | | Man | |
| --- | --- | --- | --- | --- |
| | Three or four (novice) | Five or more (experienced) | Three or four (novice) | Five or more (experienced) |
| Calories/kg | 35-38 | 44-50 | 42 | 52+ |
| Calories/lb | 16-17 | 20-23 | 19 | 24+ |
| **Protein** | | | | |
| g/kg | 2.0 | 2.2 | 2.2 | 2.5 |
| g/lb | 0.9 | 1.0 | 1.0 | 1.1 |
| **Carbohydrate** | | | | |
| g/kg | 4.5 | 6.5 | 5.5 | 7.0 |
| g/lb | 2.1 | 3.0 | 2.5 | 3.2 |
| **Fat*** | | | | |
| g/ kg | ~1.0-1.3 | ~1.0-1.77 | ~1.33 | 1.77 |
| g/lb | ~0.45-0.59 | ~0.5-0.8 | ~0.6 | 0.8 |

*Total fat varies based on total calories. To find your fat grams, determine your total calories, protein grams, and carbohydrate grams. Add your protein and carbohydrate calories (1 g protein = 4 calories, 1 g carbohydrate = 4 calories), subtract this total from the total calories, and divide by 9 (1 g fat = 9 calories). See chapter 10 for more information.

## 130-POUND (59 KG) NOVICE WOMAN
### (three or four workouts per week)

2,080 calories (35 calories/kg); 118 grams protein; 266 grams carbohydrate; 60 grams fat

| Food groups | Number of servings |
|---|---|
| Bread/starch | 6 |
| Fruit | 5 |
| Nonfat milk | 3 |
| Teaspoons of added sugar | 3 |
| Vegetable | 8 |
| Protein: | |
|   Very lean | 5 |
|   Lean | 3 |
|   Medium-fat | 1 |
| Fat | 9 |

| Food group servings | Menu |
|---|---|
| **Breakfast** | |
| 2 bread/starch | 1 cup cooked oatmeal or other cooked cereal |
| 1 milk | 1 cup (240 ml) fat-free milk |
| 2 fruit | 1/2 cup (120 ml) orange juice<br>3/4 cup (110 g) berries for cereal |
| 1 medium-fat protein | 1 whole egg, scrambled in nonstick skillet |
| 1-2 seconds cooking spray | For cooking eggs |
| 1 fat | 1 tbsp ground flaxseed sprinkled on cereal |
| | Water |
| **Snack** | |
| 1 fruit | 8 dried apricot halves |
| 2 vegetable | 1 cup (128 g) mini carrots<br>1 cup (128 g) cherry tomatoes |
| 2 fat | 12 almonds |
| | Green tea (or other tea) |

| Food group servings | Menu |
|---|---|
| **Lunch** | |
| 2 bread/starch | 2 slices whole-grain (ideally sprouted grain) bread |
| 3 vegetable | Fill sandwich with vegetable choices<br>2 cups mixed green salad |
| 3 very lean protein | 2 oz (60 g) turkey<br>1 oz (30 g) cheese |
| 3 fat | 1 fat included in cheese<br>1/8 avocado<br>1 tbsp salad dressing or 2 tbsp reduced-fat salad dressing |
| | Mustard for sandwich |
| | Water |
| **Preworkout snack** | |
| 1 milk | 1 cup (230 g) plain yogurt |
| 1 fruit | 1 small banana |
| | Water |
| **Workout** | |
| | Water |
| **Postworkout smoothie** | |
| 1 fruit | 1 1/4 cups (180 g) whole strawberries |
| 1 milk | 1 cup (240 ml) nonfat milk |
| 3 tsp added sugar | 3 tsp honey |
| 2 very lean protein | 14 g isolate whey protein |
| **Dinner** | |
| 2 bread/starch | 1 baked sweet potato |
| 3 vegetable | 1 cup (180 g) steamed asparagus<br>4 cups (112 g) mixed green salad |
| 3 lean protein | 3 oz (90 g) wild salmon, grilled |
| 3 fat | 1 tsp olive oil for salmon<br>1 tsp butter or Heart Smart margarine for potato<br>4 tbsp reduced-fat salad dressing |
| | Green tea (or other tea) |

# 130-POUND (59 KG) EXPERIENCED WOMAN
## (five or more workouts per week)

2,950 calories (50 calories/kg, the top of the range); 130 grams protein; 384 grams carbohydrate; 99 grams fat

| Food groups | Number of servings |
|---|---|
| Bread/starch | 8 |
| Fruit | 8 |
| Nonfat milk | 3 |
| Teaspoons of added sugar | 18 |
| Vegetable | 7 |
| Protein: | |
|   Very lean | 6 |
|   Lean | 4 |
|   Medium-fat | 1 |
| Fat | 16 |

| Food group servings | Menu |
|---|---|
| **Breakfast** | |
| 2 bread/starch | 2 slices whole-grain bread |
| 1 milk | 1 cup (240 ml) fat-free milk |
| 2 fruit | 1 cup (240 ml) orange juice |
| 4 tsp added sugar | 4 tsp 100% fruit spread for bread |
| 1 vegetable | 1/2 cup (28 g) sautéed mushrooms added to egg |
| 1 medium-fat protein | 1 whole egg, scrambled |
| 4 fat | 1/4 avocado, sliced and cooked with egg<br>2 tsp Heart Smart Omega margarine for cooking mushrooms and eggs |
| | Water |
| **Snack** | |
| 2 fruit | 16 dried apricot halves |
| 3 fat | 18 almonds |
| | Green tea (or other tea) |

| Food group servings | Menu |
|---|---|
| **Lunch** | |
| 3 bread/starch | 6 in. (18 cm) Subway sandwich (choose from "6 grams of fat or less" list) |
| 2 vegetable | Fill sandwich with vegetable choices |
| 2 very lean protein | 2 oz (60 g) meat included in sandwich<br>1 oz (30 g) cheese |
| 3 fat | 1 fat included in cheese<br>2 tsp olive oil or 2 tbsp salad dressing |
| | Water |
| **Preworkout snack** | |
| 1 milk | 1 cup (230 g) plain yogurt |
| 1 fruit | 3/4 cup (110 g) blueberries |
| 3 tsp added sugar | 3 tsp honey |
| | Water |
| **Workout** | |
| 8 tsp added sugar | 16 oz (480 ml) sport drink |
| | Water |
| **Postworkout smoothie** | |
| 1 fruit | 1 1/4 (180 g) cups whole strawberries |
| 1 milk | 1 cup (240 ml) nonfat milk |
| 3 tsp added sugar | 3 tsp honey |
| 3 very lean protein | 21 g isolate whey protein |
| 1 fat | 1/8 avocado |
| **Dinner** | |
| 3 bread/starch | 1 baked sweet potato<br>1/2 cup (98 g) brown rice |
| 2 fruit | 6 oz (about 30) red grapes |
| 4 vegetable | 1 cup (180 g) steamed asparagus<br>4 cups (112 g) mixed green salad |
| 4 lean protein | 4 oz (120 g) wild salmon, grilled |
| 5 fat | 1 tsp olive oil to rub on salmon<br>4 tbsp salad dressing |
| | Green tea (or other tea) |

# 180-POUND (82 KG) NOVICE MAN

## (three or four workouts per week)

3,420 calories; 180 grams protein; 450 grams carbohydrate; 100 grams fat

| Food groups | Number of servings |
|---|---|
| Bread/starch | 10 |
| Fruit | 8 |
| Nonfat milk | 3 |
| Teaspoons of added sugar | 24 |
| Vegetable | 9 |
| Protein: | |
|   Very lean | 10 |
|   Lean | 6 |
|   Medium-fat | 1 |
| Fat | 14 |

| Food group servings | Menu |
|---|---|
| **Preworkout snack** | |
| 1 milk | 1 cup (230 g) plain yogurt |
| 1 fruit | 3/4 cup (110 g) blueberries |
| 3 tsp added sugar | 3 tsp honey |
| 2 very lean protein | 14 g whey protein isolate whisked into yogurt |
| | Water |
| **Workout** | |
| 16 tsp added sugar | 32 oz (950 ml) sport drink |
| | Water |
| **Breakfast** | |
| 2 bread/starch | 2 slices whole-grain bread |
| 1 milk | 1 cup (240 ml) fat-free milk |
| 2 fruit | 1 cup (240 ml) orange juice |
| 4 tsp added sugar | 4 tsp 100% fruit spread for bread |
| 2 vegetable | 1 cup sautéed veggies to add to eggs |
| 1 medium-fat protein | 1 whole egg, scrambled |
| 2 very lean protein | 4 egg whites, cooked with whole egg |

| Food group servings | Menu |
|---|---|
| **Breakfast,** *continued* | |
| 4 fat | 1/4 avocado, sliced and cooked with eggs<br>1 tsp Heart Smart Omega margarine plus<br>1 tsp olive oil for cooking veggies and eggs |
| | Water |
| **Snack** | |
| 2 bread/starch | 8 whole-wheat crackers |
| 1 lean protein | 1 oz (30 g) cheese |
| 1 vegetable | 1 cup (124 g) celery sticks |
| 3 fat | 1 1/2 tbsp natural peanut butter |
| **Lunch** | |
| 5 bread/starch | 12-in. (36 cm) Subway sandwich (choose from "6 grams of fat or less" list) |
| 2 vegetable | Fill sandwich with vegetable choices |
| 1 fruit | Banana |
| 6 very lean protein | 4 oz (120 g) meat included in sandwich<br>2 oz (60 g) cheese |
| 3 fat | 2 fat servings included in cheese<br>1 tsp olive oil or 1 tbsp salad dressing |
| **Snack** | |
| 2 fruit | 16 dried apricot halves |
| 1 milk | 1 tall nonfat latté |
| 1 tsp added sugar | 1 tsp sugar |
| 2 fat | 12 almonds |
| **Dinner** | |
| 1 bread/starch | 1/2 baked sweet potato |
| 2 fruit | 6 oz (about 30) red grapes |
| 4 vegetable | 1 cup (180 g) steamed asparagus<br>4 cups (112 g) mixed green salad |
| 5 lean protein | 5 oz (150 g) wild salmon, grilled |
| 2 fat | 1 tsp olive oil for salmon<br>4 tbsp reduced-fat salad dressing |
| | Green tea (or other tea) |

# 180-POUND (82 KG) EXPERIENCED MAN

## (five or more workouts per week)

4,245 calories; 205 grams protein; 576 grams carbohydrate; 125 grams fat

| Food groups | Number of servings |
|---|---|
| Bread/starch | 13 |
| Fruit | 12 |
| Nonfat milk | 3 |
| Teaspoons of added sugar | 30 |
| Vegetable | 9 |
| Protein: | |
| Very lean | 13 |
| Lean | 5 |
| Medium-fat | 1 |
| Fat | 24 |

| Food group servings | Menu |
|---|---|
| **Preworkout snack** | |
| 1 milk | 1 cup (230 g) plain yogurt |
| 1 fruit | 3/4 cup (110 g) blueberries |
| 3 tsp added sugar | 3 tsp honey |
| 3 very lean protein | 21 g whey protein isolate whisked into yogurt |
| | Water |
| **Workout** | |
| 16 tsp added sugar | 32 oz (950 ml) sport drink |
| | Water |
| **Breakfast** | |
| 2 bread/starch | 2 slices whole-grain bread |
| 1 milk | 1 cup (240 ml) fat-free milk (make a smoothie with milk, juice fruit, whey protein) |
| 3 fruit | 1/2 cup (120 ml) orange juice<br>1 1/2 cups frozen fruit |
| 6 tsp added sugar | 2 tbsp 100% fruit spread for bread |
| 2 vegetable | 1 cup sautéed mushrooms and red peppers |
| 1 medium-fat protein | 1 whole egg, scrambled |
| 4 very lean protein | 4 egg whites, cooked with whole egg<br>14 g whey protein isolate (for smoothie) |

| Food group servings | Menu |
|---|---|
| **Breakfast,** *continued* | |
| 6 fat | 1/2 avocado, sliced and cooked with eggs<br>2 tsp Heart Smart Omega margarine for cooking eggs and vegetables |
| | Water |
| **Snack** | |
| 2 bread/starch | 8 whole-wheat crackers |
| 2 fruit | 2/3 cup (158 ml) Concord grape juice (make a spritzer by mixing with sparkling water) |
| 1 vegetable | 1 cup (124 g) celery sticks |
| 6 fat | 3 tbsp natural peanut butter |
| **Lunch** | |
| 5 bread/starch | 12-in. (36 cm) Subway sandwich (choose from "6 grams of fat or less" list) |
| 2 vegetable | Fill sandwich with vegetable choices |
| 1 fruit | Banana |
| 6 very lean protein | 4 oz (120 g) meat included in sandwich<br>2 oz (60 g) cheese |
| 4 fat | 2 fat servings included in cheese; 2 tsp olive oil or 2 tbsp salad dressing |
| **Snack** | |
| 2 fruit | 16 dried apricot halves |
| 1 milk | 1 tall nonfat latté |
| 2 tsp added sugar | 2 tsp sugar |
| 2 fat | 12 almonds |
| **Dinner** | |
| 4 bread/starch | 1 baked sweet potato<br>1 cup cooked quinoa |
| 3 fruit | 1 cup (124 g) raspberries and 1 cup (165 g) cubed mango; put on top of ice cream |
| 3 tsp added sugar | 1/2 cup light ice cream |
| 4 vegetable | 1 cup (180 g) steamed asparagus<br>4 cups (112 g) mixed green salad |
| 5 lean protein | 5 oz (150 g) wild salmon, grilled |
| 6 fat | 1 fat included in ice cream<br>1 tsp olive oil for salmon<br>4 tbsp salad dressing |
| Free (no calories) | 1 tbsp whipped cream to top fruit and ice cream |

VERY IMPORTANT: These calorie levels reflect the needs of people training consistently very hard. If that's not you, then these calorie levels will be too high. If that's the case, use the menu for those doing fewer workouts per week, use female calorie levels if you're a man, or use a maintenance plan from chapter 12. If you need to drop only a few calories, then cut out the added sugar everywhere except around training. Please note: For all listings of added sugar in each of these diet plans, you can choose to substitute starch. Please see the section Solving the Problem of Added Sugars in Performance and Recovery in chapter 11 before making the substitution.

## POWER PROFILE: Weight Gain

Are you a hard gainer—unable to put on any appreciable muscle weight no matter how hard you try?

That was the case of Scott E., a 44-year-old business executive who, at 6 feet, 3 inches (191 cm) and 177 pounds (80 kg), had not been able to gain weight in 20 years. To make matters worse, he had no appetite; plus he had stomach problems caused by stress, infections, and overtreatment with antibiotics. I placed him on my Power Eating building diet.

Before beginning this diet, Scott was consuming only about 2,800 calories a day and not enough vitamins, minerals, or fluids. I increased his calories to 3,560 calories daily, plus added more protein (113 g daily) and carbohydrate (570 g daily). He started supplementing with a good antioxidant, eating multiple meals throughout the day, and consuming healthier fat from fish and plant sources. He also decreased his alcohol intake.

In addition, I recommended that Scott supplement with Kleiner's Easy Muscle-Building Formula, take 400 milligrams of vitamin E, and continue taking acidophilus, a supplement that restores intestinal flora after antibiotic treatment. I also suggested that Scott try a natural supplement, Prelief, to help reduce stomach irritation.

In only six weeks, Scott's energy levels soared, and he felt energetic enough to begin a regular exercise program. He gained 15 pounds (7 kg) of pure muscle—with no increase in his waist measurement. Scott felt that the Prelief helped him eat the extra calories without stomach irritation.

As Scott put it, "In the first three weeks, I gained 14 pounds [6 kg], from 180 [82 kg] to 194 [88 kg]. To put this in perspective, I have not weighed over 184 [83 kg] in 20 years and have been trying to gain weight for the past two to three years."

What's more, most of his stomach problems were resolved.

# 14

# Cross-Training Menu Plans

If you're really interested in performance, or even high-level fitness, you probably cross-train with a variety of fitness activities. This chapter is for everyone who strength trains to enhance power for an endurance sport. Unlike the other menu plans, which are focused squarely on building strength and power and cutting fat, these menu plans will help you fine-tune your diet to build power yet still enhance endurance.

Because you're focusing on building strength and endurance, you'll use more carbohydrate to fuel your cardiorespiratory exercise. And because athletes who race don't want to add size and weight to their frames, you won't need the amount of protein that it takes to build muscle size. You want just enough to increase power and recover fully. And of course, you'll need the right amount of fat to fuel your endurance and allow for important joint cushioning and lubrication, hormonal balance, cellular recovery, anti-inflammatory functions, and brain support, for which fat is key.

## Fat Adaptation

When you exercise in an endurance event, your body starts out by burning carbohydrate, moves into fat burning for the majority of the middle of the event, and then as you tire, you return to burning carbohydrate for the final sprint to the finish. The better trained you are, the better your body is at switching from carbohydrate to fat at the beginning of the race, and the longer you will use fat for fuel before you begin to tire and return to carbohydrate. This final switch actually determines how much endurance you really have, and how much power you'll have for the last lap or final sprint to the finish line. If you could get your body to switch to fat metabolism more quickly, stay there longer, and preserve more carbohydrate for the very end of the race, you'd definitely have a competitive edge. That's the whole theory behind fat adaptation.

Although sport nutrition scientists pretty much agree on the range of carbohydrate and fat in the diets of strength athletes, the science is currently in a state of flux in terms of the diets of endurance athletes—especially those who depend on both power and endurance. The question is whether well-trained athletes could use fat adaptation to their benefit and extend endurance time before exhaustion hits.

At this point we know that fat adaptation actually happens. Some people adapt better to the diet than others, but in those who respond well, a high-fat, low-carbohydrate diet followed for five days to two weeks, along with high-intensity, long-duration exercise, can stretch the body's ability to burn fat instead of carbohydrate. The nature of the diet, only 15 percent of calories from carbohydrate and 70 percent from fat, leaves you with very low carbohydrate stores. To remedy that losing situation, scientists have created a "dietary periodization" model that has you follow the high-fat protocol with one to three days of carbohydrate restoration. At this point you flip the carbohydrate–fat ratios to 70:15 and taper your exercise. Your ability to oxidize fat for fuel drops slightly, but is still elevated well above where it would be without the fat adaptation diet strategy, and you partially regain your ability to burn carbohydrate when you need it.

Despite the fact that this all really does happen in responsive subjects, the measures of performance have been disappointing. It is not clear at all whether altering metabolic profiles actually improves performance. Some studies showed a small amount of improvement, others showed no change, and some recorded a decrement in cycling performance.

The concept of fat adaptation is still very much in the testing phase. You can try it out and see whether you are a responder, and whether you can tolerate the diet as well as the metabolic changes. I'll be honest: It's not an easy diet to follow, especially if your calorie needs are high. And because we still have no data to support the fat adaptation theory for enhanced performance, these menus focus on the well-established and scientifically supported higher-carbohydrate diet for endurance athletes.

## Protein During Training and Events

Just about anyone who is active has heard that you refuel, recover, rebuild, and grow much better if you have carbohydrate and protein soon after exercise. More recent data have begun to support the idea that the carbohydrate–protein combo prior to exercise also enhances muscle recovery and growth. But the question of whether protein is helpful during exercise when it is taken along with carbohydrate has been hanging around for at least a decade. The first studies on the use of protein, or amino acids, during exercise focused on endurance activity and the question of whether, when given during exercise, protein positively affects the brain, and the lengthening of time to exhaustion during exercise. That question has still not been answered. But as we have developed better laboratory tests for muscle protein synthesis and breakdown, the research into protein consumption with carbohydrate during endurance exercise has moved in that direction. As athletes have begun to cross-train to support their endurance activities, interest in the area of protein- carbohydrate consumption during exercise has grown as well, offering opportunity for more research to support product development.

The most recent evidence appears to lean toward positive effects from the use of some protein with carbohydrate during exercise; however, it is not definitely clear. A peer-reviewed sophisticated study investigated the impact of protein–carbohydrate coingestion during endurance exercise on muscle protein balance and synthesis. During exercise on a cycle ergometer, the subjects were given either a carbohydrate-only beverage (1 g/kg/hr carbohydrate) or a calorically identical beverage of both carbohydrate (0.8 g/kg/hr) and casein protein hydrolysate (0.2 g/kg/hr). The study demonstrated that muscle protein synthesis rates improved with either beverage beyond a fasting state, but that the addition of protein did not further augment rates of muscle protein synthesis.

A separate study examined the influence of carbohydrate–protein coingestion on running capacity toward the end of a soccer-specific intermittent exercise protocol. The subjects ran three trials while randomly consuming either a placebo, a 6.9 percent carbohydrate solution, or a solution that was 4.8 percent carbohydrate and 2.1 percent protein. All beverages were matched for color and taste. The carbohydrate–protein beverage resulted in longer run times to fatigue compared to those in the other two test trials. The subjects recovered faster between sets of intermittent exercise to better endurance capacity and perceived a lower rate of exertion during exercise when they ingested the carbohydrate–protein beverage.

A third study tested the effect of a carbohydrate–protein beverage during competitive endurance exercise in the heat. Twenty-eight cyclists competing in the eight-day Transalp mountain bike race were the subjects of the study and were randomly assigned either a carbohydrate-only placebo (76 g/L) or a carbohydrate–protein beverage (72 g/L carbohydrate; 18 g/L protein). Carbohydrate–protein supplementation significantly prevented body mass loss, enhanced body temperature regulation, and improved competitive exercise performance compared to the placebo. The combination did not have an effect on muscle damage or soreness. The flaw in this study is that the placebo and the test beverage were not of the same caloric value. The carbohydrate–protein beverage contained more calories, or more energy. So it is difficult to assess whether the total energy or the presence of protein actually made the difference in the results.

There is a practical consideration with protein supplementation during exercise: many people cannot tolerate protein or amino acids in their fluid-replacement, or sport, drinks. These commonly cause stomach upset and nausea. If that happens to you, clearly it will not improve your performance. If you tolerate the protein in your beverage during exercise, then I think it's worth trying. If you don't observe any benefits after a few weeks, then you might do well to drop it. There's no use in wasting money on something that doesn't work.

## Caffeine Works

Caffeine has been used before exercise for decades, but a new twist was presented by a study that investigated the effect of adding caffeine to a postexercise carbohydrate drink on subsequent high-intensity interval running capacity. In this study the six subjects first exercised to exhaustion to deplete their muscles of glycogen (stored carbohydrate). Immediately following the workout and at one, two, and three hours after exercise, they consumed either water, a carbohydrate-only solution (1.2 g/kg of body weight) or a similar carbohydrate solution with 8 milligrams per kilogram of body weight of caffeine added. All beverages looked and tasted the same. After four hours of recovery, the subjects performed a shuttle test (test of high-intensity running capacity) to exhaustion. All six subjects improved performance in the carbohydrate–caffeine trial compared with the other two trials. Although for years word on the street has been that this is a winning strategy for those who can tolerate caffeine, it's very good to have data to back up the common knowledge. And because the half-life of caffeine is five to seven hours, it's not really all that surprising that an efficacious dose of caffeine, an acknowledged performance-enhancing aid, helps in the second round of performance.

## Power Eating Cross-Training Diet*

| Workouts per week | Woman | | Man | |
|---|---|---|---|---|
| | Three or four (novice) | Five or more (experienced) | Three or four (novice) | Five or more (experienced) |
| Calories/kg | 35-37+ | 44-51+ | 37-41+ | 50-58+ |
| Calories/lb | 16-16.8+ | 20-23.2+ | 16.8-18.6+ | 22.7-26.4+ |
| **Protein** | | | | |
| g/kg | 1.5 | 1.8 | 1.5 | 1.8 |
| g/lb | 0.6 | 0.72-0.82 | 0.6 | 0.72-0.82 |
| **Carbohydrate** | | | | |
| g/kg | 5-7 | 6-10+ | 5-7 | 6-10+ |
| g/lb | 2.3-3.2 | 2.7-4.6+ | 2.3-3.2 | 2.7-4.6+ |
| **Fat**** | | | | |
| g/ kg | ~1.2 | ~1.8 | ~0.7 | ~1.0 |
| g/lb | ~0.55 | ~0.82 | ~0.32 | ~0.45 |

*The distribution of calories and nutrients for the cross-training plan will vary based on the volume and intensity of training in total, and from day to day. Adjust your total calories and carbohydrate intake to meet your day's needs, from rest days to long-distance, high-intensity, multiple-workout days, and as you near race day. This is a diet recommendation for daily training. Specific competition preparation and race day nutrition are highly individualized and variable. Seek expert advice from a sports nutritionist for customized planning.

**Total fat varies based on total calories. To find your fat grams, determine your total calories, protein grams, and carbohydrate grams. Add your protein and carbohydrate calories (1 g protein = 4 calories, 1 g carbohydrate = 4 calories), subtract this total from the total calories, and divide by 9 (1 g fat = 9 calories). See chapter 10 for more information.

## 130-POUND (59 KG) NOVICE WOMAN
### (three or four workouts per week)

2,128 calories (36 calories/kg); 89 grams protein; 355 grams carbohydrate; 40 grams fat

| Food groups | Number of servings |
| --- | --- |
| Bread/starch | 7 |
| Fruit | 6 |
| Nonfat milk | 3 |
| Teaspoons of added sugar | 20 |
| Vegetable | 9 |
| Protein: | |
|   Very lean | 4 |
|   Lean | 3 |
|   Medium-fat | 1 |
| Fat | 5 |

| Food group servings | Menu |
| --- | --- |
| **Breakfast** | |
| 2 bread/starch | 1 cup cooked oatmeal or other cooked cereal |
| 1 milk | 1 cup (240 ml) fat-free milk |
| 2 fruit | 1/2 (120 ml) cup orange juice<br>3/4 cup (110 g) berries for cereal |
| 1 medium-fat protein | 1 whole egg, scrambled in nonstick skillet |
| 1-2 seconds cooking spray | For cooking eggs |
| 1 fat | 1 tbsp ground flaxseed sprinkled on cereal |
| | Water |
| **Snack** | |
| 1 bread/starch | 3/4 oz (23 g) pretzels |
| 1 fruit | 4 dried apricots |
| 2 vegetable | 1 cup (128 g) mini-carrots<br>1 cup (128 g) cherry tomatoes |
| 1 fat | 6 almonds |
| | Green tea (or other tea) |

| Food group servings | Menu |
| --- | --- |
| **Lunch** | |
| 2 bread/starch | 2 slices whole-grain (ideally sprouted grain) bread |
| 1 fruit | Apple |
| 3 vegetable | Fill sandwich with vegetable choices<br>2 cups (112 g) mixed green salad |
| 2 very lean protein | 2 oz (60 g) turkey |
| 1 fat | 1/8 avocado<br>Mustard for sandwich |
| | Water |
| **Preworkout snack** | |
| 1 milk | 1 cup (230 g) plain yogurt |
| 1 fruit | 1 small banana |
| | Water |
| **Workout** | |
| 12 tsp added sugar | 32 oz (950 ml) typical sport drink |
| **Postworkout smoothie** | |
| 1 fruit | 1 1/4 cups (180 g) whole strawberries |
| 1 milk | 1 cup (240 ml) nonfat milk |
| 8 tsp added sugar | 6 tsp sugar and 2 tsp honey |
| 2 very lean protein | 14 g isolate whey protein |
| **Dinner** | |
| 2 bread/starch | 1 baked sweet potato |
| 3 vegetable | 1 cup (180 g) steamed asparagus<br>4 cups (122 g) mixed green salad |
| 3 lean protein | 3 oz (90 g) wild salmon, grilled |
| 2 fat | 1 tsp olive oil for salmon<br>2 tbsp reduced-fat salad dressing |
| | Green tea (or other tea) |

# 130-POUND (59 KG) EXPERIENCED WOMAN

## (five or more workouts per week)

2,837 calories (48 calories/kg); 106 grams protein; 473 grams carbohydrate; 60 grams fat

PLUS: 0.2 g/kg/hr protein combined with carbohydrate (added sugar) in beverage DURING exercise. In this case: 11 g protein/hr. If you prefer to try essential amino acids (EAAs) instead of whey protein isolate, the formula is 0.2 g of EAA per 1 g total protein.

| Food groups | Number of servings |
| --- | --- |
| Bread/starch | 9 |
| Fruit | 9 |
| Nonfat milk | 3 |
| Teaspoons of added sugar | 32 |
| Vegetable | 8 |
| Protein: | |
| Very lean | 5 |
| Lean | 4 |
| Medium-fat | 1 |
| Fat | 9 |

| Food group servings | Menu |
| --- | --- |
| **Breakfast** | |
| 2 bread/starch | 2 slices whole-grain bread |
| 1 milk | 1 cup (240 ml) fat-free milk |
| 2 fruit | 1 cup (240 ml) orange juice |
| 4 tsp added sugar | 4 tsp 100% fruit spread for bread |
| 2 vegetable | 1 cup sautéed mushrooms and onions added to egg |
| 1 medium-fat protein | 1 whole egg, scrambled |
| 2 fat | 1/8 avocado, spread on bread<br>1 tsp canola oil for cooking veggies and eggs |
| | Water |
| **Snack** | |
| 2 fruit | 16 dried apricot halves |
| 3 fat | 18 almonds |
| | Green tea (or other tea) |

| Food group servings | Menu |
|---|---|
| **Lunch** | |
| 3 bread/starch | 6 in. (15 cm) Subway sandwich (choose from "6 grams of fat or less" list) |
| 2 vegetable | Fill sandwich with vegetable choices |
| 2 very lean protein | 2 oz (60 g) meat included in sandwich |
| 1 fat | 1 tsp olive oil or 1 tbsp salad dressing |
| | Water |
| **Preworkout snack** | |
| 1 bread/starch | 3/4 oz (21 g) pretzels |
| 1 milk | 1 cup (230 g) plain low-fat yogurt |
| 1 fruit | 3/4 cup (110 g) blueberries |
| 3 tsp added sugar | 3 tsp honey |
| | Water |
| **Workout** | |
| 16 tsp added sugar | 32 oz (950 ml) sport drink |
| 11 g protein isolate/hr | Casein or whey protein isolate (typically 1/2 serving) |
| | Water |
| **Postworkout smoothie** | |
| 2 fruit | 1 1/4 cups (180 g) frozen whole strawberries<br>1 frozen medium banana |
| 1 milk | 1 cup (240 ml) nonfat milk |
| 9 tsp added sugar | 6 tsp sugar and 3 tsp honey |
| 3 very lean protein | 21 g isolate whey protein |
| **Dinner** | |
| 3 bread/starch | 1 baked sweet potato<br>1/2 cup brown rice |
| 2 fruit | 6 oz (about 30) red grapes |
| 4 vegetable | 1 cup (180 g) steamed asparagus<br>4 cups (112 g) mixed green salad |
| 4 lean protein | 4 oz (120 g) wild salmon, grilled |
| 3 fat | 1 tsp olive oil to rub on salmon<br>4 tbsp reduced-fat salad dressing |
| | Green tea (or other tea) |

# 180-POUND (82 KG) NOVICE MAN

## (three or four workouts per week)

3,272 calories (40 calories/kg); 123 grams protein; 491 grams carbohydrate; 91 grams fat

| Food groups | Number of servings |
|---|---|
| Bread/starch | 12 |
| Fruit | 9 |
| Nonfat milk | 3 |
| Teaspoons of added sugar | 24 |
| Vegetable | 9 |
| Protein: | |
|   Very lean | 7 |
|   Lean | 5 |
|   Medium-fat | 1 |
| Fat | 8 |

| Food group servings | Menu |
|---|---|
| **Preworkout snack** | |
| 1 milk | 1 cup (230 g) plain yogurt |
| 1 fruit | 3/4 (110 g) cup blueberries |
| 2 tbsp added sugar | 2 tbsp honey |
| 2 very lean protein | 14 g whey protein isolate whisked into yogurt |
| | Water |
| **Workout** | |
| 16 tsp added sugar | 32 oz (950 ml) sport drink |
| | Water |
| **Breakfast** | |
| 2 bread/starch | 2 slices whole-grain bread |
| 1 milk | 1 cup (240 ml) fat-free milk |
| 2 fruit | 1 cup (240 ml) orange juice |
| 4 tsp added sugar | 4 tsp 100% fruit spread for bread |
| 2 vegetable | 1 cup sautéed veggies to add to eggs |
| 1 medium-fat protein | 1 whole egg, scrambled |

| Food group servings | Menu |
|---|---|
| **Breakfast,** *continued* | |
| 1 very lean protein | 2 egg whites, cooked with whole egg |
| 2 fat | 1/4 avocado, spread on bread<br>1 tsp olive oil for cooking veggies and eggs |
| | Water |
| **Snack** | |
| 2 bread/starch | 8 whole-wheat crackers |
| 1 fruit | 3 tbsp no-sugar-added apple butter |
| 1 vegetable | 1 cup (124 g) celery sticks |
| 3 fat | 1 1/2 tbsp natural peanut butter |
| **Lunch** | |
| 5 bread/starch | 12 in. (36 cm) Subway sandwich (choose from "6 grams of fat or less" list) |
| 2 vegetable | Fill sandwich with vegetable choices |
| 1 fruit | Banana |
| 4 very lean protein | 4 oz (120 g) meat included in sandwich |
| 1 fat | 1 tsp olive oil or 1 tbsp salad dressing |
| **Snack** | |
| 2 fruit | 16 dried apricot halves |
| 1 milk | 1 tall nonfat latté |
| 1 tsp added sugar | 1 tsp sugar |
| **Dinner** | |
| 3 bread/starch | 1 baked sweet potato<br>1/2 cup brown rice |
| 2 fruit | 6 oz (about 30) red grapes |
| 4 vegetable | 1 cup (180 g) steamed asparagus<br>4 cups (112 g) mixed green salad |
| 5 lean protein | 5 oz (150 g) wild salmon, grilled |
| 2 fat | 1 tsp olive oil for salmon<br>4 tbsp reduced-fat salad dressing |
| | Green tea (or other tea) |

# 180-POUND (82 KG) EXPERIENCED MAN

## (five or more workouts per week)

4,500 calories (55 calories/kg); 147 grams protein; 654 grams carbohydrate; 144 grams fat

PLUS: 0.2 g/kg/hr protein combined with carbohydrate (added sugar) in beverage DURING exercise. In this case: 16 g protein/hr. If you prefer to try essential amino acids (EAAs) instead of whey protein isolate, the formula is 0.2 g of EAA per 1 g total protein.

| Food groups | Number of servings |
|---|---|
| Bread/starch | 15 |
| Fruit | 13 |
| Nonfat milk | 3 |
| Teaspoons of added sugar | 39 |
| Vegetable | 9 |
| Protein: | |
|   Very lean | 9 |
|   Lean | 6 |
|   Medium-fat | 1 |
| Fat | 14 |

| Food group servings | Menu |
|---|---|
| **Preworkout snack** | |
| 1 milk | 1 cup (230 g) plain yogurt |
| 1 fruit | 3/4 cup (110 g) blueberries |
| 6 tsp added sugar | 6 tsp honey |
| 3 very lean protein | 21 g whey protein isolate whisked into yogurt |
| | Water |
| **Workout** | |
| 16 tsp added sugar | 32 oz (950 ml) sport drink |
| 16 g protein isolate/hr | Casein or whey protein isolate |
| | Water |
| **Breakfast** | |
| 4 bread/starch | 2 slices whole-grain bread<br>1 cup cooked oatmeal |
| 1 milk | 1 cup (240 ml) fat-free milk (make a smoothie with milk, juice, fruit, sugar, whey protein) |

| Food group servings | Menu |
|---|---|
| **Breakfast,** *continued* | |
| 4 fruit | 1/2 cup (120 ml) orange juice<br>1 1/2 cups frozen fruit<br>2 tbsp raisins or 1/2 cup fresh fruit for oatmeal |
| 12 tsp added sugar | 2 tbsp 100% fruit spread for bread<br>2 tbsp sugar for smoothie |
| 2 vegetable | 1 cup sautéed mushrooms and red peppers |
| 1 medium-fat protein | 1 whole egg, scrambled |
| 2 very lean protein | 4 egg whites, cooked with whole egg<br>14 g whey protein isolate (for smoothie) |
| 4 fat | 1/4 avocado, sliced and cooked with eggs<br>1 tsp Heart Smart Omega margarine for cooking eggs and vegetables |
| | Water |
| **Snack** | |
| 2 bread/starch | 8 whole-wheat crackers |
| 2 fruit | 2/3 cup (158 ml) Concord grape juice (make a spritzer by mixing with sparkling water) |
| 1 vegetable | 1 cup (124 g) celery sticks |
| 4 fat | 2 tbsp natural peanut butter |
| **Lunch** | |
| 5 bread/starch | 12 in. (36 cm) Subway sandwich (choose from "6 grams of fat or less" list) |
| 2 vegetable | Fill sandwich with vegetable choices |
| 1 fruit | Banana |
| 4 very lean protein | 4 oz (120 g) meat included in sandwich |
| 1 fat | 1 tsp olive oil or 1 tbsp salad dressing |
| **Snack** | |
| 2 fruit | 16 dried apricot halves |
| 1 milk | 1 tall nonfat latté |
| 2 tsp added sugar | 2 tsp sugar |

> continued

> *continued*

| Food group servings | Menu |
|---|---|
| **Dinner** | |
| 4 bread/starch | 1 baked sweet potato<br>1 cup cooked quinoa |
| 3 fruit | 1 cup (124 g) raspberries and 1 cup (165 g) cubed mango; put on top of ice cream |
| 3 tsp added sugar | 1/2 cup light ice cream |
| 4 vegetable | 1 cup (180 g) steamed asparagus<br>4 cups (112 g) mixed green salad |
| 6 lean protein | 6 oz (180 g) wild salmon, grilled |
| 5 fat | 1 fat included in ice cream; 1 tsp olive oil for salmon; 3 tbsp salad dressing |
| Free (no calories) | 1 tbsp whipped cream to top fruit and ice cream |

# 15

# Fat-Loss Menu Plans

The diets in this chapter for losing fat are for novice and experienced exercisers, bodybuilders, athletes, and virtually anyone who wants to lose body fat in a safe, controlled manner—without losing precious muscle. Caloric levels differ for men and women because it is more difficult for women to lose fat than it is for men.

### Power Eating Fat-Loss Diet

| | Woman | | Man | |
|---|---|---|---|---|
| Workouts per week | Three or four (novice) | Five or more (experienced) | Three or four (novice) | Five or more (experienced) |
| Calories/kg | 25 | 35 | 28 | 38 |
| Calories/lb | 11.4 | 16.0 | 12.7 | 17.3 |
| **Protein** | | | | |
| g/kg | 2.2 | 2.2 | 2.2 | 2.2 |
| g/lb | 1.0 | 1.0 | 1.0 | 1.0 |
| **Carbohydrate** | | | | |
| g/kg | 2.5 | 3.5 | 3.0 | 4.0 |
| g/lb | 1.1 | 1.6 | 1.4 | 1.8 |
| **Fat*** | | | | |
| g/kg | ~0.7 | ~1.4 | ~0.8 | ~1.5 |
| g/lb | ~0.32 | ~0.64 | ~0.36 | ~0.68 |

*Total fat varies based on total calories. To find your fat grams, determine your total calories, protein grams, and carbohydrate grams. Add your protein and carbohydrate calories (1 g protein = 4 calories, 1 g carbohydrate = 4 calories), subtract this total from the total calories, and divide by 9 (1 g fat = 9 calories). See chapter 10 for more information.

## 130-POUND (59 KG) NOVICE WOMAN
### (three or four workouts per week)

1,475 calories; 130 grams protein; 148 grams carbohydrate; 40 grams fat

| Food groups | Number of servings |
|---|---|
| Bread/starch | 3 |
| Fruit | 3 |
| Nonfat milk | 3 |
| Teaspoons of added sugar | 0 |
| Vegetable | 4 |
| Protein: | |
|   Very lean | 7 |
|   Lean | 5 |
|   Medium-fat | 1 |
| Fat | 4 |

| Food group servings | Menu |
|---|---|
| **Breakfast** | |
| 1 bread/starch | 1 cup (25 g) Kashi puffed cereal |
| 1 milk | 1 cup (240 ml) fat-free milk |
| 1 fruit | 3/4 (110 g) cup blueberries for cereal |
| 1 medium-fat protein | 1 whole egg, scrambled in nonstick skillet |
| 1 very lean protein | 2 egg whites, scrambled with whole egg |
| 1 fat | 1 tbsp ground flaxseed sprinkled on cereal |
| | Water |
| **Snack** | |
| 1 vegetable | 1 cup (128 g) mini carrots |
| 1 fat | 6 almonds |
| | Green tea (or other tea) |

| Food group servings | Menu |
|---|---|
| **Lunch** | |
| 1 bread/starch | Subway Turkey Breast Wrap |
| 2 vegetables | Fill sandwich with vegetable choices |
| 4 very lean protein | 3 oz (90 g) turkey included<br>1 oz (30 g) cheese |
| 1 fat | 1 fat included in cheese |
| Free (no calories) | Dijon mustard |
| | Water |
| **Preworkout Snack** | |
| 1 milk | 1 cup (230 g) plain yogurt |
| 1 fruit | 1 small banana |
| | Water |
| **Workout** | |
| | Water |
| **Postworkout smoothie** | |
| 1 fruit | 3/4 cup (112 g) frozen whole strawberries<br>1/4 cup (60 ml) orange juice |
| 1 milk | 1 cup (240 ml) nonfat milk |
| 2 very lean protein | 14 g isolate whey protein |
| **Dinner** | |
| 1 bread/starch | 1/2 baked sweet potato |
| 1 vegetable | 1/2 cup (90 g) steamed asparagus |
| 5 lean protein | 5 oz (150 g) wild salmon, grilled |
| 1 fat | 1 tsp olive oil for salmon |
| | Green tea (or other tea) |

# 130-POUND (59 KG) EXPERIENCED WOMAN
## (five or more workouts per week)

2,065 calories; 130 grams protein; 207 grams carbohydrate; 80 grams fat

| Food groups | Number of servings |
|---|---|
| Bread/starch | 5 |
| Fruit | 4 |
| Nonfat milk | 3 |
| Teaspoons of added sugar | 0 |
| Vegetable | 8 |
| Protein: | |
| Very lean | 6 |
| Lean | 4 |
| Medium-fat | 1 |
| Fat | 11 |

| Food group servings | Menu |
|---|---|
| **Breakfast** | |
| 2 bread/starch | 2 slices whole-grain bread |
| 1 milk | 1 cup (240 ml) fat-free milk |
| 1 fruit | 1/2 cup (120 ml) orange juice |
| 2 vegetable | 1 cup sautéed vegetables for eggs |
| 1 medium-fat protein | 1 whole egg, scrambled |
| 3 fat | 1/8 avocado, spread on bread<br>1 tsp Heart Smart Omega margarine<br>1 tsp olive oil for cooking eggs and veggies |
| | Water |
| **Snack** | |
| 1 fruit | 8 dried apricot halves |
| 3 fat | 18 almonds |
| | Green tea (or other tea) |

| Food group servings | Menu |
| --- | --- |
| **Lunch** | |
| 1 bread/starch | Subway Turkey Breast Wrap |
| 2 vegetable | Fill sandwich with vegetable choices |
| 4 very lean protein | 3 oz (90 g) turkey included in sandwich<br>1 oz (30 g) cheese |
| 2 fat | 1 fat included in cheese; 1 tsp olive oil or<br>1 tbsp salad dressing |
| | Water |
| **Preworkout snack** | |
| 1 bread/starch | 3/4 oz (23 g) whole-wheat pretzels |
| 1 milk | 1 cup (230 g) plain yogurt |
| 1 fruit | 3/4 cup (110 g) blueberries |
| | Water |
| **Workout** | |
| | Water |
| **Postworkout smoothie** | |
| 1 fruit | 1 1/4 cups (180 g) whole strawberries |
| 1 milk | 1 cup (240 ml) nonfat milk |
| 2 very lean protein | 14 g whey protein isolate |
| **Dinner** | |
| 1 bread/starch | 1/2 baked sweet potato |
| 4 vegetable | 1 cup (180 g) steamed asparagus<br>4 cups (112 g) mixed green salad |
| 4 lean protein | 4 oz (120 g) wild salmon, grilled |
| 3 fat | 1 tsp olive oil for salmon<br>4 tbsp reduced-fat salad dressing |
| | Green tea (or other tea) |

# 180-POUND (82 KG) NOVICE MAN

## (three or four workouts per week)

2,290 calories; 180 grams protein; 245 grams carbohydrate; 66 grams fat

| Food groups | Number of servings |
|---|---|
| Bread/starch | 6 |
| Fruit | 5 |
| Nonfat milk | 3 |
| Teaspoons of added sugar | 0 |
| Vegetable | 9 |
| Protein:<br>  Very lean<br>  Lean<br>  Medium-fat | <br>11<br>6<br>1 |
| Fat | 8 |

| Food group servings | Menu |
|---|---|
| **Preworkout snack** | |
| 1 milk | 1 cup (230 g) plain yogurt |
| 1 fruit | 3/4 cup (110 g) blueberries |
| | Water |
| **Workout** | |
| | Water |
| **Breakfast** | |
| 1 bread/starch | 1 slice whole-grain bread |
| 1 milk | 1 cup (240 ml) fat-free milk |
| 2 fruit | 1/2 cup (120 ml) orange juice<br>1/2 cup frozen mango or other fruit |
| 2 vegetable | 1 cup sautéed vegetables for eggs |
| 1 medium-fat protein | 1 whole egg, scrambled in nonstick skillet |
| 5 very lean protein | 4 egg whites, cooked with whole egg<br>21 g whey protein isolate added to milk and<br>orange juice and blend |
| 1 fat | 1/8 avocado, spread on bread |

| Food group servings | Menu |
|---|---|
| **Breakfast,** *continued* | |
| Cooking spray | 1-2 seconds to sauté vegetables and add eggs |
| | Water |
| **Snack** | |
| 1 bread/starch | Included in the edamame or Genisoy soy crisps |
| 1 vegetable | 1 cup (124 g) celery sticks |
| 1 very lean protein | 1/2 cup (90 g) edamame or 1 serving (about 1/3 of bag) of Genisoy soy crisps |
| 2 fat | 1 tbsp natural peanut butter |
| **Lunch** | |
| 3 bread/starch | 6 in. (18 cm) Subway sandwich (choose from "6 grams of fat or less" list) |
| 2 vegetable | Fill sandwich with vegetable choices |
| 1 fruit | Banana |
| 5 very lean protein | 2 oz (60 g) included in sandwich; request double meat<br>1 oz (30 g) cheese |
| 1 fat | 1 fat included in cheese |
| Free | Dijon mustard |
| **Snack** | |
| 1 fruit | 8 dried apricot halves |
| 1 milk | 1 tall nonfat latté |
| 2 fat | 12 almonds |
| **Dinner** | |
| 1 bread/starch | 1/2 baked sweet potato |
| 1 fruit | 3 oz (about 15) red grapes |
| 4 vegetable | 1 cup (180 g) steamed asparagus<br>4 cups(112 g) mixed green salad |
| 6 lean protein | 6 oz (180 g) wild salmon, grilled |
| 2 fat | 1 tsp olive oil for salmon<br>2 tbsp reduced-fat salad dressing |
| | Green tea (or other tea) |

# 180-POUND (82 KG) EXPERIENCED MAN

## (five or more workouts per week

3,108 calories; 180 grams protein; 327 grams carbohydrate; 120 grams fat

| Food groups | Number of servings |
|---|---|
| Bread/starch | 8 |
| Fruit | 8 |
| Nonfat milk | 3 |
| Teaspoons of added sugar | 0 |
| Vegetable | 9 |
| Protein: | |
| Very lean | 10 |
| Lean | 6 |
| Medium-fat | 1 |
| Fat | 21 |

| Food group servings | Menu |
|---|---|
| **Preworkout snack** | |
| 1 milk | 1 cup (230 g) plain yogurt |
| 1 fruit | 3/4 cup (110 g) blueberries |
| | Water |
| **Workout** | |
| | Water |
| **Breakfast** | |
| 2 bread/starch | 2 slices whole-grain bread |
| 1 milk | 1 cup (240 ml) fat-free milk |
| 3 fruit | 1 cup (240 ml) orange juice<br>3/4 cup frozen berries<br>1/2 frozen medium banana |
| 2 vegetable | 1 cup sautéed vegetables with eggs |
| 1 medium-fat protein | 1 whole egg, scrambled |
| 4 very lean protein | 4 egg whites, cooked with whole egg<br>14 g whey protein isolate added to milk,<br>orange juice and fruit and blend |

| Food group servings | Menu |
|---|---|
| **Breakfast,** *continued* | |
| 4 fat | 1/4 avocado, spread on bread<br>1 tsp Heart Smart Omega margarine and<br>1 tsp olive oil for cooking vegetables and eggs |
| | Water |
| **Snack** | |
| 2 bread/starch | Included in edamame or Genisoy soy crisps |
| 1 vegetable | 1 cup (124 g) celery sticks |
| 2 very lean protein | 1 cup edamame (180 g) or 2 servings (about 2/3 of the bag) of Genisoy soy crisps |
| 6 fat | 3 tbsp natural peanut butter |
| **Lunch** | |
| 3 bread/starch | 6 in. (18 cm) Subway sandwich (choose from "6 grams of fat or less" list) |
| 2 vegetable | Fill sandwich with vegetable choices |
| 1 fruit | Banana |
| 4 very lean protein | 2 oz (60 g) meat included in sandwich; request double meat |
| 2 fat | 2 tsp olive oil or 2 tbsp salad dressing |
| **Snack** | |
| 2 fruit | 16 dried apricot halves |
| 1 milk | 1 tall nonfat latté |
| 3 fat | 18 almonds |
| **Dinner** | |
| 1 bread/starch | 1/2 baked sweet potato |
| 1 fruit | 3 oz (about 15) red grapes |
| 4 vegetables | 1 cup (180 g) steamed asparagus<br>4 cups (112 g) mixed green salad |
| 6 lean protein | 6 oz (180 g) wild salmon, grilled |
| 6 fat | 8 large black olives;<br>1 tsp olive oil for rubbing on salmon and drizzled on asparagus; 4 tbsp salad dressing |
| | Green tea (or other tea) |

## POWER PROFILE: Fat Loss

Several years ago, I was asked to work with a 28-year-old basketball player after his physical conditioning and performance had markedly diminished over a period of a year.

At our initial meeting, the 6-foot, 11-inch (211 cm) player weighed 276 pounds (125 kg) and had 23 percent body fat. Seriously concerned about his condition and his performance, he reported that he had been desperately trying to lose weight, particularly because his contract required him to maintain a certain weight and body fat; his ultimate goal was 257 pounds (166.5 kg) or 13 percent body fat.

His diet consisted of 1,700 calories, with 30 percent coming from protein, 27 percent from carbohydrate, 32 percent from fat, and 11 percent from alcohol. These are clearly not optimal percentages for an athlete, particularly one who is trying to lose weight and retain muscle.

Because of his poor diet, he was fatigued, even unable to eat when he got home from practice. What's more, he was afraid to eat, fearing that food would show up the next day on the scale. He truly was in the beginning stages of an eating disorder. And the less he ate, the higher his body-fat percentage climbed.

With only five weeks to go until his first goal-weight deadline, I placed him on the Power Eating diet for losing fat. This initially included 4,019 calories (33 calories per kilogram), 222 grams of protein, 603 grams of carbohydrate, and 80 grams of fat. In addition, he drank a gallon (4 L) of fluid a day and supplemented with 500 milligrams of vitamin E. During his workout, he sipped 48 ounces (1.4 L) of a glucose–electrolyte solution; after his workout, he consumed a serving of Kleiner's Essential Muscle-Building Formula for Men or Kleiner's Muscle-Building Formula.

After several weeks and some success, I discontinued the glucose–electrolyte solution during his aerobic workouts to enhance fat-burning during exercise because he was required to make weight by a contract deadline. This was the only major change I made. I also decreased his daily calories by 100 to activate further weight loss.

In five weeks, he made amazing progress, reaching 263.5 pounds (119.5 kg) and 12.75 percent body fat. A few weeks later, he weighed in at 261 pounds (118 kg) and 12.9 percent body fat. Both the team and the athlete were excited about the outcome, and he returned to successful full-court play.

# 16

# Getting Cut Menu Plans

To lean out—either for additional body-fat reduction or for a bodybuilding competition—tweak your diet using my Power Eating seven-day cutting diet. (It's particularly useful for bodybuilders who must lean out the week before a competition.) The distribution of nutrients for the cutting plan is based on getting enough protein and fat within the restricted number of calories. This forces a limited amount of carbohydrate, which allows for rapid weight loss. Use this approach only when absolutely necessary. Because women have more difficulty losing fat than men do, calorie levels are different for them. Stay on this diet no longer than 14 days.

## Power Eating Getting Cut Diet

| Workouts per week | Woman | | Man | |
| --- | --- | --- | --- | --- |
| | Three or four (novice) | Five or more (experienced) | Three or four (novice) | Five or more (experienced) |
| Calories/kg | 22 | 29 | 25 | 32 |
| Calories/lb | 10 | 13.2 | 11.4 | 14.5 |
| **Protein** | | | | |
| g/kg | 2.3 | 2.3 | 2.3 | 2.3 |
| g/lb | 1.05 | 1.05 | 1.05 | 1.05 |
| **Carbohydrate** | | | | |
| g/kg | 1.8 | 2.9 | 2.3 | 3.0 |
| g/lb | 0.82 | 1.32 | 1.05 | 1.36 |
| **Fat*** | | | | |
| g/kg | ~0.6 | ~0.9 | ~0.7 | ~1.2 |
| g/lb | ~0.27 | ~0.41 | ~0.32 | ~0.55 |

*Total fat varies based on total calories. To find your fat grams, determine your total calories, protein grams, and carbohydrate grams. Add your protein and carbohydrate calories (1 g protein = 4 calories, 1 g carbohydrate = 4 calories), subtract this total from the total calories, and divide by 9 (1 g fat = 9 calories). See chapter 10 for more information.

## 130-POUND (59 KG) NOVICE WOMAN

### (three or four workouts per week)

1,300 calories; 136 grams protein; 106 grams carbohydrate; 37 grams fat

| Food groups | Number of servings |
|---|---|
| Bread/starch | 1 |
| Fruit | 2 |
| Nonfat milk | 3 |
| Teaspoons of added sugar | 0 |
| Vegetable | 5 |
| Protein: | |
| Very lean | 10 |
| Lean | 4 |
| Medium-fat | 1 |
| Fat | 4 |

| Food group servings | Menu |
|---|---|
| **Breakfast** | |
| 1 bread/starch | 1 cup (25 g) Kashi puffed cereal |
| 1 milk | 1 cup ( 240 ml) fat-free milk |
| 1 fruit | 3/4 cup (110 g) blueberries for cereal |
| 1 medium-fat protein | 1 whole egg, scrambled in nonstick skillet |
| 2 very lean protein | 4 egg whites, scrambled with whole egg |
| 1 fat | 1 tbsp (12 g) ground flaxseed sprinkled on cereal |
| | Water |
| **Snack** | |
| 1 vegetable | 1 cup (128 g) mini carrots |
| 1 fat | 6 almonds |
| | Green tea (or other tea) |

| Food group servings | Menu |
|---|---|
| **Lunch** | |
| 2 vegetable | Subway grilled chicken breast and spinach salad |
| 6 very lean protein | 3 oz (90 g) chicken included in salad; request double meat |
| 1 fat | 2 tbsp (30 ml) reduced-fat dressing |
| | Water |
| **Preworkout snack** | |
| 1 milk | 1 cup (230 g) plain yogurt |
| 1 fruit | 1 small banana |
| | Water |
| **Workout** | |
| | Water |
| **Postworkout smoothie** | |
| 1 milk | 1 cup (240 ml) nonfat milk |
| 2 very lean protein | 14 g whey protein isolate, blend with milk and 3 or 4 ice cubes |
| **Dinner** | |
| 2 vegetable | 1/2 cup (90 g) steamed asparagus<br>2 cups (56 g) mixed green salad |
| 4 lean protein | 4 oz (120 g) wild salmon, grilled |
| 1 fat | 1 tsp (5 ml) olive oil for salmon |
| Free | 2 tbsp (30 ml) fat-free Italian dressing |
| | Green tea (or other tea) |

# 130-POUND (59 KG) EXPERIENCED WOMAN

## (five or more workouts per week)

1,711 calories; 136 grams protein; 171 grams carbohydrate; 54 grams fat

| Food groups | Number of servings |
|---|---|
| Bread/starch | 3 |
| Fruit | 4 |
| Nonfat milk | 3 |
| Teaspoons of added sugar | 0 |
| Vegetable | 6 |
| Protein: | |
| Very lean | 8 |
| Lean | 5 |
| Medium-fat | 1 |
| Fat | 7 |

| Food group servings | Menu |
|---|---|
| **Breakfast** | |
| 1 bread/starch | 1 slice whole-grain bread |
| 1 milk | 1 cup (240 ml) fat-free milk |
| 1 fruit | 1/2 cup (120 ml) orange juice |
| 1 medium-fat protein | 1 whole egg, scrambled in nonstick skillet |
| 2 very lean protein | 4 egg whites, cooked with whole egg |
| 1 fat | 1/8 avocado, spread on bread |
| | Water |
| **Snack** | |
| 1 fruit | 4 dried apricots |
| 1 vegetable | 1 cup (128 g) mini carrots |
| 2 fat | 12 almonds |
| | Green tea (or other tea) |

| Food group servings | Menu |
|---|---|
| **Lunch** | |
| 1 bread/starch | Subway Turkey Breast Wrap |
| 2 vegetable | Fill wrap with vegetable choices |
| 4 very lean protein | 3 oz (90 g) turkey included in wrap<br>1 oz (30 g) cheese included in wrap |
| 2 fat | 1 fat included in cheese<br>1 tsp (5 ml) olive oil or 1 tbsp (15 ml) salad dressing |
| | Water |
| **Preworkout snack** | |
| 1 milk | 1 cup (230 g) plain yogurt |
| 1 fruit | 3/4 cup (110 g) blueberries |
| | Water |
| **Workout** | |
| | Water |
| **Postworkout smoothie** | |
| 1 fruit | 3/4 cup (112 g) whole frozen strawberries |
| 1 milk | 1 cup (240 ml) fat-free milk |
| 2 very lean protein | 14 g whey protein isolate |
| **Dinner** | |
| 1 bread/starch | 1/2 baked sweet potato |
| 3 vegetable | 1/2 cup (90 g) steamed asparagus<br>4 cups (112 g) mixed green salad |
| 5 lean protein | 5 oz (150 g) wild salmon, grilled |
| 2 fat | 1 tsp (5 ml) olive oil for salmon<br>2 tbsp (30 ml) reduced-fat salad dressing |
| | Green tea (or other tea) |

# 180-POUND (82 KG) NOVICE MAN

## (three or four workouts per week)

2,045 calories; 188 grams protein; 188 grams carbohydrate; 60 grams fat

| Food groups | Number of servings |
|---|---|
| Bread/starch | 5 |
| Fruit | 3 |
| Nonfat milk | 3 |
| Teaspoons of added sugar | 0 |
| Vegetable | 6 |
| Protein: | |
| Very lean | 11 |
| Lean | 8 |
| Medium-fat | 1 |
| Fat | 8 |

| Food group servings | Menu |
|---|---|
| **Preworkout snack** | |
| 1 milk | 1 cup (230 g) plain yogurt |
| 1 fruit | 3/4 cup (110 g) blueberries |
| | Water |
| **Workout** | |
| | Water |
| **Breakfast** | |
| 1 bread/starch | 1 slice whole-grain bread |
| 1 milk | 1 cup (240 ml) fat-free milk |
| 1 fruit | 1/2 cup (120 ml) orange juice |
| 1 medium-fat protein | 1 whole egg, scrambled in nonstick skillet |
| 5 very lean protein | 4 egg whites, cooked with whole egg<br>21 g whey protein isolate, added to milk and orange juice and blend with 3 or 4 ice cubes |

| Food group servings | Menu |
|---|---|
| **Breakfast,** *continued* | |
| 1 fat | 1/8 avocado, sliced and cooked with eggs |
| | Water |
| **Snack** | |
| 2 bread/starch | Included in the edamame or Genisoy soy crisps |
| 1 vegetable | 1 cup (124 g) celery sticks |
| 2 very lean protein | 1 cup (180 g) edamame or 2 servings (about 2/3 bag) of Genisoy soy crisps |
| 2 fat | 1 tbsp (16 g) natural peanut butter |
| **Lunch** | |
| 1 bread/starch | Subway Turkey Breast Wrap |
| 2 vegetable | Fill wrap with vegetable choices |
| 4 very lean protein | 3 oz (90 g) turkey included in wrap<br>1 oz (30 g) cheese included in wrap |
| 1 fat | 1 fat included in cheese |
| Free (no calories) | Dijon mustard |
| **Snack** | |
| 1 fruit | 4 dried apricots |
| 1 milk | 1 tall nonfat latté |
| 2 fat | 12 almonds |
| **Dinner** | |
| 1 bread/starch | 1/2 baked sweet potato |
| 3 vegetable | 1/2 cup (90 g) steamed asparagus<br>4 cups (112 g) mixed green salad |
| 8 lean protein | 8 oz (240 g) wild salmon, grilled |
| 2 fat | 1 tsp (5 ml) olive oil for salmon<br>2 tbsp (30 ml) reduced-fat salad dressing |
| | Green tea (or other tea) |

# 180-POUND (82 KG) EXPERIENCED MAN

## (five or more workouts per week)

2,618 calories; 188 grams protein; 245 grams carbohydrate; 98 grams fat

| Food groups | Number of servings |
| --- | --- |
| Bread/starch | 5 |
| Fruit | 6 |
| Nonfat Milk | 3 |
| Teaspoons of added sugar | 0 |
| Vegetable | 9 |
| Protein: | |
| Very lean | 10 |
| Lean | 8 |
| Medium-fat | 1 |
| Fat | 14 |

| Food group servings | Menu |
| --- | --- |
| **Preworkout snack** | |
| 1 milk | 1 cup (230 g) plain yogurt |
| 1 fruit | 3/4 cup (110 g) blueberries |
| | Water |
| **Workout** | |
| | Water |
| **Breakfast** | |
| 1 bread/starch | 1 slice whole-grain bread |
| 1 milk | 1 cup (240 ml) fat-free milk for smoothie |
| 2 fruit | 1/2 cup (120 ml) orange juice for smoothie<br>1/2 cup frozen mango or other fruit for smoothie |
| 2 vegetable | 1 cup sautéed vegetables for eggs |
| 1 medium-fat protein | 1 whole egg, scrambled |
| 4 very lean protein | 4 egg whites, cooked with whole egg 14 g whey protein isolate, added to milk, orange juice, and fruit and blend with ice cubes |

| Food group servings | Menu |
|---|---|
| **Breakfast, *continued*** | |
| 4 fat | 1/4 avocado, spread on bread<br>1 tsp (4 g) Heart Smart Omega margarine and<br>1 tsp (5 ml) olive oil for cooking vegetables and<br>eggs |
| | Water |
| **Snack** | |
| 2 bread/starch | Included in edamame or Genisoy soy crisps |
| 1 vegetable | 1 cup (124 g) celery sticks |
| 2 very lean protein | 1 cup (180 g) edamame or 2 servings (about 2/3<br>bag) of Genisoy soy crisps |
| 4 fat | 2 tbsp (32 g) natural peanut butter |
| **Lunch** | |
| 1 bread/starch | Subway Turkey Breast Wrap |
| 2 vegetable | Fill wrap with vegetable choices |
| 4 very lean protein | 3 oz (90 g) turkey included in wrap<br>1 oz (30 g) cheese included in wrap |
| 1 fat | 1 fat included in cheese |
| Free (no calories) | Dijon mustard |
| **Snack** | |
| 2 fruit | 8 dried apricots |
| 1 milk | 1 tall nonfat latté |
| 2 fat | 12 almonds |
| **Dinner** | |
| 1 bread/starch | 1/2 baked sweet potato |
| 1 fruit | 3 oz (90 g, or about 15) red grapes |
| 4 vegetable | 1 cup (180 g) steamed asparagus<br>4 cups (112 g) mixed green salad |
| 8 lean protein | 8 oz (240 g) wild salmon, grilled |
| 3 fat | 8 large black olives<br>1 tsp (5 ml) olive oil for salmon<br>2 tbsp (30 ml) reduced-fat Italian salad dressing |
| | Green tea (or other tea) |

## Special Advice to Competitors

Many strength athletes worry about being too full just as they go into competition. However, it's critical to have enough fluid, calories, and nutrients to feel strong and look great. Probably the best way to do this is to supplement your diet with liquid meal replacements. These will charge you up but pass through your digestive system more quickly than solid foods.

Whatever meal-replacement brand and product you choose, make sure it is third party tested for purity. The company should guarantee that it is absolutely clean! This is not the time to get caught with a positive reading on a doping test. Protein and meal-replacement supplements are notorious for being intentionally or unintentionally spiked with performance-enhancing aids.

Because each serving of a meal replacement is about the same number of calories as a small meal or snack, you should drink it 90 minutes to two hours before your competition to feel your best during the contest. If you feel comfortable, you can also add some low-fiber foods throughout the day to increase your nutritional intake and avoid the boredom of just drinking. Then, eat a variety of foods after the competition to round out your nutrition for the day.

# 17

# Power Eating Recipes

Although there are many supplements on the market, I always like to use fresh ingredients whenever possible. These recipes were designed for the strength-training clients and teams I have worked with over many years. Try them all to find out which ones are your favorites. They've been created for busy people, so each recipe should only take about five minutes to prepare and five minutes to cook. If you've been a reader of earlier editions of *Power Eating*, you'll notice that some of the recipes have been updated, using new formulations and new ingredients. And there are some awesome new ones that I know you're going to love!

# Power Drinks

## Kleiner's Essential Muscle-Building Formula for Women

    1 cup (240 ml) nonfat milk

    1/4 cup (60 ml) calcium-fortified orange juice

    1/4 cup (37 g) frozen strawberries

    14 g whey protein isolate

Blend until smooth.

*One serving contains:*

| Nutrients | Food Group Servings |
|---|---|
| 224 calories | 1 fruit serving |
| 29 g carbohydrate | 3 very lean protein servings |
| 27 g protein | 1 nonfat milk serving |
| 0 fat | |
| <1 g dietary fiber | |

## Kleiner's Essential Muscle-Building Formula for Men

    1 cup (240 ml) nonfat milk

    1/2 cup (120 ml) calcium-fortified orange juice

    1 tbsp (21 g) honey

    1/4 cup (37 g) frozen strawberries

    21 g whey protein isolate

Blend until smooth.

*One serving contains:*

| Nutrients | Food Group Servings |
|---|---|
| 360 calories | 1 1/2 fruit servings |
| 54 g carbohydrate | 4 very lean protein servings |
| 36 g protein | 1 nonfat milk serving |
| 0 fat | 4 tsp (20 g) added sugar |
| 1 g dietary fiber | |

## Kleiner's Easy Muscle-Building Formula

1 cup (240 ml) nonfat milk

1 packet instant breakfast

1 banana

1 tbsp (16 g) peanut butter

(Optional: Add 25 g whey protein isolate and 100 calories.)

Blend until smooth.

*One serving contains:*

| Nutrients | Food Group Servings |
|---|---|
| 438 calories | 1 nonfat milk serving |
| 70 g carbohydrate | 2 fruit servings |
| 17 g protein | 1 very lean protein serving |
| 10 g fat | 2 fat servings |
| 6 g fiber | 6 tsp (30 g) added sugar |

## Kleiner's Muscle-Building Formula

1 cup (150 g) frozen strawberries

1 cup (230 g) nonfat strawberry yogurt

15 g whey protein isolate

1 tbsp (21 g) honey

1 cup (240 ml) nonfat milk

1 cup (240 ml) calcium-fortified orange juice

Blend until smooth.

*One serving contains:*

| Nutrients | Food Group Servings |
|---|---|
| 529 calories | 3 fruit servings |
| 100 g carbohydrate | 2 very lean protein servings |
| 31 g protein | 2 nonfat milk servings |
| 1 g fat | 6 tsp (30 g) added sugar |
| 4 g dietary fiber | |

## Kleiner's Muscle Formula Plus

24 g bovine colostrum or whey protein isolate

1 cup (150 g) frozen unsweetened strawberries

1 medium banana

1 cup (240 ml) nonfat vanilla soy milk fortified with calcium and vitamins A and D

1 cup (240 ml) orange juice fortified with calcium and vitamin C

Blend until smooth.

*One serving contains:*

| Nutrients | Food Group Servings |
|---|---|
| 436 calories | 4 fruit servings |
| 86 g carbohydrate | 3 very lean protein servings |
| 27 g protein | 1 nonfat milk serving |
| 0 g fat | 3 tsp (15 g) added sugar |
| 8 g dietary fiber | |

## Kleiner's Muscle Formula Plus Light

21 g bovine colostrum or whey protein isolate

1 cup (150 g) frozen unsweetened strawberries

1/2 medium banana

1 cup (240 ml) nonfat vanilla soy milk fortified with calcium and vitamins A and D

1/2 cup (120 ml) orange juice fortified with calcium and vitamin C

Blend until smooth.

*One serving contains:*

| Nutrients | Food Group Servings |
|---|---|
| 316 calories | 2 1/2 fruit servings |
| 58 g carbohydrate | 3 very lean protein servings |
| 26 g protein | 1 nonfat milk serving |
| 0 g fat | 3 tsp (15 g) added sugar |
| 6 g dietary fiber | |

## Bone-Builder Smoothie

1 cup (240 ml) nonfat milk

1/2 cup (120 ml) calcium-fortified orange juice

1/2 cup (115 g) nonfat vanilla yogurt

1 cup (150 g) mixture of frozen mango, blueberries, strawberries

1 tbsp (15 g) nonfat dry milk powder

14 g whey protein isolate

Blend until smooth.

*One serving contains:*

| Nutrients | Food Group Servings |
|---|---|
| 440 calories | 3 fruit servings |
| 80 g carbohydrate | 2 very lean protein servings |
| 30 g protein | 2 nonfat milk servings |
| 0 g fat | 3 tsp (15 g) added sugar |
| 5 g dietary fiber | |

## Mocha Breakfast Smoothie

1 cup (240 ml) nonfat milk

1/2 cup (120 ml) strongly brewed coffee

2 tbsp (32 g) natural peanut butter

1/2 large banana

1 envelope chocolate instant breakfast mix

10 ice cubes

Blend until smooth.

*One serving contains:*

| Nutrients | Food Group Servings |
|---|---|
| 485 calories | 1 fruit serving |
| 62 g carbohydrate | 3 very lean protein servings |
| 21 g protein | 2 nonfat milk servings |
| 17 g fat | 3 fat servings |
| 5 g dietary fiber | 4 tsp (20 g) added sugar |

## Soyful Smoothie (Lactose Free)

1/3 block soft tofu (5 oz, or 150 g)

3/4 cup (112 g) frozen strawberries

1/2 medium banana

1/2 cup (120 ml) vanilla nonfat soy milk fortified with vitamins A and D and calcium

1/2 cup (120 ml) calcium-fortified orange juice

2 tsp (14 g) honey

Cream tofu in blender until smooth. Add the next five ingredients and blend until smooth.

*One serving contains:*

| Nutrients | Food Group Servings |
|---|---|
| 321 calories | 3 fruit servings |
| 61 g carbohydrate | 1 medium-fat protein serving |
| 11 g protein | 1/2 nonfat milk serving |
| 5 g fat | 2 tsp (10 g) added sugar |
| 4 g dietary fiber | |

## Phytochemical Phenomenon II

1 cup (150 g) frozen mixture of mango and papaya

1/2 medium kiwifruit, peeled and quartered

1/2 cup (115 g) plain nonfat yogurt

1/3 cup (79 ml) pomegranate juice

2/3 cup (158 ml) pineapple juice

1 cup (240 ml) nonfat milk or unflavored soy milk

Blend until smooth.

*One serving contains:*

| Nutrients | Food Group Servings |
|---|---|
| 383 calories | 5 fruit servings |
| 83 g carbohydrate | 3 very lean protein servings |
| 16 g protein | 1 1/2 nonfat milk servings |
| 1 g fat | |
| 4 g dietary fiber | |

## Zesty Citrus Smoothie

This smoothie will help replenish fluids and electrolytes, particularly on hot days.

**2 in. (6 cm) piece of fresh ginger**

**1 cup (148 g) lemon sorbet**

**2 cups (480 ml) cold unflavored sparkling water**

**2 tbsp (30 ml) fresh lemon juice**

**1 tbsp (15 ml) lime juice**

**1/8 tsp salt**

**2 tbsp (30 g) sugar***

**15 ice cubes**

**Zest of 1 large lemon (about 2 tbsp, or 30 g)**

*If you prefer a sweeter drink, add more sugar, agave syrup, or stevia.

Grate the ginger and squeeze the juice from the grated ginger. Blend the ginger juice with the remaining ingredients until the mixture reaches the consistency of a frozen margarita drink. For a lower-calorie beverage, make one recipe for two servings.

*One serving contains:*

**Nutrients**
150 calories
38 g carbohydrate
1 g protein
0 g fat
1 g dietary fiber

**Food Group Servings**
9 1/2 tsp (48 g) added sugar

## Piña Colada Smoothie

    1 cup (240 ml) nonfat milk

    1 serving vanilla instant breakfast powder

    6 oz (170 g) low-fat piña colada yogurt (or other coconut and pineapple yogurt)

    1/2 cup (120 ml) crushed pineapple in natural juice

    2 tbsp (30 ml) light coconut milk

    1/2 tsp (3 ml) rum extract

    4 ice cubes

Blend until smooth.

*One serving contains:*

| Nutrients | Food Group Servings |
|---|---|
| 455 calories | 1 fruit serving |
| 82 g carbohydrate | 3 nonfat milk servings |
| 21 g protein | 1 fat serving |
| 5 g fat | 6 tsp (30 g) added sugar |
| 1 g dietary fiber | |

## Antioxidant Advantage

    1 cup (240 ml) nonfat milk

    1/3 cup (79 ml) Concord grape juice

    1 tbsp (15 ml) lime juice

    1/2 cup (115 g) plain nonfat yogurt

    1/2 cup (75 g) frozen strawberries

    1/4 cup (37 g) frozen blueberries

    5 g creatine monohydrate

Blend until smooth.

*One serving contains:*

| Nutrients | Food Group Servings |
|---|---|
| 255 calories | 2 fruit servings |
| 50 g carbohydrate | 1 very lean protein |
| 18 g protein | 1 1/2 nonfat milk servings |
| 0 g fat | 3 g dietary fiber |

## Morning Pick-Me-Up

2 tsp (10 g) chai tea leaves

2 cups (480 ml) nonfat milk

1/3 cup (40 g) nonfat dry milk powder

1 1/2 tbsp (32 g) honey

1/8 tsp (0.5 g) nutmeg

4 ice cubes

Simmer the tea in milk for 5 to 8 minutes. Cool in the refrigerator. Pour the milk into a blender, straining out the tea leaves. Add the remaining ingredients. Blend until smooth.

*One serving contains:*

| Nutrients | Food Group Servings |
|---|---|
| 350 calories | 3 nonfat milk servings |
| 62 g carbohydrate | 6 tsp (30 g) added sugar |
| 25 g protein | |
| 1 g fat | |
| 0 g dietary fiber | |

## Caribbean Crush

11.5 oz (340 ml, or 1 can) papaya juice

1/3 cup crushed pineapple in natural juice

1/2 banana

21 g whey protein isolate

6 ice cubes

Blend until smooth.

*One serving contains:*

| Nutrients | Food Group Servings |
|---|---|
| 364 calories | 4 1/2 fruit servings |
| 69 g carbohydrate | 3 very lean protein servings |
| 23 g protein | |
| 1 g fat | |
| 4 g dietary fiber | |

## Apple Pie à la Mode

1 cup (240 ml) unfiltered apple juice

1/2 cup (115 g) unsweetened applesauce

1/3 cup (48 g) vanilla nonfat frozen yogurt

2 tbsp (30 g) toasted wheat germ

1/3 cup (40 g) nonfat dry milk powder

10 g whey protein isolate

Blend until smooth.

*One serving contains:*

| Nutrients | Food Group Servings |
|---|---|
| 399 calories | 3 fruit servings |
| 74 g carbohydrate | 2 very lean protein servings |
| 25 g protein | 1 nonfat milk serving |
| 2 g fat | 3 tsp (15 g) added sugar |
| 4 g dietary fiber | |

## Lemon-Lime Zinger Sport Drink

To fuel and hydrate your body, drink this power booster within two hours before exercise. It's also a great fluid replenisher during or after exercise or anytime during an active day.

1 in. (3 cm) piece of fresh ginger

2 cups (480 ml) cold unflavored sparkling water

1 tbsp (15 ml) lemon juice

2 tsp (10 ml) lime juice

2 tbsp (30 g) sugar

Scant 1/8 tsp (0.75 g) salt

Grate the ginger and squeeze out the juice. Blend the ginger juice with the remaining ingredients for 20 seconds. Serve immediately.

*One serving contains:*

| Nutrients | Food Group Servings |
|---|---|
| 109 calories | 7 tsp (35 g) added sugar |
| 28 g carbohydrate | |
| 0 g protein | |
| 0 g fat | |
| 0 g dietary fiber | |

# Anti-Inflammatory Recovery Shake Recipes

I use the USANA Nutrimeal here because it is a nicely designed meal replacement that boosts your total nutrition, is guaranteed pure, and allows for the nutritional profile that I desire. Whatever brand you use, look for a guarantee of purity.

Combine the following ingredients in a blender, blend on high speed, and enjoy.

## Apple Ginger Spinach Berry

> 1 cup (240 ml) all-natural 100% apple juice
>
> 1 tbsp fresh chopped ginger (approx. 1 in., or 6 cm, piece)
>
> 2 cups (56 g) baby spinach
>
> 1/2 cup (72 g) fresh or frozen blueberries
>
> 3 scoops chocolate whey USANA Nutrimeal
>
> 1 scoop whey protein isolate

Makes 2 servings.

*One serving contains (includes apple juice):*

| Nutrients | Food Group Servings |
|---|---|
| 323 calories | 2 fruit servings |
| 48 g carbohydrate | 2 1/2 very lean protein servings |
| 21 g protein | 1/2 nonfat milk serving |
| 3 g fat | 3 tsp (15 g) added sugar |
| 7 g fiber | 1/2 fat serving |

## Raspberry Plum Basil

1 cup (240 ml) water or 100% natural juice (apple, berry, etc.)

1/2 cup (75 g) fresh or frozen raspberries

2 medium plums, sliced

1 tbsp fresh basil (1 tsp dried)

3 scoops vanilla USANA Nutrimeal

1 scoop whey protein isolate

Makes 2 servings.

*One serving contains (includes apple juice):*

| Nutrients | Food Group Servings |
|---|---|
| 370 calories | 2 1/2 fruit servings |
| 61 g carbohydrate | 2 1/2 very lean protein servings |
| 21 g protein | 1/2 nonfat milk serving |
| 4 g fat | 3 tsp (15 g) added sugar |
| 7 g fiber | 1/2 fat serving |

## Banana Beet Orange

1 cup (240 m) water or 100% all-natural orange juice

1 tsp (2.4 g) cinnamon

1/4 tsp (0.6 g) ground nutmeg

1 small banana

1/2 cup beets, chopped (about two or three beets)

3 scoops vanilla USANA Nutrimeal

1 scoop whey protein isolate

Makes 2 servings.

*One serving contains (includes orange juice):*

| Nutrients | Food Group Servings |
|---|---|
| 318 calories | 2 fruit servings |
| 52 g carbohydrate | 2 1/2 very lean protein servings |
| 22 g protein | 1/2 nonfat milk serving |
| 3 g fat | 3 tsp (15 g) added sugar |
| 5 g fiber | 1/2 fat serving |

## Almond Peach

1 cup (240 ml) water or almond milk

1 cup frozen peaches

1 tbsp (16 g) nut butter

1 tsp (2.4 g) cinnamon

3 scoops vanilla USANA Nutrimeal

1 scoop whey protein isolate

Makes 2 servings.

*One serving contains (includes almond milk):*

| Nutrients | Food Group Servings |
|---|---|
| 275 calories | 1/2 fruit servings |
| 30 g carbohydrate | 2 1/2 very lean protein servings |
| 22 g protein | 1/2 nonfat milk serving |
| 10 g fat | 3 tsp (15 g) added sugar |
| 7 g fiber | 2 fat serving |

# Pump Up Your Power Drink

You can create your own designer drink by adding certain natural ingredients and nutritional supplements. Here's a rundown:

**Fiber.** With a goal of 25 to 35 grams per day, getting enough fiber is often difficult. Commercial juices and smoothies are usually devoid of fiber, but they don't have to be. Increase the fiber content of your power drinks by using fruit, fruit with skins or seeds, ground flaxseed, or wheat germ. You can also eat whole-wheat crackers or breads with your drink to easily increase fiber.

**Protein.** Protein powders boost the protein content of your drink when you don't want to increase any other nutrients. If you just want to add protein, use whey or soy protein isolate.

**Energy.** To pack in energy and nutrients, instant breakfast and meal-replacement powders work well. If you are lactose intolerant, choose a lactose-free energy-boosting supplement powder and meal replacements.

**Creatine monohydrate.** If you participate in power sports or strength train, add creatine to your diet to enhance your performance. Especially after exercise, a power drink is a great way to get in one of your four daily 5-milligram doses.

# Power Breakfasts

## Indian Breakfast Salad

This delicious salad is served as a side dish in India but makes a fast and fabulous breakfast. It is spiced with cardamom, but because cardamom is expensive, you may prefer to use cinnamon.

**1/2 tsp (2 g) butter**

**2 tbsp (14 g) slivered almonds**

**2 medium bananas, thinly sliced**

**4 tbsp (61 g) low-fat plain yogurt**

**3 tbsp (45 g) light sour cream**

**1 tbsp (21 g) honey**

**1/8 tsp (0.25 g) ground cardamom or 1/4 tsp (0.6 g) ground cinnamon**

1. Melt the butter in a small nonstick skillet over medium heat. Toast almonds, stirring frequently, until golden, about 3 minutes.

2. Meanwhile, in a medium bowl, mix bananas with yogurt, sour cream, honey, and cardamom. Add almonds and enjoy.

Makes 2 servings.

*One serving contains:*

| Nutrients | Food Group Servings |
| --- | --- |
| 250 calories | 2 fruit servings |
| 42 g carbohydrate | 1 lean protein serving |
| 6 g protein | 1 fat serving |
| 8 g fat | 3 tsp (15 g) added sugar |
| 4 g dietary fiber | |

## Breakfast Parfait

2 cups (480 g) fat-free Greek yogurt

1 cup (110 g) muesli

1 1/4 cups (180 g) fresh berries

2 tbsp flaxseed meal (13 g ground flaxseeds)

2 tbsp toasted chopped nuts (your choice)

1. In two 16 oz (480 ml) glass or plastic cups, layer the ingredients by adding 1/4 of the yogurt, 1/4 of the muesli, 1/4 of the flaxseed meal, and 1/4 of the berries.

2. Repeat step 1, reserving a dollop of the yogurt for the top, and top with 1/2 the chopped nuts.

Makes 2 servings.

*One serving contains:*

| Nutrients | Food Group Servings |
|---|---|
| 340 calories | 2 bread serving |
| 50 g carbohydrate | 1/2 fruit serving |
| 24 g protein | 1 milk serving |
| 7 g fat | 3 very lean protein servings |
| 8 g dietary fiber | 1 fat serving |

## Peach Melba Yogurt Pops

These delicious pops can be prepared the night before to make a great light breakfast that you can easily hit the road with on a warm summer morning. If you don't want to bother with adding the sticks, just poke a fork into the pop when you're ready to eat.

**1 cup (247 g) sliced canned peaches in light syrup**

**1 cup (230 g) low-fat raspberry yogurt**

**1 cup (240 ml) orange juice**

1. Blend ingredients until smooth. Pour into four 10 oz (300 ml) plastic cups. Place in the freezer.
2. When mixture is partly frozen, insert sticks or plastic spoons.

Makes 2 servings.

*One serving contains:*

| Nutrients | Food Group Servings |
|---|---|
| 280 calories | 2 fruit servings |
| 64 g carbohydrate | 1 nonfat milk serving |
| 6 g protein | 5 tsp (25 g) added sugar |
| 1 g fat | |
| 3 g dietary fiber | |

## Orange Cinnamon French Toast

This toast takes only slightly longer to prepare than the standard version that pops out of the toaster.

**2 large eggs, lightly beaten**

**2 tbsp (30 ml) orange juice**

**1/4 tsp (0.6 g) ground cinnamon**

**4 slices whole-wheat bread**

**Vegetable cooking spray**

1. In a shallow bowl, combine eggs, orange juice, and cinnamon.
2. Spray a nonstick skillet and heat over medium heat for 1 to 2 minutes, until hot. Dip bread into the mixture to coat both sides. Place bread slices in the skillet, pouring any extra egg mixture over them. Cook for about 2 minutes on each side or until browned.

Makes 2 servings.

*One serving contains:*

| Nutrients | Food Group Servings |
|---|---|
| 220 calories | 2 bread servings |
| 28 g carbohydrate | 1 medium-fat protein serving |
| 12 g protein | |
| 7 g fat | |
| 4 g dietary fiber | |

## Pineapple Cheese Danish

4 slices raisin bread

4 tbsp (62 g) canned unsweetened crushed pineapple, drained

1/2 cup (4 oz, or 120 g) part-skim ricotta cheese

1 tsp (5 g) brown sugar

Dash ground cinnamon

1. Spread each slice of bread with 1 oz (30 g) of cheese and top with pineapple. Combine brown sugar and cinnamon and sprinkle on top of the pineapple.
2. Broil in toaster oven or under the broiler until sugar starts to bubble, about 2 minutes.

Makes 2 servings.

*One serving contains:*

| Nutrients | Food Group Servings |
|---|---|
| 246 calories | 2 bread servings |
| 35 g carbohydrate | 1/3 fruit serving |
| 11 g protein | 1/2 medium-fat protein serving |
| 7 g fat | 1/2 fat serving |
| 3 g dietary fiber | |

## Fruit 'n' Cheese

1 small red apple, cored and sliced

1 small d'Anjou or Bartlett pear, cored and sliced

2 oz (60 g) thinly sliced cheddar cheese

4 slices whole-wheat toast

1. Place apple and pear slices on bread and cover with cheese to make open-face sandwiches.
2. Place under broiler or in toaster oven for 2 to 3 minutes or until cheese melts and bubbles.

Makes 2 servings.

*One serving contains:*

| Nutrients | Food Group Servings |
|---|---|
| 322 calories | 2 bread servings |
| 47 g carbohydrate | 1 fruit serving |
| 13 g protein | 1 medium-fat protein serving |
| 12 g fat | 1 fat serving |
| 7 g dietary fiber | |

## Asparagus, Spinach, and Feta Omelet

1 cup (240 ml) pure egg whites

1 whole egg

4 asparagus spears, trimmed

1/2 cup (14 g) fresh baby spinach leaves (chopped)

1 oz (30 g) low-fat feta cheese

Canola oil spray

Ground black pepper (to taste)

Sea salt (to taste)

Wash and chop baby spinach. Whisk egg and egg whites together. Lightly spray frying pan with canola oil and heat. When pan is hot, pour in egg mixture; when egg mix bubbles, flip with spatula.

Lower the heat by 50 percent, and place asparagus spears and spinach leaves evenly on one half of the omelet. Crumble feta over the top and season with a little salt and pepper. Continue cooking until egg mixture is almost cooked.

Using a flat, wide-lipped spatula, fold the uncovered half omelet over spinach, asparagus, and feta. Place the spatula on top of omelet for 15 seconds (this allows the feta to melt). Serve immediately.

Makes 2 servings.

*One serving contains:*

| Nutrients | Food Group Servings |
|---|---|
| 294 calories | 1 vegetable serving |
| 5 g carbohydrate | 2 very lean protein servings |
| 41 g protein | 2 medium-fat protein servings |
| 10 g fat | |
| 2 g dietary fiber | |

Recipe created by Shar Sault. Used with permission.

# Easy Main Courses

## Chicken in Orange Sauce With Pistachios

8 skinless, boneless chicken breast halves

4 tbsp (34 g) cake flour

1 1/2 cups (360 ml) fresh orange juice

1/4 cup (60 ml) white wine

1/4 cup (60 ml) white wine vinegar

1/2 cup (120 ml) minced shallots

2 tbsp (30 g) brown sugar

2 tbsp (30 ml) olive oil

2 tbsp (24 g) unsalted butter, cut into small pieces

3 tbsp (63 g) honey

8 orange slices and 8 tbsp (62 g) unsalted pistachio nuts to garnish

Salt and pepper to taste

Wax paper

1. Trim chicken breasts and pound thick ends under wax paper to cook evenly. Combine salt, pepper, and cake flour. Dust on chicken breasts.
2. In a saucepan, bring orange juice, wine, vinegar, shallots, and brown sugar to a boil. Simmer and reduce to about 1 cup. Keep warm.
3. Heat olive oil in a large skillet over medium heat. Sauté chicken breasts in batches until springy to the touch, 4 minutes per side. Transfer to an ovenproof casserole dish and set aside.
4. Remove sauce from heat and whisk in cold butter pieces. Pour over chicken and keep chicken warm in oven set at 250 degrees F (121 degrees C). Chicken may be chilled or frozen at this point.
5. To serve, thoroughly reheat chicken in oven at 325 degrees F (163 degrees C), basting well with the sauce.
6. Heat honey with 2 tbsp (30 ml) of the orange sauce. Sprinkle each breast with 1 tbsp (8 g) of pistachios. Coat orange slice to garnish chicken.

Makes 8 servings.

*One serving contains:*

| Nutrients | Food Group Servings |
|---|---|
| 334 calories | 4 very lean protein servings |
| 22 g carbohydrate | 2 fat servings |
| 30 g protein | 1/2 fruit serving |
| 13 g fat | 1 tsp (5 g) added sugar |
| 2 g dietary fiber | |

Here are two recipes that give you the mood-boosting effects of omega-3 fat and the metabolism-boosting benefits of cayenne pepper. If you can stand the heat, add cayenne to your diet on a daily basis to help you stay lean, but not mean.

## Pan-Fried Cajun Catfish

1/2 cup (69 g) cornmeal
1 tsp (0.3 g) dried parsley flakes
1/2 tsp (1 g) paprika
1/8 tsp (0.2 g) cayenne pepper (or to taste)
1/8 tsp (0.2 g) white pepper
1/8 tsp (0.2 g) black pepper
1/2 tsp (3 g) salt
1/4 tsp (0.4 g) thyme
1/2 tsp (1.4 g) garlic powder
1/4 tsp (0.6 g) onion powder
1 egg
2 1/2 tbsp (37 ml) water
12 oz (360 g) catfish fillets
Nonstick cooking spray
Lemon wedges

1. Mix together the cornmeal, herbs, and spices in a flat dish. In a separate dish, beat the egg with the water.
2. Heat a nonstick frying pan over medium-high heat for 30 seconds. Generously spray the pan with cooking spray. Dip each fillet in the egg–water mixture and then coat generously in the cornmeal mixture. Place skin side down in the frying pan for 5 to 6 minutes, or until the bottom is golden brown. Turn the fish and cook another 6 to 7 minutes. Turn again if needed and remove promptly. Watch the fish closely as it cooks. Do not let the oil smoke or the coating burn. Fish should be tender inside, crisp and brown on the outside. Serve hot with lemon wedges.

Makes 3 servings.

*One serving contains:*

| Nutrients | Food Group Servings |
|---|---|
| 281 calories | 4 lean protein servings |
| 18 g carbohydrate | 1 bread serving |
| 25 g protein | |
| 11 g fat | |
| 2 g dietary fiber | |

## Lemon Sole With Mustard Sauce

This is a great fish recipe for those who don't love fish, as well as for those who do.

**1 lb (480 g) lemon sole fillets**
**1/4 cup (60 ml) lemon juice**
**1/4 cup (60 ml) white wine**
**1 tsp (5 ml) cornstarch dissolved in 1/8 cup (30 ml) cold water**
**1 cup (240 ml) water**
**1/4 cup (60 ml) apple juice**
**2 tsp (10 ml) dry white wine**
**1 tsp (3 g) minced garlic**
**1 tbsp (15 ml) lime juice sweetened with 1 tsp (5 g) sugar**
**2 tsp (10 g) prepared yellow mustard**
**1 tsp (5 ml) Worcestershire sauce**
**1/8 tsp (0.2 g) cayenne pepper (or to taste)**

1. Place the fish, lemon juice, and 1/4 cup (60 ml) white wine in a pan and bake at 400 degrees F (200 degrees C) for 20 minutes, or until the fish is flaky and white.
2. Combine the dissolved cornstarch, water, apple juice, dry white wine, and garlic in a saucepan. Heat over medium heat to thicken, stirring often.
3. In a small bowl, whisk together the sweetened lime juice, mustard, Worcestershire sauce, and cayenne pepper. Add the mustard mixture to the cornstarch mixture and whisk until well blended. Allow the mixture to continue cooking until thickened.
4. Place the fish on a platter, pour the mustard sauce over it, and serve.

Makes 4 servings.

*One serving contains:*

| Nutrients | Food Group Servings |
|---|---|
| 170 calories | 1/2 fruit serving |
| 6 g carbohydrate | 4 very lean protein servings |
| 26 g protein | |
| 2 g fat | |
| 0 g dietary fiber | |

## Tuna Supreme

This is great in a salad or in a wrap. In less than 5 minutes you can make tuna interesting enough to look forward to every day. I always double the ingredients when I make this meal so that I know I always have plenty on hand every day. Preparation and forward planning makes life so much easier when maintaining a great nutrition plan. Serves two.

**2 celery sticks, finely diced (add leaves)**

**1/2 red pepper, diced**

**1/2 red onion, finely diced**

**1/2 cup (120 ml) finely chopped parsley**

**2 7 oz cans (400 g total) tuna in spring water (drained)**

**1/2 cup (73 g) corn kernels**

**2 tbsp (20g) low-fat mayonnaise**

**1/2 tsp (2.5 g) Dijon mustard**

**Fresh ground pepper to season**

1. First prepare and finely dice celery, pepper, red onion, and parsley.
2. Drain tuna and place into a bowl.
3. Add all chopped ingredients; then add corn, pepper, mayonnaise, and mustard.
4. Mix together well, making sure the mayonnaise and mustard are dispersed evenly throughout.
5. Serve on rice cakes, with a salad, or in a tortilla wrap.

This meal is quick 'n' easy, tastes great, and is full of protein.

*One serving contains:*

| Nutrients | Food Group Servings |
|---|---|
| 292 calories | 3 vegetable servings |
| 18 g carbohydrate | 7 very lean protein servings |
| 55 g protein | 1/2 fat serving |
| 4 g fat | |
| 3 g dietary fiber | |

Recipe created by Shar Sault. Used with permission.

## Mediterranean Brussels Sprouts With Tuna

Brussels sprouts are one of the most nutritious vegetables you can add to your plan. They belong to the cruciferous family and are rich in vitamins C and E, folate, beta-carotene, and iron, and contain a unique spectrum of phytonutrients and fiber.

When sprayed with a little olive oil and seasoned with fresh herbs, garlic, and spices, these brussels sprouts are simply delicious. Serves four.

1 tbsp (15 ml) virgin olive oil or canola oil spray

1 red pepper, sliced into 2 in. (6 cm) long, thin strips

2 cloves garlic, finely chopped

3 cans (7 oz each; 600 g total) albacore tuna chunks in spring water (drained)

1 cup (225 g) Roma tomatoes, peeled and chopped

1 tsp (5 g) brown or raw sugar

1 2/3 cups (375 g) brussels sprouts, washed well and sliced in halves or quarters

1/2 cup (about 24) pitted kalamata olives, sliced

2 tbsp (30 ml each) fresh basil and cilantro, both finely chopped

Cracked black pepper, to taste

Pine nuts to garnish (optional)

1. Heat oil in frying pan or wok, and stir-fry pepper and garlic for 2 to 3 minutes.

2. Add tuna, Roma tomatoes, sugar, brussels sprouts, olives, and fresh herbs.

3. Cover and cook for 5 to 7 minutes. Stir frequently.

4. Season with pepper and serve immediately. Sprinkle pine nuts as garnish (optional).

*One serving contains:*

| Nutrients | Food Group Servings |
|---|---|
| 291 calories | 4 vegetable servings |
| 20 g carbohydrates | 5 very lean protein servings |
| 37 g protein | 1/2 fat serving |
| 7 g fat | |
| 5 g fiber | |

Recipe created by Shar Sault. Used with permission.

# Five-Minute Tuna Cakes

Our household should have shares in a tuna cannery with the amount of tuna we consume. These tuna cakes are fast, delicious, and nutritious! They can be eaten hot or cold, and served with salad or vegetables. Make up a large batch of these tuna cakes and store them in the freezer. They come in really handy when you want a fast meal! Makes eight cakes.

**2 7 oz (400 g) cans of albacore tuna in spring water, drained**

**1 onion, finely chopped**

**1 tbsp fresh ginger (1 inch or 2.5 cm root), finely chopped**

**1 clove garlic, finely chopped**

**2 tbsp (30 ml) chopped cilantro**

**2 tbsp (30 ml) chopped parsley**

**1 whole egg**

**Canola oil spray**

**Freshly ground black pepper**

1. Heat frying pan and spray lightly with oil.
2. Add onion, ginger, and garlic in and cook for 1 minute, stirring frequently.
3. Remove from heat. Cool.
4. Place tuna into a bowl.
5. Add coriander, parsley, black pepper, and the cooked onion mixture. Add egg and mix well to combine.
6. Shape into small cakes.
7. Heat fry pan used earlier. Spray lightly with oil.
8. Place patties in pan and cook on high for 2 to 3 minutes on each side until brown. Tuna cakes should be moist and a little pink in the center when cooked.

*One serving contains:*

| Nutrients | Food Group Servings |
|---|---|
| 79 calories | 2 very lean protein servings |
| 2 g carbohydrate | |
| 14 g protein | |
| 2 g fat | |
| <1 g fiber | |

Recipe created by Shar Sault. Used with permission.

# Ready-to-Serve Vegetables

## Irene's Marinated Broccoli

This is the easiest recipe to prepare for yourself or for entertaining. It makes the best-tasting raw broccoli you could imagine! It's great alone, or you could add the optional dip for a special occasion. If you drain well, the fat content will be lower.

1 bunch broccoli, cut into small florets (about 3 cups, or 213 g)

1/4 cup (60 ml) cider or wine vinegar

3/4 cup (180 ml) virgin olive oil

2 cloves garlic, split (or more if desired)

1 tsp (5 g) sugar

2 tsp (2 g) fresh dill

Marinade

Put broccoli in resealable bag and cover with marinade. Marinate in bag, refrigerated, overnight. Drain.

Optional Dip*

2 cups (448 g) light canola mayonnaise (also works with half mayo and half plain yogurt, the way I actually make it at home)

1 1/2 tsp (3 g) curry powder

1 tsp (5 g) ketchup

1/4 tsp (1 ml) Worcestershire sauce

Mix together. Serve with drained broccoli. Makes 6 servings.

*One serving without dip contains:*

| Nutrients | Food Group Servings |
|---|---|
| 90 calories | 1/2 vegetable serving |
| 2 g carbohydrate | 2 fat servings |
| 1 g protein | |
| 9 g fat | |
| 1 g dietary fiber | |

*Add 1 fat serving for every 1 tbsp (15 ml) dip

## Alotta Onions Soup

Whenever I've shared this recipe with anyone, the description has always started out with "a lot of onions." The water and electrolyte content makes it a great fluid replacer after exercise. This recipe, which serves only two or three, is pared down from the army-sized version we make at home.

2 cloves fresh garlic, minced

1 tbsp (15 ml) canola oil

1/2 tbsp (7 ml) sesame oil

1 1/2 large yellow onions, thinly sliced

6 cups (1.4 L) water

1 1/2 tbsp (22 ml) soy sauce

1/4 tsp (1 ml) freshly ground black pepper

4-6 tsp (8-12 g) freshly grated Parmesan cheese

1. Sauté the garlic in the oils in a shallow nonstick pan over medium heat until slightly soft, about 3 to 5 minutes. Add onions and cook, stirring occasionally, until slightly caramelized, about 20 minutes.

2. Transfer the onions and garlic to a soup pot. Add the water, soy sauce, and pepper. Bring to a low boil over high heat; then reduce the heat to low and simmer uncovered for 15 minutes.

3. Serve in full bowls sprinkled with 2 tsp (4 g) of Parmesan cheese.

Makes 3 servings.

*One serving contains:*

**Nutrients**
109 calories
8 g carbohydrate
2 g protein
8 g fat
1 g dietary fiber

**Food Group Servings**
1 1/2 vegetable servings
1 1/2 fat servings

# Great Grains

## Easy Energy Couscous

4 tbsp (27 g) slivered almonds

4 tbsp (40 g) golden raisins

12 dried apricots, quartered

8 dried figs, quartered

1/2 tsp (1.2 g) cinnamon

1/2 cup (120 ml) fresh orange juice

1 1/2 cups (360 ml) water

1/4 tsp (1 ml) salt

1 tbsp (12 g) butter

1 cup (173 g) whole-wheat couscous

1. Place the almonds, raisins, apricots, and figs in a bowl with the cinnamon. Cover with the orange juice and refrigerate for a minimum of 30 minutes and up to overnight.

2. In a saucepan, bring the water, salt, and butter to a boil. Stir in the couscous. Cover and simmer over low heat for 5 minutes. Remove from heat and let stand 5 minutes. Fluff the couscous lightly with a fork.

3. Transfer the fruit and nut mixture to a saucepan and warm thoroughly over medium-low heat. Turn into a mixing bowl and add the cooked couscous. Mix well. Couscous can be served warm or cold.

Makes 6 servings.

*One serving contains:*

| Nutrients | Food Group Servings |
|---|---|
| 258 calories | 2 fruit servings |
| 49 g carbohydrate | 1 bread serving |
| 5 g protein | 1 fat serving |
| 5 g fat | |
| 7 g dietary fiber | |

# Seashore Buckwheat

2/3 cup whole-wheat pasta shells (70 g)

1 tbsp (15 ml) canola oil

1 cup (70 g) sliced mushrooms

1 small onion, diced

2 cups (480 ml) chicken stock

1 whole egg, slightly beaten

1 cup (164 g) preroasted buckwheat kernels or groats

Pinch of white pepper and salt to taste

1. Cook the pasta shells until al dente according to package directions; drain and set aside.
2. Heat the oil in a nonstick pan over medium heat. Add the mushrooms and onion and sauté until the onion is translucent, about 7 minutes. Set aside.
3. Heat the stock to boiling. In a small mixing bowl, combine the egg with the buckwheat until the kernels are coated. Turn the buckwheat into a medium-sized skillet. Stir the egg and buckwheat mixture over medium-high heat for 3 to 4 minutes until it is hot and slightly toasted and the egg-coated kernels are well separated. Reduce the heat to low and carefully stir in the boiling stock, sautéed mushrooms and onions, and pepper and salt. Cover tightly and simmer 10 to 12 minutes, or until the buckwheat kernels are tender and all the liquid has been absorbed.
4. Turn into an oven-safe casserole dish and mix in the pasta shells. Place uncovered under an oven broiler for 3 to 5 minutes, just to brown the top. Watch closely and remove promptly.

Makes 4 servings.

*One serving contains:*

| Nutrients | Food Group Servings |
|---|---|
| 232 calories | 2 bread servings |
| 39 g carbohydrate | 2 vegetable servings |
| 9 g protein | 1/2 very lean protein serving |
| 6 g fat | 1/2 fat serving |
| 5 g dietary fiber | |

# Appendix A

# Three-Day Food Record

Choose at least three days that will represent your typical schedule (workdays and nonworkdays, training days and rest days, or home days and travel days), and record your food intake for those days in a 24-hour diet log. You can make copies of the diet log that follows. Try to record the food as you eat it or just afterward; it is often difficult to remember in the evening exactly what you ate eight hours before. Record everything you eat and drink, including water, and be as detailed as possible.

When you are finished recording, translate all the foods from a single day into food groups, and then into calories and grams of protein, carbohydrate, and fat by plugging them into the diet analysis table that follows. Use the food group tables from chapter 10 to get the nutrient details about each food group.

You can do this yourself by hand, the old-fashioned way, and really learn the details of your diet. Online and mobile apps vary in content, data quality, and ease of use, but they keep improving. Whichever works for you is the better choice. Recording your diet and training is one of the best ways to change old habits into new habits.

# 24-Hour Diet Log

| Time of day | Food eaten | Description | Quantity | Location | Why you ate |
|---|---|---|---|---|---|
| | | | | | |
| | | | | | |
| | | | | | |
| | | | | | |
| | | | | | |
| | | | | | |
| | | | | | |
| | | | | | |
| | | | | | |
| | | | | | |
| | | | | | |
| | | | | | |
| | | | | | |
| | | | | | |

From S. Kleiner and M. Greenwood-Robinson, 2014, *Power eating,* 4th ed. (Champaign, IL: Human Kinetics).

# Diet Analysis Table

Diet record date: _____

| Food groups | Number of servings | Carbohydrate (g) | Protein (g) | Fat (g) | Calories |
|---|---|---|---|---|---|
| Bread/starch | | | | | |
| Fruit | | | | | |
| Nonfat milk | | | | | |
| Low-fat milk | | | | | |
| Teaspoons of added sugar | | | | | |
| Vegetable | | | | | |
| Very lean protein | | | | | |
| Lean protein | | | | | |
| Medium-fat protein | | | | | |
| Fat protein | | | | | |
| **Totals** | | | | | |

From S. Kleiner and M. Greenwood-Robinson, 2014, *Power eating*, 4th ed. (Champaign, IL: Human Kinetics).

# Appendix B

# Restaurant Guide and Healthy Fast Food

Dining out does not have to mean diet disaster. You can take control of your menu and your meals at restaurants. The trick is to have a game plan before you go.

To start with, choose a restaurant that serves nutritious choices: chicken, fish, salads, baked potatoes, and steamed vegetables, to name just a few. Avoid all-you-can-eat buffets and restaurants that offer only high-calorie, high-fat foods. Before arriving at the restaurant, decide what you'll order, and how you'd like it prepared—grilled chicken, baked or grilled fish, or lean red meat, for example.

Beware of fat hiding in certain restaurant foods. Sauces, condiments, butter, oil, mayonnaise, creams, and rich cheeses all add a lot of unhealthy fat to appetizers, entrees, and side dishes. Ask the serving staff to leave out high-fat ingredients. Another option is to make a substitution, such as a baked potato for French fries.

Request that sauces, salad dressings, and sour cream be served on the side so you can control the amount you use. Request that a menu item be prepared using an alternative method, such as broiling instead of frying.

Be inquisitive! Ask questions about foods on the menu. Be specific! How is the food prepared? What are the ingredients? To help you, consult the following menu dictionary, which shows what to choose and what to avoid.

# MENU DICTIONARY

| Choose | Avoid |
|---|---|
| **Entrees** | |
| In their own juices | Fried |
| Boiled | Sauteed |
| Grilled | Au gratin |
| Baked | Buttery, buttered |
| Roasted | Creamed, cream sauce |
| Poached | Hollandaise |
| Lean meats (round, sirloin, tenderloin, flank steak, filet mignon) | Parmesan |
| Garden fresh | Marinated (in oil) |
| Tomato juice | Casserole |
| | Gravy |
| | Hash |
| | Potpie |
| | Crispy |
| **Appetizers** | |
| Steamed seafood (e.g., mussels, clams, crabs, lobsters, or shrimp) | Swimming in butter |
| Raw or steamed vegetables | Cheese |
| Vegetable antipasto | |
| **Soups** | |
| Gazpacho, consommé, broth-type | Creamed |
| **Vegetables** | |
| Fresh, raw, or steamed | Fried |
| Baked potato or yams | Heavily buttered, creamed, or in cheese sauce |
| **Salads** | |
| With clear or reduced-fat dressings | With meat, bacon, cheese, or croutons |
| | With creamy dressings |

## MENU DICTIONARY, *continued*

| Choose | Avoid |
|---|---|
| **Breads** | |
| Dry (no butter) | Baked with butter, shortening, or cheese |
| Whole grain or sprouted grain with seeds | Sweet rolls |
| **Sandwiches** | |
| Tuna, chicken, turkey, seafood, or lean cooked beef | Processed lunch meats, hard cheese, fried foods |
| | Sandwiches with sauces, gravies, mayonnaise, or bacon |
| **Desserts** | |
| Fruit, sorbet, sherbet, low-fat ice creams and frozen yogurt, angel food cake, and other specially made low-fat and low-sugar items | Commercial pies, cakes, pastries, ice cream, and candies |

# Top 10 Fast-Food Restaurants and Best Choices

The establishments listed in this section have made an effort to stand above the crowd. And then, of course, sometimes you just can't do any better than one of the big fast-food chains. So here are my top choices and the best menu options.

Menus and recipes change so quickly that nutrition information in a book is outdated in a heartbeat. All of these restaurants have nutrition information available both on the premises and online.

The following are in alphabetical order (not best to worst).

**Au Bon Pain**

Best choices: whole grains, salads, small plates, fresh fruit, vegetarian options

**Chipotle**

Best choices: burrito bowls, fresh (often locally sourced) produce, low-sodium options

**Einstein Brothers Bagels**

Best choices: Good Grains Bagel, high-fiber Veg Out, reduced-fat shmears, hummus, peanut butter, half or whole-sized salad

**McDonald's (sometimes it's the only place you've got)**

Best choices: Grilled Chicken Classic and wraps (skip the mayo or sauce), salad, Egg McMuffin

**Noah's Bagels:**

Best choices: Bagel Thin sandwiches, egg sandwiches, fresh fruit and vegetables, salads, and "Smart Choices"

**Panera Bread**

Best choices: whole grains, fresh fruit, full or half-size portions, salads, vegetarian options

**Qdoba**

Best choices: Craft 2–Naked Burrito (customize your size and ingredients), fresh produce, vegetarian choices

**Subway**

Best choices: all items with 6 grams of fat or less on a wheat roll with extra veggies and double protein on a 6-inch roll (Skip the mayo and use mustard, vinegar, and oil. Chicken salad is also a winner.)

**Taco Del Mar**

Best choices: fresh produce, fish, whole grains, chicken burrito, vegetarian options

**Wendy's**

Best choices: baked potato topped with chili, broccoli, and chives (Skip the sour cream, cheese, and Buttery Best Spread.)

# Works Consulted

Abramowicz, W.N., et al. 2005. Effects of acute versus chronic L-carnitine L-tartrate supplementation on metabolic responses to steady state exercise in males and females. *International Journal of Sport Nutrition and Exercise Metabolism* 15: 386-400.

Achten, J. et al. 2004. Higher dietary carbohydrate content during intensified running training results in better maintenance of performance and mood state. *Journal of Applied Physiology* 96: 1331-1340.

Akermark, C., I. Jacobs, M. Rasmusson, and J. Karlsson. 1996. Diet and muscle glycogen concentration in relation to physical performance in Swedish elite ice hockey players. *International Journal of Sport Nutrition* 6: 272-284.

Alkhenizan, A.H., et al. 2004. The role of vitamin E in the prevention of coronary events and stroke. Meta-analysis of randomized controlled trials. *Saudi Medical Journal* 25: 1808-1814.

Allen, J.D., et al. 1998. Ginseng supplementation does not enhance healthy young adults' peak aerobic exercise performance. *Journal of the American College of Nutrition* 17: 462-466.

American Dietetic Association. 1995. Position of the American Dietetic Association: Phytochemicals and functional foods. *Journal of the American Dietetic Association* 95: 493-496.

American Dietetic Association. 1998. Position of the American Dietetic Association: Use of nutritive and non-nutritive sweeteners. *Journal of the American Dietetic Association* 98: 580-588.

American Dietetic Association. 2009. Position of the American Dietetic Association: Functional Foods. *Journal of the American Dietetic Association* 98: 735-746.

American Institute for Cancer Research. (n.d.). Coconut water: Health or hype? Retrieved from http://preventcancer.aicr.org/site/News2?page=NewsArticle&id=19168&news_iv_ctrl=2303.

Anderson, G.H., et al. 2002. Inverse association between the effect of carbohydrates on blood glucose and subsequent short-term food intake in young men. *American Journal of Clinical Nutrition* 76: 1023-1030.

Anderson, J.W., et al. 2009. Health benefits of dietary fiber. *Nutrition Reviews* 67: 188-205.

Andersson, B., X. Xuefan, M. Rebuffe-Scrive, K. Terning, et al. 1991. The effects of exercise training on body composition and metabolism in men and women. *International Journal of Obesity* 15: 75-81.

Anomasiri, W., et al. 2004. Low dose creatine supplementation enhances sprint phase of 400 meters swimming performance. *Journal of the Medical Association of Thailand* 87: S228-S232.

Antonio, J., 2000. The effects of Tribulus terrestris on body composition and exercise performance in resistance-trained males. *International Journal of Sports Nutrition and Exercise Metabolism* 10: 208-215.

Antonio, J., et al. 1999. Glutamine: A potentially useful supplement for athletes. *Canadian Journal of Applied Physiology* 24: 1-14.

Applegate, L. 1992. Protein power. *Runner's World*, June, 22-24.

Armstrong, L.E. 2002. Caffeine, body fluid-electrolyte balance, and exercise performance. *International Journal of Sport Nutrition and Exercise Metabolism* 12: 189-206.

Aulin, K.P., et al. 2000. Muscle glycogen resynthesis rate in humans after supplementation of drinks containing carbohydrates with low and high molecular masses. *European Journal of Applied Physiology* 81: 346-351.

Avery, N.G., et al. 2003. Effects of vitamin E supplementation on recovery from repeated bouts of resistance exercise. *Journal of Strength and Conditioning Research* 17: 801-809.

Azadbakht, L., et al. 2007. Soy inclusion in the diet improves features of the metabolic syndrome: A randomized crossover study in postmenopausal women. *American Journal of Clinical Nutrition* 85: 735-741.

Bachman, J.G., L.D. Johnston, and P.M. O'Malley. 2011. *Monitoring the future: Questionnaire responses from the nation's high school seniors, 2010.* Ann Arbor, MI: Institute for Social Research.

Backhouse, S.H., et al. 2005. Effect of carbohydrate and prolonged exercise on affect and perceived exertion. *Medicine & Science in Sports & Exercise* 37: 1768-1773.

Bahrke, M.S., et al. 1994. Evaluation of the ergogenic properties of ginseng. *Sports Medicine* 18: 229-248.

Bahrke, M.S., et al. 2004. Abuse of anabolic androgenic steroids and related substances in sport and exercise. *Current Opinion in Pharmacology* 4: 614-620.

Balon, T.W., J.F. Horowitz, and K.M. Fitzsimmons. 1992. Effects of carbohydrate loading and weight-lifting on muscle girth. *International Journal of Sports Nutrition* 2: 328-334.

Balsom, P.D., et al. 1998. Carbohydrate intake and multiple sprint sports: With special reference to football (soccer). *International Journal of Sports Medicine* 20: 48-52.

Baranov, A.I. 1982. Medicinal uses of ginseng and related plants in the Soviet Union: Recent trends in the Soviet literature. *Journal of Ethnopharmacology* 6: 339-353.

Barth, C.A., and U. Behnke. 1997. Nutritional physiology of whey components. *Nahrung* 41: 2-12.

Bazzarre, T.L., et al. 1992. Plasma amino acid responses of trained athletes to two successive exhaustive trials with and without interim carbohydrate feeding. *Journal of the American College of Nutrition* 11 (5): 501-511.

Bean, A. 1996, February 23. Here's to your immunity. *Runner's World.*

Bellisle, F., and C. Perez. 1994. Low-energy substitutes for sugars and fats in the human diet: Impact on nutritional regulation. *Neuroscience Behavioral Review* 18: 197-205.

Belza, A., et al. 2007. Body fat loss achieved by stimulation of thermogenesis by a combination of bioactive food ingredients: A placebo-controlled, double-blind 8-week intervention in obese subjects. *International Journal of Obesity* 31: 121-130.

Bemben, M.G., et al. 2005. Creatine supplementation and exercise performance: Recent findings. *Sports Medicine* 35: 107-125.

Bent, S., et al. 2006. Saw palmetto for benign prostatic hyperplasia. *New England Journal of Medicine* 354: 557-566.

Benton, D., et al. 2001. The influence of phosphatidylserine supplementation on mood and heart rate when faced with an acute stressor. *Nutritional Neuroscience* 4: 169-178.

Biolo, G., et al. 1997. An abundant supply of amino acids enhances the metabolic effect of exercise on muscle protein. *American Journal of Physiology* 273: E122-E129.

Bird, S.P., et al. 2006. Effects of liquid carbohydrate/essential amino acid ingestion on acute hormonal response during a single bout of resistance exercise in untrained men. *Nutrition* 22: 367-375.

Birketvedt, G.S., et al. 2005. Experiences with three different fiber supplements in weight reduction. *Medical Science Monitor* 11: P15-P18.

Bjorntorp, P. 1991. Importance of fat as a support nutrient for energy: Metabolism of athletes. *Journal of Sports Sciences* 9: 71-76.

Blankson, H., et al. 2000. Conjugated linoleic acid reduces body fat mass in overweight and obese humans. *Journal of Nutrition* 130: 2943-2948.

Blomstrand, E. 2006. A role for branched-chain amino acids in reducing central fatigue. *Journal of Nutrition* 136: 544S-547S.

Blomstrand, E., et al. 2006. Branched-chain amino acids activate key enzymes in protein synthesis after physical exercise. *Journal of Nutrition* 136: 269S-273S.

Bloomer, R.J., et al. 2000. Effects of meal form and composition on plasma testosterone, cortisol, and insulin following resistance exercise. *International Journal of Sport Nutrition and Exercise Metabolism* 10: 415-424.

Blumenthal, M. (Ed.). 1998. *The complete German Commission E monographs.* Austin, TX: American Botanical Council.

Blumenthal Mark. (2000) Herbal Medicine: Expanded Commission E Monographs. *American Botanical Council, Integrative Medicine Communications*: 174.

Borsheim, E., et al. 2002. Essential amino acids and muscle protein recovery from resistance exercise. *American Journal of Physiology, Endocrinology, and Metabolism* 4(283): E648-E657.

Borsheim, E., et al. 2004. Effect of an amino acid, protein, and carbohydrate mixture on net muscle protein balance after resistance exercise. *International Journal of Sport Nutrition and Exercise Metabolism* 14: 255-271.

Boullata, J.I., et al. 2003. Anaphylactic reaction to a dietary supplement containing willow bark. *The Annals of Pharmacotherapy* 37: 832-835.

Brass, E.P. 2004. Carnitine and sports medicine: Use or abuse? *Annals of the New York Academy of Sciences* 1033: 67-78.

Bremner, K., et al. 2002. The effect of phosphate loading on erythrocyte 2,3-bisphosphoglycerate levels. *Clinica Chimica Acta* 323: 111-114.

Brilla, L.R., and V. Conte. 1999. Effects of zinc-magnesium (ZMA) supplementation on muscle attributes of football players. *Medicine & Science in Sports & Exercise* 31 (Suppl. 5): Abstract No. 483.

Brilla, L.R., and T.F. Haley. 1992. Effect of magnesium supplementation on strength training in humans. *Journal of the American College of Nutrition* 11: 326-329.

Brown, G.A., et al. 2000. Effects of anabolic precursors on serum testosterone concentrations and adaptations to resistance training in young men. *International Journal of Sports Nutrition and Exercise Metabolism* 10: 340-359.

Brown, J., M.C. Crim, V.R. Young, and W.J. Evans. 1994. Increased energy requirements and changes in body composition with resistance training in older adults. *The American Journal of Clinical Nutrition* 60: 167-175.

Bryner, R.W., R.C. Toffle, I.H. Ullrich, and R.A. Yeager. 1997. The effects of exercise intensity on body composition, weight loss, and dietary composition in women. *Journal of the American College of Nutrition* 16: 68-73.

Bucci, L.R. 2000. Selected herbals and human exercise performance. *The American Journal of Clinical Nutrition* 72 (Suppl. 2): 624S-636S.

Buckley, J.D., et al. 1998. Effect of an oral bovine colostrum supplement (Intact) on running performance. Abstract, 1998 Australian Conference of Science and Medicine in Sport, Adelaide, South Australia.

Buckley, J.D., et al. 1999. Oral supplementation with bovine colostrum (Intact) increases vertical jump performance. Abstract, 4th Annual Congress of the European College of Sport Science, Rome.

Bujko, J., et al. 1997. Benefit of more but smaller meals at a fixed daily protein intake. *Zeitschrift Fur Ernahrungswissenschaft* 36: 347-349.

Burke, E.R. 1999. *D-ribose: What you need to know.* Garden City Park, NY: Avery.

Burke, L.E., et al. 2008. A randomized clinical trial of a standard versus vegetarian diet for weight loss: The impact of treatment preference. *International Journal of Obesity* 32: 166–176.

Burke, L.M. 1997. Nutrition for post-exercise recovery. *International Journal of Sports Nutrition* 1: 214-224.

Burke, L.M., et al. 1998. Carbohydrate intake during prolonged cycling minimizes effect of glycemic index of preexercise meal. *Journal of Applied Physiology* 85: 2220-2226.

Butteiger, D.N., M. Cope, P. Liu, R. Mukherjea, E. Volpi, B.B. Rasmussen, and E.S. Krul. 2012, October 13. A soy, whey and caseinate blend extends postprandial skeletal muscle protein synthesis in rats. *Clinical Nutrition* [Epub ahead of print]. pii: S0261-5614(12)00216-6. doi: 10.1016/j.clnu.2012.10.001.

Butterfield, G., et al. 1991. Amino acids and high protein diets. In D. Lamb and M. Williams (Eds.), *Perspectives in exercise science and sports medicine.* Vol. 4, pp. 87-122. Madison, WI: Brown & Benchmark.

Calder, A., et al. 2011. A review on the dietary flavonoid kaempferol. *Mini Reviews in Medicinal Chemistry* 11: 298-344.

Campbell, B.I., et al. 2004. The ergogenic potential of arginine. *Journal of the International Society of Sports Nutrition* 1: 35-38.

Campbell, W.W., M.C. Crim, V.R. Young, et al. 1995. Effects of resistance training and dietary protein intake on protein metabolism in older adults. *American Journal of Physiology* 268: E1143-E1153.

Campbell, W.W., et al. 1999. Effects of an omnivorous diet compared with a lactoovovegetarian diet on resistance-training-induced changes in body composition and skeletal muscle in older men. *American Journal of Clinical Nutrition* 70: 1032-1039.

Carli, G., et al. 1992. Changes in exercise-induced hormone response to branched chain amino acid administration. *European Journal of Applied Physiology* 64: 272-277.

Carlson, J.J., et al. 2011. Dietary fiber and nutrient density are inversely associated with the metabolic syndrome in US adolescents. Journal of the American Dietetic Association 111: 1688-1695.

Castell, L.M. 1996. Does glutamine have a role in reducing infections in athletes? *European Journal of Applied Physiology* 73: 488-490.

Center for Science in the Public Interest. 2006. Choosing safer beef to eat. Retrieved from www.cspinet.org/foodsafety/saferbeef.html.

Chandler, R.M., H.K. Byrne, J.G. Patterson, and J.L. Ivy. 1994. Dietary supplements affect the anabolic hormones after weight-training exercise. *Journal of Applied Physiology* 76: 839-845.

Charley, H. 1982. *Food science.* New York: John Wiley & Sons.

Chilibeck, P.D., et al. 2004. Effect of creatine ingestion after exercise on muscle thickness in males and females. *Medicine & Science in Sports & Exercise* 36: 1781-1788.

Chilibeck, P.D., et al. 2005. Creatine monohydrate and resistance training increase bone mineral content and density in older men. *The Journal of Nutrition, Health & Aging* 9: 352-353.

Clancy, S.P., P.M. Clarkson, M.E. DeCheke, et al. 1994. Effects of chromium picolinate supplementation on body composition, strength, and urinary chromium loss in football players. *International Journal of Sport Nutrition* 4: 142-153.

Clark, N. 1993. Athletes with amenorrhea. *The Physician and Sportsmedicine* 21: 45-48.

Clarkson, P.M. 1991. Nutritional ergogenic aids: Chromium, exercise, and muscle mass. *International Journal of Sport Nutrition* 1: 289-293.

Clarkson, P.M. 1996. Nutrition for improved sports performance: Current issues on ergogenic aids. *Sports Medicine* 21: 393-401.

Coleman, E. 1997. Carbohydrate unloading: A reality check. *The Physician and Sportsmedicine* 25: 97-98.

Collomp, K. 1991. Effects of caffeine ingestion on performance and anaerobic metabolism during the Wingate Test. *International Journal of Sports Medicine* 12: 439-443.

Collomp, K., A. Ahmaidi, M. Audran, and C. Prefaut. 1992. Benefits of caffeine ingestion on sprint performance in trained and untrained swimmers. *European Journal of Applied Physiology* 64: 377-380.

Colson, S.N., et al. 2005. Cordyceps sinensis- and Rhodiola rosea-based supplementation in male cyclists and its effect on muscle tissue oxygen saturation. *Journal of Strength and Conditioning Research* 19: 358-363.

Conjugated linoleic acid overview. 2001, March 1. Professional monographs: Herbal, mineral, vitamin, nutraceuticals. Westlake Village, CA: Intramedicine.

Convertino, V.A., et al. 1996. ACSM position stand. Exercise and fluid replacement. *Medicine & Science in Sports & Exercise* 28: i-vii.

Coyle, E.F. 1991. Timing and method of increased carbohydrate intake to cope with heavy training, competition and recovery. *Journal of Sports Sciences* 9 Spec No: 29-51.

Coyle, E.F. 1995. Fat metabolism during exercise. *Sports Science Exchange* 8: 1-7.

Coyle, E.F. 1997. Fuels for sport performance. In D. Lamb and R. Murray (Eds.), *Perspectives in exercise science and sports medicine.* Carmel, IN: Cooper.

Craciun, A.M., et al. 1998. Improved bone metabolism in female elite athletes after vitamin K supplementation. *International Journal of Sports Medicine* 19: 479-484.

Daley, C.A., A. Abbott , P.S. Doyle, G.A. Nader, and S. Larson. (2010, March). A review of fatty acid profiles and antioxidant content in grass-fed and grain-fed beef. *Nutrition Journal* 9: 10. doi: 10.1186/1475-2891-9-10

Dalton, R.A., et al. 1999. Acute carbohydrate consumption does not influence resistance exercise performance during energy restriction. *International Journal of Sport Nutrition* 9: 319-332.

Davis, J.M., et al. 1999. Effects of branched-chain amino acids and carbohydrate on fatigue during intermittent, high-intensity running. *International Journal of Sports Medicine* 20: 309-314.

Delzenne, N.M., et al. 2011. Modulation of the gut microbiota by nutrients with prebiotic properties: Consequences for host health in the context of obesity and metabolic syndrome. *Microbial Cell Factories* 10 (Suppl. 1): S10.

DeMarco, H.M., et al. 1999. Pre-exercise carbohydrate meals: Application of glycemic index. *Medicine & Science in Sports & Exercise* 31: 164-170.

Deschenes, M.R., and W.J. Kraemer. 1989. The biochemical basis of muscular fatigue. *National Strength and Conditioning Association Journal* 11: 41-44.

Diepvens, K., et al. 2006. Metabolic effects of green tea and of phases of weight loss. *Physiology & Behavior* 87: 185-191.

Diepvens, K., et al. 2007. Obesity and thermogenesis related to the consumption of caffeine, ephedrine, capsaicin, and green tea. *American Journal of Physiology* 292: R77-R85.

Dimeff, R.J. 1993. Steroids and other performance enhancers. In R.N. Matzen and R.S. Lang (Eds.), *Clinical preventive medicine*. St. Louis: Mosby-Year Book, Inc.

Dimeff, R.J. May 19, 1996. Drugs and sports: Prescription and non-prescription. Presented at Sports Medicine for the Rheumatologist, American College of Rheumatology, Phoenix, Arizona.

Doherty, M., et al. 2005. Effects of caffeine ingestion on rating of perceived exertion during and after exercise: A meta-analysis. *Scandinavian Journal of Medicine & Science in Sports* 15: 69-78.

Dowling, E.A., et al. 1996. Effect of Eleutherococcus senticosus on submaximal and maximal performance. *Medicine & Science in Sports & Exercise* 28: 482-489.

Dulloo, A.G. 1999. Efficacy of a green tea extract rich in catechin polyphenols and caffeine in increasing 24-h energy expenditure and fat oxidation in humans. *The American Journal of Clinical Nutrition* 70: 1040-1045.

Earnest, C.P., et al. 2004. Effects of a commercial herbal-based formula on exercise performance in cyclists. *Medicine & Science in Sports & Exercise* 36: 504-509.

Engels, H.J., et al. 1997. No ergogenic effects of ginseng (Panax C.A. Meyer) during graded maximal aerobic exercise. *Journal of the American Dietetic Association* 97: 1110-1115.

Ergogenic aids: Reported facts and claims. 1997, Winter. *Scan's Pulse Supplement*: 15-19.

Essen-Gustavsson, B., and P.A. Tesch. 1990. Glycogen and triglyceride utilization in relation to muscle metabolic characteristics in men performing heavy-resistance exercise. *European Journal of Applied Physiology* 61: 5-10.

Evans, W. 1996, April 28. The protective role of antioxidants in exercise induced oxidative stress. Keynote address, 13th Annual SCAN Symposium, Scottsdale, Arizona.

Fairfield, K.M., and R.H. Fletcher. 2002. Vitamins for chronic disease prevention in adults. *Journal of the American Medical Association* 287: 3116-3126.

Fawcett, J.P., S.J. Farquhar, R.J. Walker, et al. 1996. The effect of oral vanadyl sulfate on body composition and performance in weight-training athletes. *International Journal of Sport Nutrition* 6: 382-390.

Fedor, D., and D.S. Kelley. 2009. Prevention of insulin resistance by n-3 polyunsaturated fatty acids. *Current Opinion in Clinical Nutrition and Metabolic Care* 12: 138-146.

Ferreira, M., et al. 1997. Effects of conjugated linoleic acid supplementation during resistance training on body composition and strength. *Journal of Strength and Conditioning Research* 11: 280.

Fogelholm, M. 1992. Micronutrient status in females during a 24-week fitness-type exercise program. *Annals of Nutrition and Metabolism* 36: 209-218.

Fogt, D.L., et al. 2000. Effects of post exercise carbohydrate-protein supplement on skeletal muscle glycogen storage. *Medicine & Science in Sports & Exercise* 2 (Suppl.): Abstract No. 131.

Foley, D. 1984, April. Best health bets from the B team. *Prevention*, 62-67.

Frentsos, J.A., and J.R. Baer. 1997. Increased energy and nutrient intake during training and competition improves elite triathletes' endurance performance. *International Journal of Sport Nutrition* 7: 61-71.

Frey-Hewitt, K.M., K.M. Vranizan, D.M. Dreon, and P.D. Wood. 1990. The effect of weight loss by dieting or exercise on resting metabolic rate in overweight men. *International Journal of Obesity* 14: 327-334.

Friedl, K.E., R.J. Moore, L.E. Martinez-Lopez, et al. 1994. Lower limit of body fat in healthy active men. *Journal of Applied Physiology* 77: 933-940.

Galgani, J.E., et al. 2010. Effect of dihydrocapsiate on resting metabolic rate in humans. *American Journal of Clinical Nutrition* 92: 1089-1093.

Gaullier, J.M., et al. 2007. Six months supplementation with conjugated linoleic acid induces regional-specific fat mass decreases in overweight and obese. *British Journal of Nutrition* 97: 550-560.

Gerster, H. 1989. The role of vitamin C in athletic performance. *Journal of the American College of Nutrition* 8: 636-643.

Gerster, H. 1991. Function of vitamin E in physical exercise: A review. *Zeitschrift fur Ernahrungswissenschaft* 30: 89-97.

Gibala, M. 2009. Molecular responses to high-intensity interval exercise. *Applied Physiology, Nutrition, and Metabolism* 34 (3): 428-432. doi: 10.1139/H09-046.

Gillette, C.A., R.C. Bullough, and C.L. Melby. 1994. Postexercise energy expenditure in response to acute aerobic or resistive exercise. *International Journal of Sport Nutrition* 4: 347-360.

Gillman, M.W., L.A. Cupples, D. Gagnon, et al. 1995. Protective effect of fruits and vegetables on development of stroke in men. *Journal of the American Medical Association* 273: 1113-1117.

Giovannucci, E., A. Ascherio, E.B. Rimm, et al. 1995. Intake of carotenoids and retinol in relation to risk of prostate cancer. *Journal of the National Cancer Institute* 87: 1767-1776.

Gisolfi, C.V., et al. 1992. Guidelines for optimal replacement beverages for different athletic events. *Medicine & Science in Sports & Exercise* 24: 679-687.

Goldfarb, A.H. 1999. Nutritional antioxidants as therapeutic and preventive modalities in exercise-induced muscle damage. *Canadian Journal of Applied Physiology* 24: 249-266.

Goldstein, E.R., et al. 2010. International Society of Sports Nutrition position stand: caffeine and performance. *Journal of the International Society of Sports Nutrition* 7: 5.

Gornall, J., and R.G. Villani. 1996. Short-term changes in body composition and metabolism with severe dieting and resistance exercise. *International Journal of Sport Nutrition* 6: 285-294.

Goulet, E.D., et al. 2005. Assessment of the effects of eleutherococcus senticosus on endurance performance. *International Journal of Sport Nutrition and Exercise Metabolism* 15: 75-83.

Graef, J.L., et al. 2009. The effects of four weeks of creatine supplementation and high-intensity interval training on cardiorespiratory fitness: A randomized controlled trial. *Journal of the International Society of Sports Nutrition* 6: 18.

Green, A.L., E. Hultman, I.A. MacDonald, D.A. Sewell, and P.L. Greenhaff. 1996. Carbohydrate ingestion augments skeletal muscle creatine accumulation during creatine supplementation in humans. *American Journal of Physiology* 271: E821-E826.

Green, N.R., and A.A. Ferrando. 1994. Plasma boron and the effects of boron supplementation in males. *Environmental Health Perspective Supplement* 7: 73-77.

Groeneveld, G.J., et al. 2005. Few adverse effects of long-term creatine supplementation in a placebo-controlled trial. *International Journal of Sports Medicine* 26: 307-313.

Gross, M., et al. 1991. Ribose administration during exercise: Effects on substrates and products of energy metabolism in healthy subjects and a patient with myoadenylate deaminase deficiency. *Klinische Wochenschrift* 69: 151-155.

Haaz, S., et al. 2006. Citrus aurantium and synephrine alkaloids in the treatment of overweight and obesity: An update. *Obesity Reviews* 7: 79-88.

Habeck, M. 2002. A succulent cure to end obesity. *Drug Discovery Today* 7: 280-281.

Haff, G.G., et al. 1999. The effect of carbohydrate supplementation on multiple sessions and bouts of resistance exercise. *Journal of Strength and Conditioning Research* 13: 111-117.

Haff, G.G., et al. 2000. Carbohydrate supplementation attenuates muscle glycogen loss during acute bouts of resistance exercise. *International Journal of Sport Nutrition and Exercise Metabolism* 10: 326-339.

Harberson, D.A. 1988. Weight gain and body composition of weightlifters: Effect of high-calorie supplementation vs. anabolic steroids. In W.E. Garrett Jr. and T.E. Malone (Eds.). *Report of the Ross Laboratories Symposium on muscle development: Nutritional alternatives to anabolic steroids.* Columbus, OH: Ross Laboratories, 72-78.

Hargreaves, M. 2000. Skeletal muscle metabolism during exercise in humans. *Clinical and Experimental Pharmacology and Physiology* 27: 225-228.

Hartung, G.H., J.P. Foreyt, R.S. Reeves, et al. 1990. Effect of alcohol dose on plasma lipoprotein subfractions and lipolytic enzyme activity in active and inactive men. *Metabolism* 39: 81-86.

Hasler, C.M. 1996. Functional foods: The western perspective. *Nutrition Reviews* 54 (11 Part 2): S6-S10.

Hassmen, P., et al. 1994. Branched-chain amino acid supplementation during 30-km competitive run: Mood and cognitive performance. *Nutrition* 10: 405-410.

Haub, M.D., et al. 2002. Effect of protein source on resistive-training-induced changes in body composition and muscle size in older men. *American Journal of Clinical Nutrition* 76: 511-517.

Hymowitz, T. 2007. History of soy. National Soybean Research Laboratory. Retrieved from www.nsrl.uiuc.edu/aboutsoy/history.html

Health, M.K. (Ed.). 1982. *Diet manual, including a vegetarian meal plan* (6th ed.). Loma Linda, CA: Seventh Day Adventist Dietetic Association.

Heaney, R.P. 1993. Protein intake and the calcium economy. *Journal of the American Dietetic Association* 93: 1259-1260.

Hegewald, M.G., et al. 1991. Ribose infusion accelerates thallium redistribution with early imaging compared with late 24-hour imaging without ribose. *Journal of the American College of Cardiology* 18: 1671-1681.

Heinonen, O.J. 1996. Carnitine and physical exercise. *Sports Medicine* 22: 109-132.

Hemila, H. 1996. Vitamin C and common cold incidence: A review of studies with subjects under heavy physical stress. *International Journal of Sports Medicine* 17: 379-383.

Henderson, S., et al. 2005. Effects of coleus forskohlii supplementation on body composition and hematological profiles in mildly overweight women. *Journal of the International Society of Sports Nutrition* 2: 54-62.

Herbert, V., and K.C. Dos. 1994. Folic acid and vitamin $B_{12}$. In M. Shils, J. Olson, and M. Shike (Eds.), *Modern nutrition in health and disease.* Philadelphia: Lea & Febiger, 1430-1435.

Hickson, J.F., et al. 1987. Nutritional intake from food sources of high school football athletes. *Journal of the American Dietetic Association* 87: 1656-1659.

Hitchins, S., et al. 1999. Glycerol hyperhydration improves cycle time trial performance in hot, humid conditions. *European Journal of Applied Physiology and Occupational Physiology* 80: 494-501.

Hoffman, J.R., et al. 2004. Effects of beta-hydroxy beta-methylbutyrate on power performance and indices of muscle damage and stress during high-intensity training. *Journal of Strength and Conditioning Research* 1: 747-752.

Holt, S.H., et al. 1999. The effects of high-carbohydrate vs high-fat breakfasts on feelings of fullness and alertness, and subsequent food intake. *International Journal of Food Sciences and Nutrition* 50: 13-28.

The hoopla about hoodia. 2006. Retrieved from www.bestdietforme.com.

Hulmi, J.J., et al. 2005. Protein ingestion prior to strength exercise affects blood hormones and metabolism. *Medicine & Science in Sports & Exercise* 37: 1990-1997.

Irving, B.A., et al. 2008. Effect of exercise training intensity on abdominal visceral fat and body composition. *Medicine & Science in Sports & Exercise* 40: 1863-1872.

Ivy, J.L. 2002. Early postexercise muscle glycogen recovery is enhanced with a carbohydrate- protein supplement. *Journal of Applied Physiology* 93: 1337-1344.

Ivy, J.L., et al. 1988. Muscle glycogen storage after different amounts of carbohydrate ingestion. *Journal of Applied Physiology* 65: 2018-2023.

Jackman, M., P. Wendling, D. Friars, et al. 1994. Caffeine ingestion and high-intensity intermittent exercise. Abstract. Personal communication with Larry Spriet, University of Guelph, Ontario, Canada.

Jacobsen, B.H. 1990. Effect of amino acids on growth hormone release. *The Physician and Sportsmedicine* 18: 68.

Jäger, R. et al. 2008. The effects of creatine pyruvate and creatine citrate on performance during high intensity exercise. *Journal of the International Society of Sports Nutrition* 5: 4.

Jamurtas, A.Z., et al. 2011. The effects of low and high glycemic index foods on exercise performance and beta-endorphin responses. *Journal of the International Society of Sports Nutrition* 8: 15.

Jennings, E. 1995. Folic acid as a cancer-preventing agent. *Medical Hypotheses* 45: 297-303.

Ji, L.L. 1996. Exercise, oxidative stress, and antioxidants. *The American Journal of Sports Medicine* 24: S20-S24.

Kalman, D., et al. 1999. The effects of pyruvate supplementation on body composition in overweight individuals. *Nutrition* 15: 337-340.

Kanarek, R. 1997. Psychological effects of snacks and altered meal frequency. *British Journal of Nutrition* 77 (Suppl.): S105-S118.

Kanter, M.M., et al. 1995. Antioxidants, carnitine and choline as putative ergogenic aids. *International Journal of Sport Nutrition* 5: S120-S131.

Kanter, M.M., L.A. Nolte, and J.O. Holloszy. 1993. Effects of an antioxidant vitamin mixture on lipid peroxidation at rest and postexercise. *Journal of Applied Physiology* 74: 965-969.

Kaplan, S.A., et al. 2004. A prospective, 1-year trial using saw palmetto versus finasteride in the treatment of category III prostatitis/chronic pelvic pain syndrome. *Journal of Urology* 171: 284-288.

Kelly, G.S. 2001. Conjugated linoleic acid: A review. *Alternative Medicine Review* 6: 367-382.

Keim, N.L., T.F Barbieri, M.D. Van Loan, and B.L. Anderson. 1990. Energy expenditure and physical performance in overweight women: Response to training with and without caloric restriction. *Metabolism* 39: 651-658.

Keim, N.L., A.Z. Belko, and T.F. Barbieri. 1996. Body fat percentage and gender: Associations with exercise energy expenditure, substrate utilization, and mechanical work efficiency. *International Journal of Sport Nutrition* 6: 356-369.

Keith, R.E., K.A. O'Keefe, D.L. Blessing, and G.D. Wilson. 1991. Alterations in dietary carbohydrate, protein, and fat intake and mood state in trained female cyclists. *Medicine & Science in Sports & Exercise* 2: 212-216.

Kendrick, Z.V., M.B. Affrime, and D.T. Lowenthal. 1993. Effect of ethanol on metabolic responses to treadmill running in well-trained men. *Journal of Clinical Pharmacology* 33: 136-139.

Kennedy A, et al. 2010. Antiobesity mechanisms of action of conjugated linoleic acid. *Journal of Nutritional Biochemistry* 21 (3): 171-179.

Kerksick, C., et al. 2001. Bovine colostrum supplementation on training adaptations II: Performance. Abstract presented at Federation of American Societies for Experimental Biology (FASEB) meeting, Orlando, FL, March 31-April 4.

Kim, S.H., et al. 2005. Effects of Panax ginseng extract on exercise-induced oxidative stress. *The Journal of Sports Medicine and Physical Fitness* 45: 178-182.

Kingsley, M.I., et al. 2005. Effects of phosphatidylserine on oxidative stress following intermittent running. *Medicine & Science in Sports & Exercise* 37: 1300-1306.

Kingsley, M.I., et al. 2006. Effects of phosphatidylserine on exercise capacity during cycling in active males. *Medicine & Science in Sports & Exercise* 38: 64-71.

Kirkendall, D.T. 1998. Fluid and electrolyte replacement in soccer. *Clinics in Sports Medicine* 17: 729-738.

Kleiner, S.M. 1991. Performance-enhancing aids in sport: Health consequences and nutritional alternatives. *Journal of the American College of Nutrition* 10: 163-176.

Kleiner, S.M. 1999. Water: An essential but overlooked nutrient. *Journal of the American Dietetic Association* 99: 200-206.

Kleiner, S.M. 2000. Bodybuilding. In C.A. Rosenbloom (Ed.), *Sports nutrition: A guide for the professional working with active people* (3rd ed.). Chicago: SCAN, American Dietetic Association.

Kleiner, S.M., et al. 1989. Dietary influences on cardiovascular disease risk in anabolic steroid-using and non-using bodybuilders. *Journal of the American College of Nutrition* 8: 109-119.

Kleiner, S.M., et al. 1990. Metabolic profiles, diet, and health practices of championship male and female bodybuilders. *Journal of the American Dietetic Association* 90: 962-967.

Kleiner, S.M., et al. 1994. Nutritional status of nationally ranked elite bodybuilders. *International Journal of Sport Nutrition* 1: 54-69.

Koopman, R., et al. 2009. Ingestion of a protein hydrolysate is accompanied by an accelerated in vivo digestion and absorption rate when compared with its intact protein. *American Journal of Clinical Nutrition* 90: 106-115.

Kraemer, W.J., et al. 1998. Hormonal responses to consecutive days of heavy-resistance exercise with or without nutritional supplementation. *Journal of Applied Physiology* 85: 1544-1555.

Kreider, R.B. 1999. Dietary supplements and the promotion of muscle growth. *Sports Medicine* 27: 97-110.

Kreider, R.B. 2000. Nutritional considerations of overtraining. In J.R. Stout and J. Antonio (Eds.), *Sport supplements: A complete guide to physique and athletic enhancement.* Baltimore: Lippincott, Williams & Wilkins.

Kreider, R.B. 2003. Effects of creatine supplementation on performance and training adaptations. *Molecular and Cellular Biochemistry* 244: 89-94.

Kreider, R.B. 2007. Effects of ingesting protein with various forms of carbohydrate following resistance-exercise on substrate availability and markers of anabolism, catabolism, and immunity. *Journal of the International Society of Sports Nutrition* 4: 18.

Kreider, R.B., R. Klesges, K. Harmon, et al. 1996. Effects of ingesting supplements designed to promote lean tissue accretion on body composition during resistance training. *International Journal of Sport Nutrition* 6: 234-246.

Kreider, R.B., V. Miriel, and E. Bertun. 1993. Amino acid supplementation and exercise performance: Analysis of the proposed ergogenic value. *Sports Medicine* 16: 190-209.

Kreider, R., et al. 1998a. Effects of conjugated linoleic acid (CLA) supplementation during resistance training on bone mineral content, bone mineral density, and markers of immune stress. *FASEB Journal* 12: A244.

Kreider, R.B., et al. 1998b. Effects of creatine supplementation on body composition, strength, and sprint performance. *Medicine & Science in Sports & Exercise* 30: 73-82.

Kreider, R.B., et al. (Eds.). 1998c. *Overtraining in sport.* Champaign, IL: Human Kinetics.

Kreider, R.B., et al. 1999a. Effects of calcium b-hydroxy b-methylbutyrate (HMB) supplementation during resistance-training on markers of catabolism, body composition and strength. *International Journal of Sports Medicine* 22: 1-7.

Kreider, R.B., et al. 1999b. Effects of protein and amino-acid supplementation on athletic performance. *Sportscience* 3. Retrieved from http://sportscie.org/jour/9901/rbk.html.

Kreider, R.B., et al. 2000. Nutrition in exercise and sport. In T. Wilson and N. Temple (Eds.), *Frontiers in nutrition.* Totowa, NJ: Humana Press.

Kreider, R.B., et al. 2001. Bovine colostrum supplementation on training adaptations

I: Body composition. Abstract presented at Federation of American Societies for Experimental Biology (FASEB) meeting, Orlando, FL, March 31-April 4.

Kreider, R.B., et al. 2007. Effects of ingesting protein with various forms of carbohydrate following resistance-exercise on substrate availability and markers of anabolism, catabolism, and immunity. *Journal of the International Society of Sports Nutrition* 4: 18.

Krieder, R.B., et al. 2010. Research and recommendations. *Journal of the International Society of Sports Nutrition* 7: 7.

Krochmal, R., et al. 2004. Phytochemical assays of commercial botanical dietary supplements. *Evidence-Based Complementary and Alternative Medicine* 1: 305-313.

Laaksonen, R., et al. 1995. Ubiquinone supplementation and exercise capacity in trained young and older men. *European Journal of Applied Physiology* 72: 95-100.

Lamb, D.R., K.F. Rinehardt, R.L. Bartels, et al. 1990. Dietary carbohydrate and intensity of interval swim training. *The American Journal of Clinical Nutrition* 52: 1058-1063.

Lambert, C.P., M.G. Flynn, J.B. Boone, et al. 1991. Effects of carbohydrate feeding on multiple-bout resistance exercise. *Journal of Applied Sport Science Research* 5: 192-197.

Lambert, C.P., et al. 2004. Macronutrient considerations for the sport of bodybuilding. *Sports Medicine* 34: 317-327.

Lambert, M.I., et al. 1993. Failure of commercial oral amino acid supplements to increase serum growth hormone concentrations in male body-builders. *International Journal of Sport Nutrition* 3: 298-305.

Lands, L.C., et al. 1999. Effect of supplementation with cysteine donor on muscular performance. *Journal of Applied Physiology* 87: 1381-1385.

Lane, L. 1999, September 17. Nutritionist calls for tighter regulation of supplements. CNN.com News.

Langfort, J., et al. 1997. The effect of a low-carbohydrate diet on performance, hormonal and metabolic responses to a 30-s bout of supramaximal exercise. *European Journal of Applied Physiology and Occupational Physiology* 76: 128-133.

Layman, D.K. 2002. Role of leucine in protein metabolism during exercise and recovery. *Canadian Journal of Applied Physiology* 27: 646-663.

Lee, E.C., et al. 2010. Ergogenic effects of betaine supplementation on strength and power performance. *Journal of the International Society of Sports Nutrition* 7: 27

Lefavi, R.G., R.A. Anderson, R.E. Keith, et al. 1992. Efficacy of chromium supplementation in athletes: Emphasis on anabolism. *International Journal of Sport Nutrition* 2: 111-122.

Leiper, J.B., et al. 2000. Improved gastric emptying rate in humans of a unique glucose polymer with gel-forming properties. *Scandinavian Journal of Gastroenterology* 35: 1143-1149.

Lemon, P.W.R. 1991. Effect of exercise on protein requirements. *Journal of Sports Sciences* 9: 53-70.

Lemon, P.W.R. 1994, November 11-12. Dietary protein and amino acids. Presented at Nutritional Ergogenic Aids Conference sponsored by the Gatorade Sports Institute, Chicago.

Lemon, P.W.R. 2000. Beyond the zone: Protein needs of active individuals. *Journal of the American College of Nutrition* 19: 513S-521S.

Lemon, P.W.R., et al. 1992. Protein requirements and muscle mass/strength changes during intensive training in novice bodybuilders. *Journal of Applied Physiology* 73: 767-775.

Lemon, P.W., et al. 2002. The role of protein and amino acid supplements in the athlete's diet: Does type or timing of ingestion matter? *Current Sports Medicine Reports* 1: 214-221.

Li, J.J., et al. 2008. Anti-obesity effects of conjugated linoleic acid, docosahexaenoic acid, and eicosapentaenoic acid. *Molecular Nutrition & Food Research* 52: 631-645.

Liang, M.T., et al. 2005. Panax notoginseng supplementation enhances physical performance during endurance exercise. *Journal of Strength and Conditioning Research* 19: 108-114.

Liberti, L.E., et al. 1978. Evaluation of commercial ginseng products. *Journal of Pharmaceutical Sciences* 67: 1487-1489.

Liese, A.D., et al. 2005. Dietary glycemic index and glycemic load, carbohydrate and fiber intake, and measures of insulin sensitivity, secretion, and adiposity in the Insulin Resistance Atherosclerosis Study. *Diabetes Care* 12: 2832-2838.

Lim, S., H. Won, Y. Kim, M. Jang, K.R. Jyothi, Y. Kim, P. Dandona, J. Ha, and S.S. Kim, 2011. Antioxidant enzymes induced by repeated intake of excess energy in the form of high-fat, high-carbohydrate meals are not sufficient to block oxidative stress in healthy lean individuals. *British Journal of Nutrition* 106 (10): 1544-1551. doi: 10.1017/S0007114511002091.

Linde, K., et al. 2006, January 25. Echinacea for preventing and treating the common cold. *Cochrane Database of Systematic Reviews*: CD000530.

Little, J.P., et al. 2010. A practical model of low-volume high-intensity interval training induces mitochondrial biogenesis in human skeletal muscle: Potential mechanisms. *Journal of Physiology* 588: 1011-1022.

Loucks, A.B. 2007. Low energy availability in the marathon and other endurance sports. *Sports Medicine* 37: 348-352.

Louis-Sylvestre, J., et al. 2003. Highlighting the positive impact of increasing feeding frequency on metabolism and weight management. *Forum of Nutrition* 56: 126-128.

Lowe, B. 2000. Powerful products. *Nutritional Outlook* 3: 37-43.

Lowery, L., et al. 2006. Protein and overtraining: Potential applications for free-living athletes. *Journal of the International Society of Sports Nutrition* 3: 42-50.

Ludwig, D.S., et al. 2001. Relation between consumption of sugar-sweetened drinks and childhood obesity: A prospective, observational analysis. *Lancet* 357: 505-508.

Luhovyy, B.L., et al. 2007. Whey proteins in the regulation of food intake and satiety. *Journal of the American College of Nutrition* 26: 704S-712S.

Lukaski, H.C. 2000. Magnesium, zinc, and chromium nutriture and physical activity. *American Journal of Clinical Nutrition* 72 (Suppl. 2): 585S-593S.

Lukaszuk, J.M., et al. 2005. Effect of a defined lacto-ovo-vegetarian diet and oral creatine monohydrate supplementation on plasma creatine concentration. *Journal of Strength and Conditioning Research* 19: 735-740.

MacLean, D.B., and L.G. Luo. 2004. Increased ATP content/production in the hypothalamus may be a signal for energy-sensing of satiety: Studies of the anorectic mechanism of a plant steroidal glycoside. *Brain Research* 1020: 1-11.

Maki, K.C., et al. 2009. Green tea catechin consumption enhances exercise-induced abdominal fat loss in overweight and obese adults. *Journal of Nutrition* 139: 264-270.

Malm, C., et al. 1996. Supplementation with ubiquinone-10 causes cellular damage during intense exercise. *Acta Physiologica Scandinavica* 157: 511-512.

Manabe, I. 2011. Chronic inflammation links cardiovascular, metabolic and renal diseases. *Circulation Journal* 75: 2739-2748.

Manore, M.M. 2000a. Effect of physical activity on thiamine, riboflavin, and vitamin B-6 requirements. *American Journal of Clinical Nutrition* 72: 598S-606S.

Manore, M.M. 2000b. *Sports nutrition for health and performance.* Champaign, IL: Human Kinetics.

Manore, M.M., J. Thompson, and M. Russo. 1993. Diet and exercise strategies of a world-class bodybuilder. *International Journal of Sport Nutrition* 3: 76-86.

Manson, J.E., W.C. Willett, M.J. Stampfer, et al. 1994. Vegetable and fruit consumption and incidence of stroke in women. *Circulation* 89: 932.

Marette, A., et al. 2001. Prevention of skeletal muscle insulin resistance by dietary cod protein in high fat-fed rats. *American Journal of Physiology, Endocrinology, and Metabolism* 281: E62-E71.

Marquezi, M.L., et al. 2003. Effect of aspartate and asparagine supplementation on fatigue determinants in intense exercise. *International Journal of Sport Nutrition and Exercise Metabolism* 13: 65-75.

Matthan, N.R. 2007. Effect of soy protein from differently processed products on cardiovascular disease risk factors and vascular endothelial function in hypercholesterolemic subjects. *American Journal of Clinical Nutrition* 85: 960-966.

Maughan, R.J., and D.C. Poole. 1981. The effects of a glycogen-loading regimen on the capacity to perform anaerobic exercise. *European Journal of Applied Physiology* 46: 211-219.

Mazer, E. 1981, July. Biotin—The little known lifesaver. *Prevention*, 97-102.

McAfee, A.J., E.M. McSorley, G.J. Cuskelly, A.M. Fearon, B.W. Moss, J.A. Beattie, J.M. Wallace, M.P. Bonham, and J.J. Strain. 2011. Red meat from animals offered a grass diet increases plasma and platelet n-3 PUFA in healthy consumers. *British Journal of Nutrition* 105 (1): 80-89. doi: 10.1017/S0007114510003090.

McAnulty, S.R., et al. 2005. Effect of resistance exercise and carbohydrate ingestion on oxidative stress. *Free Radical Research* 39: 1219-1224.

McNaughton, L.R., et al. 1997. Neutralize acid to enhance performance. *Sportscience Training & Technology.* Retrieved from www.sportsci.org/traintech/buffer/lrm.htm.

McNulty, S.R., et al. 2005. Effect of alpha-tocopherol supplementation on plasma homocysteine and oxidative stress in highly trained athletes before and after exhaustive exercise. *The Journal of Nutritional Biochemistry* 16: 530-537.

Mendel, R.W., et al. 2005. Effects of creatine on thermoregulatory responses while exercising in the heat. *Nutrition* 21: 301-307.

Mero, A. 1999. Leucine supplementation and intensive training. *Sports Medicine* 27: 347-358.

Meydani, M., et al. 1993. Protective effect of vitamin E on exercise-induced oxidative damage in young and older adults. *American Journal of Physiology* 264 (5 Part 2): R992-998.

Miller, W.C., M.G. Niederpruem, J.P. Wallace, and A.K. Lindeman. 1994. Dietary fat, sugar, and fiber predict body fat content. *Journal of the American Dietetic Association* 94: 612-615.

Montain, S.N., et al. 2006. Exercise associated hyponatraemia: Quantitative analysis to understand the aetiology. *British Journal of Sports Medicine* 40: 98-106.

Morifuji, M., et al. 2005. Dietary whey protein downregulates fatty acid synthesis in the liver, but upregulates it in skeletal muscle of exercise-trained rats. *Nutrition* 21: 1052-1058.

Mosoni, L., et al. 2003. Type and timing of protein feeding to optimize anabolism. *Current Opinion in Clinical Nutrition and Metabolic Care* 6: 301-306.

Nagao, T., et al. 2005. Ingestion of a tea rich in catechins leads to a reduction in body fat and malondialdehyde-modified LDL in men. *American Journal of Clinical Nutrition* 81: 122-129.

National Cholesterol Education Program. 2006. *ATP III guidelines at-a-glance quick desk reference.* Washington, DC: USDHHS, Public Health Service, NIH, NHLBI.

National Research Council. 1989. *Diet and health: Implications for reducing chronic disease risk.* Washington, DC: National Academy Press.

National Research Council, Food and Nutrition Board. 1989. *Recommended dietary allowances* (10th ed.). Washington, DC: National Academy Press.

Nazar, K., et al. 1996. Phosphate supplementation prevents a decrease of triiodothyronine and increases resting metabolic rate during low energy diet. *Journal of Physiology and Pharmacology* 47: 373-383.

Nelson, G. 2001, September/October. American Heart Association calls for eating fish twice per week—What's a vegetarian to do? *Vegetarian Journal.* http://www.vrg.org/journal/vj2001sep/2001sepomega3.htm.

Nestle, M. 2012, June 19. Debunking the health claims of genetically modified foods. *The Atlantic Monthly.* http://www.theatlantic.com/health/archive/2012/06/debunking-the-health-claims-of-genetically-modified-foods/258665/.

The new diet pills: Fairly but not completely safe. 1996. *Harvard Heart Letter* 7: 1-2.

Newhouse, I.J., et al. 2000. The effects of magnesium supplementation on exercise performance. *Clinical Journal of Sport Medicine* 10: 195-200.

Neychev, V.K. 2005. The aphrodisiac herb Tribulus terrestris does not influence the androgen production in young men. *Journal of Ethnopharmacology* 101: 319-323.

Nicholas, C.W., et al. 1999. Carbohydrate-electrolyte ingestion during intermittent high-intensity running. *Medicine & Science in Sports & Exercise* 31: 1280-1286.

Nielsen, F.H., et al. 2004. A moderately high intake compared to a low intake of zinc depresses magnesium balance and alters indices of bone turnover in postmenopausal women. *European Journal of Clinical Nutrition* 58: 703-710.

Nissen, S., R. Sharp, M. Ray, et al. 1996. Effect of leucine metabolite beta-hydroxy betamethylbutyrate on muscle metabolism during resistance-exercise training. *Journal of Applied Physiology* 81: 2095-2104.

Noakes, M., et al. 2004. Meal replacements are as effective as structured weight-loss diets for treating obesity in adults with features of metabolic syndrome. *Journal of Nutrition* 134: 1894-1899.

Noakes, T.D., et al. 2005. Three independent biological mechanisms cause exercise-associated hyponatremia: Evidence from 2,135 weighed competitive athletic performances. *Proceedings of the National Academy of Sciences of the United States* 102: 18550-18550.

Norris LE, et al. 2009. Comparison of dietary conjugated linoleic acid with safflower oil on body composition in obese postmenopausal women with type 2 diabetes mellitus. *American Journal of Clinical Nutrition* 90: 468-476.

Oakley, G.P., M.J. Adams, and C.M. Dickinson. 1996. More folic acid for everyone, now. *Journal of Nutrition* 126: 751S-755S.

O'Connor, D.M., et al. 2003. The effects of beta-hydroxy-beta-methylbutyrate (HMB) and HMB/creatine supplementation on indices of health in highly trained athletes. *International Journal of Sport Nutrition and Exercise Metabolism* 13: 184-197.

Olney, J. 1996, December 29. Transcript from *60 Minutes*. New York: CBS.

Parcells, A.C., et al. 2004. Cordyceps Sinensis (CordyMax Cs-4) supplementation does not improve endurance exercise performance. *International Journal of Sport Nutrition and Exercise Metabolism* 14: 236-242.

Parker, A.G., et al. 2011. The effects of IQPLUS Focus on cognitive function, mood and endocrine response before and following acute exercise. *Journal of the International Society of Sports Nutrition* 8: 16.

Parrott, S. 1999, October 14. Herbs said harmful before surgery. AOL News.

Peake, J., et al. 2004. Neutrophil activation, antioxidant supplements and exercise-induced oxidative stress. *Exercise Immunology Review* 10: 129-141.

Peyrot des Gachons, C., et al. 2011. Unusual pungency from extra-virgin olive oil is attributable to restricted spatial expression of the receptor of oleocanthal. *The Journal of Neuroscience* 31: 999-1009.

Phillips, S.M. 2009. The role of milk- and soy-based protein in support of muscle protein synthesis and muscle protein accretion in young and elderly persons. *Journal of the American College of Nutrition* 28: 343-354.

Phillips, S.M., et al. 2005. Dietary protein to support anabolism with resistance exercise in young men. *Journal of the American College of Nutrition* 24: 134S-139S.

Phillips, S.M., et al. 2009. Effects on mixed muscle protein synthesis at ingestion. *Journal of Applied Physiology* 107: 987-992.

Pieralisi, G. 1991. Effects of standardized ginseng extract combined with dimethylaminoethanol bitartrate, vitamins, minerals, and trace elements on physical performance during exercise. *Clinical Therapeutics* 13: 373-382.

Pline, K.A., et al. 2005. The effect of creatine intake on renal function. *The Annals of Pharmacotherapy* 39: 1093-1096.

Plourde M, et al. 2008. Conjugated linoleic acids: Why the discrepancy between animal and human studies? *Nutrition Reviews* 66 (7): 415-421.

Poortmans, J.R., et al. 2000. Do regular high protein diets have potential health risks on kidney function in athletes? *International Journal of Sport Nutrition and Exercise Metabolism* 10: 28-38.

Ramel, A., et al. 2008. Beneficial effects of long-chain n-3 fatty acids included in an energy-restricted diet on insulin resistance in overweight and obese European young adults. *Diabetologia* 51: 1261-1268.

Rehrer, N.J. 2001. Fluid and electrolyte balance in ultra-endurance sport. *Sports Medicine* 31: 701-715.

Reilly, T. 1997. Energetics of high-intensity exercise (soccer) with particular reference to fatigue. *Journal of Sports Science* 15: 257-263.

Richards, J.B., et al. 2007. Higher serum vitamin D concentrations are associated with longer leukocyte telomere length in women. *American Journal of Clinical Nutrition* 86: 1420-1425.

Riserus, U., et al. 2001. Conjugated linoleic acid (CLA) reduced abdominal adipose tissue in obese middle-aged men with signs of the metabolic syndrome: A randomised controlled trial. *International Journal of Obesity and Related Metabolic Disorders* 25: 1129-1135.

Robergs, R.A. 1998. Glycerol hyperhydration to beat the heat? *Sportscience Training & Technology.* Retrieved from http://www.sportsci.org/traintech/glycerol/rar.htm.

Roberts, M.D., et al. 2011. Ingestion of a high-molecular-weight hydrothermally modified waxy maize starch alters metabolic responses to prolonged exercise in trained cyclists. *Nutrition* 27: 659-665.

Rolls, B.J., et al. 1988. The specificity of satiety: The influence of foods of different macronutrient content on the development of satiety. *Physiology and Behavior* 43: 145-153.

Rosse, A.R., et al. 2010. Effects of capsinoid ingestion on energy expenditure and lipid oxidation at rest and during exercise. *Nutrition & Metabolism* 7: 65.

Rowlands, D.S., et al. 2011. Effect of high-protein feeding on performance and nitrogen balance in female cyclists. *Medicine & Science in Sports & Exercise* 43: 44-53.

Roy, B.D., et al. 2002. The influence of post-exercise macronutrient intake on energy balance and protein metabolism in active females participating in endurance training. *International Journal of Sport Nutrition and Exercise Metabolism* 12: 172-188.

Roy, B.D., et al. 2005. Creatine monohydrate supplementation does not improve functional recovery after total knee arthroplasty. *Archives of Physical Medicine and Rehabilitation* 86: 1293-1298.

Sachan, D.S., et al. 2005. Decreasing oxidative stress with choline and carnitine in women. *Journal of the American College of Nutrition* 24: 172-176.

Sandsa, A.L., et al. 2009. Consumption of the slow-digesting waxy maize starch leads to blunted plasma glucose and insulin response but does not influence energy expenditure or appetite in humans. *Nutrition Research* 29: 383-390.

Sapone, A., et al. 2011. Divergence of gut permeability and mucosal immune gene expression in two gluten-associated conditions: celiac disease and gluten sensitivity. *BMC Medicine* 9: 23.

Sarubin, A. 2000. *The health professional's guide to popular dietary supplements.* Chicago: The American Dietetic Association, 184-188.

Saunders, M.J., et al. 2005. Effects of a carbohydrate/protein gel on exercise performance in male and female cyclists. *Journal of the International Society of Sports Nutrition* 2(1): 1-30.

Schabort, E.J., et al. 1999. The effect of a preexercise meal on time to fatigue during prolonged cycling exercise. *Medicine & Science in Sports & Exercise* 31: 464-471.

Schardt, D. 2006. Soyonara? *Nutrition Action Health Letter* 33(8): 1-7.

Schenk, S., et al. 2003. Different glycemic indexes of breakfast cereals are not due to glucose entry into blood but to glucose removal by tissue. *American Journal of Clinical Nutrition* 78: 742-748.

Schoenfeld, B. 2011. Does cardio after an overnight fast maximize fat loss? *Journal of the National Strength and Conditioning Association* 33(1): 23-25.

Schwalfenberg, G.K. 2012. The alkaline diet: Is there evidence that an alkaline pH diet benefits health? *Journal of Environmental and Public Health* 727630.

Seaton, T.B., S.L. Welle, M.K. Warenko, and R.G. Campbell. 1986. Thermic effect of medium and long chain triglycerides in man. *The American Journal of Clinical Nutrition* 44: 630-634.

Seidle, R., et al. 2000. A taurine and caffeine-containing drink stimulates cognitive performance and well-being. *Amino Acids* 19: 635-642.

Shaw, S.D., D. Brenner, M.L. Berger, D.O. Carpeter, C.S. Hong, and K. Kannan. 2006. PCBs, PCDD/Fs, and organochlorine pesticides in farmed Atlantic salmon from Maine, eastern Canada, and Norway, and wild salmon from Alaska. *Environmental Science & Technology* 40 (17): 5347-5354.

Shugarman, A.E. 1999. Trends in the sports nutrition industry. *Nutraceuticals World* 2: 56-59.

Simko, M.D., and J. Jarosz. 1990. Organic foods: Are they better? *Journal of the American Dietetic Association* 90: 367-370.

Singh, A., et al. 1994. Exercise-induced changes in immune function: Effects of zinc supplementation. *Journal of Applied Physiology* 76: 2298-2303.

Slavin, J.L. 1991. Assessing athletes' nutritional status. *The Physician and Sportsmedicine* 19: 79-94.

Smart waters. 2000. BevNet. Retrieved from www.bevnet.com/reviews/smartwater/index/asp.

Snitker, S., et al. 2009. Effects of novel capsinoid treatment on fatness and energy metabolism in humans: Possible pharmacogenetic implications. *American Journal of Clinical Nutrition* 89: 45-50.

Somer, E. 1996, May. Maximum energy: How to eat and exercise for it. *Working Woman*, 72-76.

Speechly, D.P., et al. 1999. Greater appetite control associated with an increased frequency of eating in lean males. *Appetite* 33: 285-297.

Spriet, L.L. 1995. Caffeine and performance. *International Journal of Sport Nutrition* 5: S84-S99.

Spriet, L.L., et al. 2004. Nutritional strategies to influence adaptations to training. *Journal of Sports Sciences* 22: 127-141.

St-Onge, M-P. 2005. Dietary fats, teas, dairy, and nuts: Potential functional foods for weight control. *American Journal of Clinical Nutrition* 81: 7-15.

St-Onge, M-P., and Bosarge, A. 2008. Weight-loss diet that includes consumption of medium-chain triacylglycerol oil leads to a greater rate of weight and fat mass loss than does olive oil. *American Journal of Clinical Nutrition* 87: 621-626.

St-Onge, M-P., et al. 2007. Supplementation with soy-protein-rich foods does not enhance weight loss. *Journal of the American Dietetic Association* 107: 500-505.

Stanko, R.T., et al. 1996. Inhibition of regain in body weight and fat with addition of 3-carbon compounds to the diet with hyperenergetic refeeding after weight reduction. *International Journal of Obesity Related Metabolic Disorders* 20: 925-930.

Steinmetz, K.A., et al. 1996. Vegetables, fruit, and cancer prevention: A review. *Journal of the American Dietetic Association* 96: 1027-1039.

Stephens, F.B., et al. 2006a. An acute increase in skeletal muscle carnitine content alters fuel metabolism in resting human skeletal muscle. *The Journal of Clinical Endocrinology & Metabolism* 91: 5013-5018.

Stephens, F.B., et al. 2006b. Insulin stimulates L-carnitine accumulation in human skeletal muscle. *The FASEB Journal* 20: 377-379.

Stephens, F.B., et al. 2007. Carbohydrate ingestion augments L-carnitine retention in humans. *Journal of Applied Physiology* 102: 1065-1070.

Stephens, F.B., et al. 2007a. New insights concerning the role of carnitine in the regulation of fuel metabolism in skeletal muscle. *Journal of Physiology* 581: 431-444.

Stephens, F.B., et al. 2007b. A threshold exists for the stimulatory effect of insulin on plasma L-carnitine clearance in humans. *American Journal of Physiology, Endocrinology and Metabolism* 292: E637-E641.

Stewart, A.M. 1999. Amino acids and athletic performance: A mini-conference in Oxford. *Sportscience Training & Technology.* Retrieved from www.sportsci.org/jour/9902/ams.html.

Stone, N. 1996. AHA medical/scientific statement on fish consumption, fish oil, lipids, and coronary heart disease. Retrieved from www.americanheart.org.

Stout, J.R., et al. 2008. Effects of 28 days of beta-alanine and creatine monohydrate supplementation on physical working capacity at neuromuscular fatigue threshold. Journal of the International Society of Sports Nutrition (5)21: 1550-2783.

Stout, J.R., et al. 2001. Effects of resistance exercise and creatine supplementation on myasthenia gravis: A case study. *Medicine & Science in Sports & Exercise* 33: 869-872.

Stuessi, C., et al. 2005. L -Carnitine and the recovery from exhaustive endurance exercise: A randomised, double-blind, placebo-controlled trial. *European Journal of Applied Physiology* 95: 431-435.

Szlyk, P.C., R.P. Francesconi, M.S. Rose, et al. 1991. Incidence of hypohydration when consuming carbohydrate-electrolyte solutions during field training. *Military Medicine* 156: 399-402.

Taku, K., et al. 2007. Soy isoflavones lower serum total and LDL cholesterol in humans: A meta-analysis of 11 randomized controlled trials. *American Journal of Clinical Nutrition* 85: 1148-1156.

Talanian, J.I., et al. 2007. Two weeks of high-intensity aerobic interval training increases the capacity for fat oxidation during exercise in women. *Journal of Applied Physiology* 102: 1439-1447.

Tarnopolsky, M.A. 1998. Influence of differing macronutrient intakes on muscle glycogen resynthesis after resistance training. *Journal of Applied Physiology* 84: 890-896.

Tarnopolsky, M.A., et al. 1992. Evaluation of protein requirements for trained strength athletes. *Journal of Applied Physiology* 73: 1986-1995.

Tarnopolsky, M.A., et al. 1997. Postexercise protein-carbohydrate supplements increase muscle glycogen in men and women. *Journal of Applied Physiology* 83: 1877-1883.

Thomas, D.E., et al. 1991. Carbohydrate feeding before exercise: Effect of glycemic index. *International Journal of Sports Medicine* 12: 180-186.

Thornton, J.S. 1990. How can you tell when an athlete is too thin? *The Physician and Sportsmedicine* 18: 124-133.

Tiidus, P.M., et al. 1995. Vitamin E status and response to exercise training. *Sports Medicine* 20: 12-23.

The triad. 2006. Retrieved from www.femaleathletetriad.org.

Trimmer, R., et al. 2005. Effects of two naturally occurring aromatase inhibitors on male hormonal and blood chemistry profiles. *Journal of the International Society of Sports Nutrition* 2: 14.

Trumbo, P., et al. 2001. Dietary reference intakes. *Journal of the American Dietetic Association* 101 (3): 294-301.

Tsang. G. 2006. Which sweeteners are safe? Retrieved from www.healthcastle.com/sweeteners.shtml.

Tullson, P.C., et al. 1991. Adenine nucleotide synthesis in exercising and endurance-trained skeletal muscle. *American Journal of Physiology* 261 (2 Part 1): C342-347.

Tyler, V.E. 1987. *The new honest herbal: A sensible guide to the use of herbs and related remedies.* Philadelphia: George F. Stickley Co.

U.S. Department of Agriculture. 1998, August 11. USDA urges consumers to use food thermometer when cooking ground beef patties. Washington, DC: USDA.

U.S. Department of Agriculture and U.S. Department of Health and Human Services. 1995. Nutrition and your health: Dietary guidelines for Americans. Washington, DC: Government Printing Office.

Van Someren, K.A., et al. 2005. Supplementation with beta-hydroxy-beta-methylbutyrate (HMB) and alpha-ketoisocaproic acid (KIC) reduces signs and symptoms of exercise-induced muscle damage in man. *International Journal of Sport Nutrition and Exercise Metabolism* 15: 413-424.

Van Zyl, C.G., et al. 1996. Effects of medium-chain triglyceride ingestion on fuel metabolism and cycling performance. *Journal of Applied Physiology* 80: 2217-2225.

Vanhatalo, A., et al. 2010. Acute and chronic effects of dietary nitrate supplementation on blood pressure and the physiological responses to moderate-intensity and incremental Exercise. *American Journal of Physiology—Regulatory, Integrative and Comparative Physiology* 299: R1121–R1131.

Viitala, P.E., et al. 2004a. The effects of antioxidant vitamin supplementation on resistance exercise induced lipid peroxidation in trained and untrained participants. *Lipids in Health and Disease* 3: 14.

Viitala, P.E., et al. 2004b. Vitamin E supplementation, exercise and lipid peroxidation in human participants. *European Journal of Applied Physiology* 93: 108-115.

Vitamin drink. 2000. *Nutritional Outlook* 3: 70.

Vitamin E pills: Now it's thumbs down. 2005. Consumer Reports. 70(7): 55.Volpe, S.L., et al. 2001. Effect of chromium supplementation and exercise on body composition, resting metabolic rate and selected biochemical parameters in moderately obese women following an exercise program. *Journal of the American College of Nutrition* 20: 293-306.

Wagner, D.R. 1999. Hyperhydrating with glycerol: Implications for athletic performance. *Journal of the American Dietetic Association* 99: 207-212.

Wagner, D.R., et al. 1992. Effects of oral ribose on muscle metabolism during bicycle ergometer exercise in AMPD-deficient patients. *Annals of Nutrition and Metabolism* 35: 297-302.

Wagner, J.C. 1991. Enhancement of athletic performance with drugs: An overview. *Sports Medicine* 12: 250-265.

Walberg, J.L., et al. 1988. Macronutrient content of a hypoenergy diet affects nitrogen retention and muscle function in weight lifters. *International Journal of Sports Medicine* 9: 261-266.

Walberg-Rankin, J.L. 1994, November 11-12. Ergogenic effects of carbohydrate intake during long- and short-term exercise. Presented at Nutritional Ergogenic Aids Conference sponsored by the Gatorade Sports Institute, Chicago.

Walberg-Rankin, J.L. 1995. Dietary carbohydrate as an ergogenic aid for prolonged and brief competitions in sport. *International Journal of Sport Nutrition* 5: S13-S28.

Walberg-Rankin, J.L., et al. 1994. The effect of oral arginine during energy restriction in male weight lifters. *Journal of Strength and Conditioning Research* 8: 170-177.

Wall, B.T., et al. 2011. Chronic oral ingestion of L-carnitine and carbohydrate increases muscle carnitine content and alters muscle fuel metabolism during exercise in humans. *Journal of Physiology* 589: 963-973.

Walton, R.G., R. Hudak, and R.J. Green-Waite. 1993. Adverse reactions to aspartame: Double-blind challenge in patients from a vulnerable population. *Biological Psychiatry* 34: 13-17.

Ward, R.J., et al. 1999. Changes in plasma taurine levels after different endurance events. *Amino Acids* 16 (1): 71-77.

Wardlaw, G.M., P.M. Insel, and M.F. Seyler. 1994. *Contemporary nutrition.* St. Louis: Mosby-Year Book, Inc.

Washington State Department of Agriculture. 1995. Organic food standards. Organic Food Program, Food Safety and Animal Health Division.

Watras, A.C., et al. 2007. The role of conjugated linoleic acid in reducing body fat and preventing holiday weight gain. *International Journal of Obesity* 31: 481-487.

Watson S. 2006. Diet pills: What you need to know. Retrieved from http://health.howstuffworks.com/diet-pill.htm.

Wein, D., et al. 2011. To eat or not to eat: the truth behind exercising on an empty stomach. *National Strength and Conditioning Association's Performance Training Journal* 10: 25-26.

Wesson, M., L. McNaughton, P. Davies, and S. Tristram. 1988. Effects of oral administration of aspartic acid salts on the endurance capacity of trained athletes. *Research Quarterly for Exercise and Sport* 59: 234-239.

Wilborn, C.D., et al. 2004a. Effects of methoxyisoflavone, ecdysterone, and sulfopolysaccharide (CSP3) supplementation during training on body composition and training adaptations. White paper from Exercise and Sport Nutrition Laboratory, Texas A&M University, Waco.

Wilborn, C.D., et al. 2004b. Effects of zinc magnesium aspartate (ZMA) supplementation on training adaptations and markers and anabolism and catabolism. *Journal of the International Society of Sports Nutrition* 1: 12-20.

Williams, C. 1995. Macronutrients and performance. *Journal of Sports Sciences* 13: S1- S10.

Williams, M.H. 2005. Dietary supplements and sports performance: Minerals. *Journal of the International Society of Sports Nutrition* 2: 43-49.

Williams, M.B., et al. 2003. Effects of recovery beverages on glycogen restoration and endurance exercise performance. *Journal of Strength and Conditioning Research* 17: 12-19.

Williams, M.H. 1989. Vitamin supplementation and athletic performance. *International Journal for Vitamin and Nutrition Research* (Suppl.) 30: 163-191.

Williams, M.H., et al. 1998. *The ergogenics edge.* Champaign, IL: Human Kinetics.

Williams, M.H., et al. 1999. *Creatine: The power supplement.* Champaign, IL: Human Kinetics.

Wilmore, J.H., and D.L. Costill. 1994. *Physiology of sport and exercise.* Champaign, IL: Human Kinetics, 392-395.

Winters, L.R., R.S. Yoon, H.J. Kalkwarf, J.C. Davies, et al. 1992. Riboflavin requirements and exercise adaption in older women. *The American Journal of Clinical Nutrition* 56: 526-532.

Wu, C-L., et al. 2010. Sodium bicarbonate supplementation prevents skilled tennis performance decline after a simulated match. *Nutrition* 7: 33.

Xu, Q., et al. 2009. Multivitamin use and telomere length in women. *American Journal of Clinical Nutrition* 89: 1857-1863.

Yaspelkis, B.B., et al. 1999. The effect of a carbohydrate-arginine supplement on postexercise carbohydrate metabolism. *International Journal of Sports Nutrition* 9: 241-250.

Yates, D. 2007, May 16. Soy estrogens and breast cancer: Research offers overview. News Bureau, University of Illinois. Retrieved from www.news.uiuc.edu/news/07/0516helferich.html.

Youl Kang, H., et al. 2002. Effects of ginseng ingestion on growth hormone, testosterone, cortisol, and insulin-like growth factor 1 responses to acute resistance exercise. *Journal of Strength and Conditioning Research* 16: 179-183.

Zawadzki, K.M., B.B. Yaselkis, and J.L. Ivy. 1992. Carbohydrate-protein complex increases the rate of muscle glycogen storage after exercise. *Journal of Applied Physiology* 72: 1854-1859.

Zhang, M., et al. 2004. Role of taurine supplementation to prevent exercise-induced oxidative stress in healthy young men. *Amino Acids* 26: 203-207.

Zhou, S., et al. 2005. Muscle and plasma coenzyme Q10 concentration, aerobic power and exercise economy of healthy men in response to four weeks of supplementation. *The Journal of Sports Medicine and Physical Fitness* 45: 337-346.

Ziegenfuss, T.N., et al. 2006. Safety and efficacy of a commercially available, naturally occurring aromatase inhibitor in healthy men. *Journal of the International Society of Sports Nutrition* 2: 28.

# Index

*Note:* The italicized *f* and *t* following page numbers refer to figures and tables, respectively.

## A

adaptogens 205
added sugar 58-59, 100, 224, 237-238, 247, 257
adenosine triphosphate (ATP) 4-5, 172-173, 192
aerobic exercise 23-25, 73-74, 236, 242
age, protein and 22-23
ALA. *See* alpha-linoleic acid
Alaska seafood 79*t*
alcohol 101-102, 122-124
Almond Peach shake 311
Alotta Onions Soup 325
alpha-linoleic acid (ALA) 77-78, 81
amino acids
  BCAA 27, 43-44, 182
  in protein 4, 27-28, 27*t*, 30, 36-37, 39-44, 72, 182, 193-194
  supplemental 27, 43-44, 182, 194-195, 197*t*
anabolic state 27-28, 67
anabolic steroids 50, 96, 163, 164*t*, 195, 201
androstenedione 163, 195, 197*t*
anemia 158
antifat diet strategies 97-102
anti-inflammatory botanicals 210-212
anti-inflammatory foods 240-241
anti-inflammatory recovery shakes 309-311
Antioxidant Advantage 306
antioxidants 61-62, 81-82, 85, 306
  inflammation and 134-135
  supplements and 130-138, 132*t*-134*t*
Apple Ginger Spinach Berry shake 309
Apple Pie à la Mode 308
arginine 43, 180, 197*t*
Ashley, Mike 96
Asparagus, Spinach, and Feta Omelet 317
ATP. *See* adenosine triphosphate

## B

Banana Beet Orange shake 310
banned substances 164, 165*t*
basal metabolic rate (BMR) 87
BCAAs. *See* branched-chain amino acids
B-complex vitamins 34, 38, 129, 138-145, 139*t*-140*t*, 197*t*
beef 35-36, 35*t*
bee pollen 195, 197*t*
beetroot juice 202-203, 203*t*, 215*t*
Benardot, Dan 97
benign prostatic hypertrophy (BPH) 209
beta-alanine 180-182, 197*t*
beta-carotene 132*t*, 135, 138, 146
beta-hydroxy-beta-methylbutyrate (HMB) 182, 197*t*
beverages
  to avoid 122
  sugar in 224

bioelectrical impedance analysis (BIA) 89
biological value (BV) 40
biotin 140*t*, 143-144
bloat 212
BMR. *See* basal metabolic rate
bodybuilders
  cheat day and 106
  competitive strategy of 96
  diet of 7-9
  female 8
  Power Eating plan adjusted for 228-229
body-composition testing 89
body dysmorphia 91-92
body-fat percentage 90-92
body weight, water and 121-122
Bone-Builder Smoothie 303
boron 151*t*, 161, 178
botanicals
  anti-inflammatory 210-212
  beetroot juice 202-203, 203*t*, 215*t*
  bloat and 212
  buchu 201, 215*t*
  burdock 206-207, 215*t*
  canaigre 207, 215*t*
  cayenne 204, 215*t*
  citrus aurantium 207, 215*t*
  coleus forskohlii 207, 215*t*
  cordyceps 207, 215*t*
  damiana 208, 215*t*
  that do not meet marketing claims 206-209
  echinacea 204, 215*t*
  ephedra 209, 215*t*
  flavonols 212
  fo-ti 201, 215*t*
  ginger 211
  ginseng 204-205, 215*t*
  gotu kola 208, 215*t*
  green tea 104-105, 206, 215*t*
  guarana 202, 215*t*
  hoodia 208-209, 215*t*
  maté 202, 215*t*
  that meet marketing claims 201-202
  mood-boosting 210
  pau d'arco 210, 215*t*
  that possibly meet marketing claims 202-206, 203*t*
  potentially harmful 209
  precautions 214
  rating of 215*t*
  safety of 199-201
  sassafras 210, 215*t*
  saw palmetto 209, 215*t*
  tribulus terrestris 209, 215*t*
  turmeric 211
  yohimbe 210, 215*t*

bovine colostrum  190
BPH. *See* benign prostatic hypertrophy
brain health  80, 145
branched-chain amino acids (BCAAs)  27, 43-44,
     182, 197*t*
bread  56*t*-57*t*, 59-60, 65*t*, 222
breakfast  101, 237, 312-317
Breakfast Parfait  313
Bucci, Luke  205
buchu  201, 215*t*
burdock  206-207, 215*t*
BV. *See* biological value

# C

caffeine  166-169, 197*t*, 202, 206, 268
calcium  8, 15, 149*t*, 154-157, 156*t*-157*t*
calories  6, 12, 225-226, 234-236
Campbell, Wayne W.  21
canaigre  207, 215*t*
cancer
     laetrile effect and  164-166
     phytochemicals and  61, 61*t*
     prevention  15, 17, 30, 33, 61-62, 61*t*, 69, 77-78,
          82, 111-112, 135, 142, 203
capsaicin  105, 204
capsinoid  105, 204
carbohydrate
     caffeine and  168
     creatine and  175-176
     dieting and  29, 88, 98-99, 237
     fat and  7, 11, 48, 51
     fiber and  7, 52-55, 53*t*-54*t*, 69
     fruit and  56*t*-57*t*, 60-63, 61*t*, 65*t*
     gels  177
     gluten and  71
     glycemic load of  55-58, 56*t*-57*t*, 67, 69, 100
     importance of  237-238
     intake of  49-50, 59-64, 227
     loading  70
     mental muscle and  72
     for muscle building  48-50
     nutrition principles  6-7, 67
     protein and  20-21, 29, 67-68, 88, 169-172,
          237, 267
     in recovery nutrition  66-70
     right types of  50-51, 237-238
     sources  64, 65*t*-66*t*
     strength training and  74
     sugar  58-59, 67, 100, 102, 224, 237-238, 247, 257
     supplements  49-50
     timed intake of  26, 64, 66-70
     vegetables and  56*t*-57*t*, 60-62, 61*t*, 65*t*
     for workouts  47-72, 53*t*-54*t*, 56*t*-57*t*, 61*t*, 65*t*-66*t*
carbohydrate–protein sport drinks  169-172,
     197*t*, 267
Caribbean Crush  307
carnitine  48, 182-184, 197*t*
casein  40-42
catechins  104-105
catecholamines  131

cayenne  204, 215*t*
cereal  56*t*-57*t*, 59-60, 65*t*, 224
cheating, on diet  106-107
Chicken in Orange Sauce With Pistachios  318
chili peppers  105
chloride  150*t*
chocolate  84-85
cholesterol  74, 78, 84
     HDL  59, 75, 76*t*, 77, 82, 159
     LDL  75, 76*t*, 77, 82
choline  140*t*, 144-145, 183
chondroitin sulfate  185-186, 197*t*
chromium  151*t*, 178
chromium picolinate  178
circumference measurements  89-90
citrus aurantium  207, 215*t*
CLA. *See* conjugated linoleic acid
coconut water  118
coenzyme Q10 (CoQ10)  134*t*, 137, 184, 197*t*
coleus forskohlii  207, 215*t*
colostrum  190
competition
     bodybuilders' strategy for  96
     body weight, water and  121-122
     liquid meal replacements for  298
conjugated linoleic acid (CLA)  184-185, 197*t*
copper  133*t*
CoQ10. *See* coenzyme Q10
cordyceps  207, 215*t*
CP. *See* creatine phosphate
crash dieting  87-88
creatine  172-176, 197*t*, 242
creatine phosphate (CP)  4-5, 172
cross-training, Power Eating plans for  265-278
cutting  226, 289-308

# D

dairy products  8, 14, 37, 45*t*, 84, 154-155
damiana  208, 215*t*
dark-meat poultry  34
dehydration  8, 111-114, 113*t*, 121
dehydroepiandrosterone (DHEA)  195, 197*t*
DHA. *See* docosahexaenoic acid
DHEA. *See* dehydroepiandrosterone
dietary reference intakes (DRIs)  6, 82, 131
diets
     analysis of  17
     antifat strategies  97-102
     bodybuilders'  7-9
     carbohydrate and  29, 88, 98-99, 237
     cheating during  106-107
     crash  87-88
     fad  88
     from heavy to light  237
     high-protein, low-carbohydrate  29, 88, 237
     leucine and  28
     sport supplements and  196
     varied  8-9
dimethylglycine (DMG)  196, 197*t*
disease prevention  111-112

diuretics 152, 160, 242
DMG. *See* dimethylglycine
docosahexaenoic acid (DHA) 14, 77-80
drinking schedule 114, 115*t*
drinks, power 300-311
DRIs. *See* dietary reference intakes
drugs
    banned 164, 165*t*
    NSAIDS 81, 85, 185

# E
Easy Energy Couscous 326
echinacea 204, 215*t*
eggs 11, 14, 37-38, 42, 84, 144, 190
eicosapentaenoic acid (EPA) 77-80
electrolytes 114, 117-122, 152, 176-178
electrolyzed water 117-118
endurance
    caffeine and 167
    protein and 23
energy bars 63-64
EPA. *See* eicosapentaenoic acid
ephedra 209, 215*t*
essential fats 77-82, 79*t*, 98
exercise
    aerobic 23-25, 73-74, 236, 242
    alcohol affecting 123-124
    antioxidant supplements and 137-138
    drinking schedule for 114, 115*t*
    fasting and 100-101
    fat burning and 73-74, 93-96
    protein functions in 24
    strength training 21-22, 73-74
    timing of 237

# F
fad diets 88
fast-food nutrition 230
fasting 100-101, 243
fat
    adaptation 265-266
    bodybuilders and 8
    carbohydrate and 7, 11, 48, 51
    chocolate and 84-85
    essential 77-82, 79*t*, 98
    facts 74-75, 76*t*
    in food 75-77
    as fuel 73-74
    high-performance 240
    intake recommendations 81-83, 227-228
    management of 73-85
    monounsaturated 76-77, 82, 98
    omega-3 14, 29-31, 33, 77-81, 79*t*, 98, 103
    omega-6 77-78, 80-81
    polyunsaturated 76-77, 82
    portions 223
    protein and 11, 20-21, 103
    saturated 76, 82-83
    substitutes and replacers 83
    trans 77, 84

fat burning 20-21, 48, 51, 80
    antifat diet strategies for 97-102
    cheating on diet and 106-107
    crash dieting and 87-88
    exercise and 73-74, 93-96
    food for 99-105
    goal 88-93
    water and 110
fatty acids 76
female athlete triad 90-91
female bodybuilders 8
fiber
    carbohydrate and 7, 52-55, 53*t*-54*t*, 69
    in power drinks 311
    sources 53*t*-54*t*, 81
filtration, water 115
fish
    nutrition information 79*t*
    oil supplements 78-81
    protein in 14, 29-34, 79*t*, 103
    recipes 319-323
    salmon 33-34, 33*t*, 79*t*
    tuna 31-32, 321-323
fitness water 117
Five-Minute Tuna Cakes 323
flavonoids 85
flavonols 85, 212
flaxseed 81
fluid restriction 8
fluoride 151*t*
folic acid 139*t*-140*t*, 142-143
food. *See also* plan, food
    anti-inflammatory 240-241
    combinations of 9
    fast 230
    for fat burning 99-105
    fat in 75-77
    functional 13, 213
    neurobiology of 1
    organic 16-17
    supplements compared with 62, 99, 162, 196
    timing of 9, 10*t*
fortified water 117
fo-ti 201, 215*t*
fractionated starch 68-69, 175
free radicals 131, 161
fruit 8, 224
    carbohydrate and 56*t*-57*t*, 60-63, 61*t*, 65*t*
    portions 222
Fruit 'n' Cheese 316
fuel
    fat as 73-74
    for muscle 4-5
    for workouts 47-72, 53*t*-54*t*, 56*t*-57*t*, 61*t*, 65*t*-66*t*
functional foods 13, 213

# G
Gainers Fuel 1000 178-179
gamma butyrolactone (GBL) 196, 197*t*

gastrointestinal health 81
GBL. *See* gamma butyrolactone
gels, carbohydrate 177
getting cut 226, 289-308
GH. *See* growth hormone
ginger 211
ginseng 204-205, 215*t*
glucosamine sulfate 185-186, 197*t*
glucose 5, 43, 47
glucose–electrolyte solutions 176-178, 197*t*
glutamine 186, 197*t*
gluten 71
glycemic load 55-58, 56*t*-57*t*, 67, 69, 100
glycerol 186-187, 197*t*
glycogen 5, 47, 67, 69, 89
glycolysis 5
glycolytic system 5
gotu kola 208, 215*t*
grade, beef 35-36
grains 56*t*-57*t*, 71, 224
    recipes 326-327
    refined 60
    sources of 65*t*
    whole 60, 69-70
green tea 104-105, 206, 215*t*
grocery shopping list 231
growth hormone (GH) 164, 170, 180, 201
guarana 202, 215*t*

**H**
Haff, Greg 177
HDL cholesterol. *See* high-density lipoprotein
healing 81
heat stress 113, 113*t*
heme iron 34, 38-39
hemoglobin 5, 157-159
herbal water 117
herbs 199. *See also* botanicals
high-density lipoprotein (HDL) cholesterol 59,
    75, 76*t*, 77, 82, 159
high-intensity interval training (HIIT) 20,
    94-95, 181, 229, 236
high-performance fat 240
high-protein, low-carbohydrate diets 29, 88,
    237
HIIT. *See* high-intensity interval training
HMB. *See* beta-hydroxy-beta-methylbutyrate
homocysteine 142
honey 68
hoodia 208-209, 215*t*
hydration 8, 64
    alcohol and 122-124
    dehydration and 8, 111-114, 113*t*, 121
    drinking schedule 114, 115*t*
    hyperhydration 121
    juice and 120-121, 224
    sport drinks and 10*t*, 49, 66*t*, 118-120, 169-
        172
    water and 17, 89, 109-122, 115*t*, 125
    for workouts 109-125

hyperhydration 121

**I**
illness prevention 111-112
Indian Breakfast Salad 312
inflammation 12, 80-81, 134-135, 210-212,
    240-241, 309-311
inosine 193, 197*t*
inositol 144
insoluble fiber 52
insulin 28, 41, 48, 52, 67, 72, 103, 170-171
International Olympic Committee (IOC) 164,
    165*t*
iodine 150*t*
Irene's Marinated Broccoli 324
iron
    absorption 34, 38-39
    heme 34, 38-39
    supplements 14-15, 39, 150*t*, 157-159
    women and 14, 158-159
isoleucine 43

**J**
Johnston, Carol 20
joint lubrication 111
juice 120-121, 224

**K**
ketosis 188
Kleiner's Easy Muscle-Building Formula 301
Kleiner's Essential Muscle-Building Formula for
    Men 300
Kleiner's Essential Muscle-Building Formula for
    Women 300
Kleiner's Muscle-Building Formula 301
Kleiner's Muscle Formula Plus 68, 302
Kleiner's Muscle Formula Plus Light 302

**L**
lactic acid 5, 153
lactose 41, 156
laetrile effect 164-166
LDL cholesterol. *See* low-density lipoprotein
lean meat 35-36, 35*t*, 83
legumes 66*t*
Lemon, Peter W. 26
Lemon-Lime Zinger Sport Drink 308
Lemon Sole With Mustard Sauce 320
leptin 103
leucine 27-28, 43-44, 191
lignin 81
linoleic acid 77
lipids 134*t*
liquid meal replacements 298
low-carbohydrate, high-protein diets 29, 88,
    237
low-density lipoprotein (LDL) cholesterol 75,
    76*t*, 77, 82
lycopene 62

# M

magnesium 150*t*, 160, 194, 197*t*
main courses, recipes for 318-323
maintenance, plans for 245-253
major minerals 149*t*-150*t*
manganese 134*t*
maté 202, 215*t*
maximal heart rate (MHR) 94-95
MCT oil. *See* medium-chain triglyceride oil
meals
    replacements for 298
    timing of 9, 10*t*, 237, 240
meat. *See also* fish
    lean 35-36, 35*t*, 83
    preparation 36, 84
    red 8, 34-36, 35*t*
Mediterranean Brussels Sprouts With Tuna 322
medium-chain triglyceride oil (MCT oil) 187-188, 197*t*
men
    body dysmorphia in 91-92
    endurance, protein and 23
    Kleiner's Essential Muscle-Building Formula for 300
    Power Eating plans for 250-253, 260-263, 274-278, 294-297
mental muscle 72
mental performance 111
menus. *See* Power Eating plans
mercury 30-31
metabolic rate 87-88, 93, 97, 104, 234-235
MFP factor 38
MHR. *See* maximal heart rate
milk 14, 105, 154-156, 156*t*, 221, 224
Milo of Crotona 11
minerals
    antioxidants 131, 133*t*-134*t*
    deficiencies 8
    major 149*t*-150*t*
    performance and 148-162, 149*t*-151*t*, 156*t*-157*t*
    supplements 14, 39, 129-162, 132*t*-134*t*, 149*t*-151*t*
    trace 150*t*-151*t*
Mocha Breakfast Smoothie 303
molybdenum 151*t*
monounsaturated fat 76-77, 82, 98
mood 28, 210
Morning Pick-Me-Up 307
multivitamin 14, 129-130, 160
muscle
    cramps 113-114
    fuel for 4-5
    maintained 93-94, 225-226
    mental 72
    protein for 11-12, 19-44, 27*t*, 45*t*, 98
    water and 111-112
muscle building
    calorie needs for 226
    carbohydrate for 48-50

    night eating and 243
    for power 3-4, 11-12
    Power Eating plans for 255-264
    protein and 20, 24
    sport supplements for 163-196, 164*t*-165*t*, 191*t*, 197*t*
myoglobin 5, 157

# N

N-acetylcysteine (NAC) 188, 197*t*
neurobiology, of food 1
niacin 139*t*, 141-142
night eating 243
nitrates 203, 203*t*
nitric oxide (NO) 180
nitrogen 21, 23
NO. *See* nitric oxide
nonsteroidal anti-inflammatory drugs (NSAIDS) 81, 85, 185
nutrients per food group serving 220, 220*t*
nutrition
    fast-food 230
    fish 79*t*
    for power 5-9, 10*t*
    principles, carbohydrate 6-7, 67
    recovery 66-70, 239
nuts 45*t*

# O

oleocanthal 81
olive oil 81, 104
omega-3 fatty acids 14, 29-31, 33, 77-81, 79*t*, 98, 103
omega-6 fatty acids 77-78, 80-81
Orange Cinnamon French Toast 315
organic food 16-17
overtraining 28
oxidative system 5
oxygen-enriched water 117

# P

Pan-Fried Cajun Catfish 319
pantothenic acid 140*t*, 143
pasta 59-60, 66*t*
pau d'arco 210, 215*t*
PC. *See* phosphatidylcholine
PDCAAS. *See* protein digestibility corrected amino acid score
Peach Melba Yogurt Pops 314
peak, planning 233-243
PER. *See* protein efficiency rating
performance
    antioxidant supplements and 138
    minerals and 148-162, 149*t*-151*t*, 156*t*-157*t*
    strength-training, protein and 21-22
pesticide contamination 30, 33, 201
phenylalanine 43
Phosphagain 178-179
phosphagen system 4-5
phosphate loading 153-154

phosphatidylcholine (PC) 145
phosphatidylserine (PS) 145, 189, 197*t*
phospholipids 74-75
phosphorus 149*t*
physique maintenance, menu plans for 245-253
Phytochemical Phenomenon II 304
phytochemicals 61-62, 61*t*, 304
Piña Colada Smoothie 306
Pineapple Cheese Danish 316
plan, food 9-10. *See also* Power Eating plans
plant sterols 196, 197*t*
polyunsaturated fat 76-77, 82
portions 34-35, 221-224
potassium 149*t*, 152
power
    drinks 300-308
    fuel for 4-5
    functional foods and 13
    muscle building for 3-4, 11-12
    nutrition principles for 5-9, 10*t*
    organic food and 16-17
    sports, caffeine and 167-168
    supplements and 13-14
Power Eating
    goal of 69
    introduction to 3-17
    for vegetarians 14-15, 17
Power Eating plans
    for bodybuilders 228-229
    cross-training 265-278
    development of 217-231
    for getting cut 226, 289-298
    grocery shopping list for 231
    for men 250-253, 260-263, 274-278, 294-297
    for muscle building 255-264
    nutrients per food group serving and 220, 220*t*
    overview of 217-218
    personalized 225-228
    for physique maintenance 245-253
    portions 221-224
    sticking to 229-230
    for weight gain 264
    for women 246-249, 256-259, 270-273, 290-293
Power Eating recipes
    anti-inflammatory recovery shakes 309-311
    breakfast 312-317
    fish 319-323
    grains 326-327
    main courses 318-323
    overview of 299
    power drinks 300-308
    vegetables 324-325
powerlifters 226, 242-243
prebiotic 70, 81, 104
probiotics 103-104
protein
    for aerobic exercise 23-25

age and 22-23
amino acids in 4, 27-28, 27*t*, 30, 36-37, 39-44, 72, 182, 193-194
bottom line on 42-43
carbohydrate and 20-21, 29, 67-68, 88, 169-172, 237, 267
cross-training and 266-268
endurance and 23
fat and 11, 20-21, 103
fish 14, 29-34, 79*t*, 103
functions, in exercise 24
individual requirements for 24-26, 226-227, 236
mood and 28
for muscle 11-12, 19-44, 27*t*, 45*t*, 98
portions 223
proper levels of 23-24
quality 39-40
red meat 8, 34-36, 35*t*
sleep and 28
sources 45*t*
soy 14, 28, 42, 45*t*, 61*t*, 190-191, 304
sport supplements 189-191, 191*t*, 197*t*, 267
strength and 11-12, 21-22
timed intake of 26-28, 27*t*
types 39-42
uncoupling 104
vegetarians and 36-39
whey 28, 40-41, 189-191
protein digestibility corrected amino acid score (PDCAAS) 40
protein efficiency rating (PER) 40
PS. *See* phosphatidylserine
pyridoxine 140*t*, 143
pyruvic acid 194, 197*t*

**Q**
quercetin 191, 197*t*

**R**
Raspberry Plum Basil shake 310
RDAs. *See* recommended dietary allowances
recipes. *See* Power Eating recipes
recommended dietary allowances (RDAs) 6
recovery nutrition 66-70, 239
red meat 8, 34-36, 35*t*
refined grains 60
resting metabolic rate (RMR) 87-88, 93, 97, 234-235
riboflavin 139*t*, 141
ribose 192, 197*t*
rice 59-60
Riley, Pat 72
RMR. *See* resting metabolic rate

**S**
salmon 33-34, 33*t*, 79*t*
sassafras 210, 215*t*
saturated fat 76, 82-83

saw palmetto  209, 215*t*
scales  89
Seashore Buckwheat  327
seeds  45*t*, 81
selenium  133*t*, 161-162
serotonin  28, 72
shopping list  231
skinfold measurements  89
sleep  28, 173
soda loading  153-154
sodium  118-122, 149*t*, 152, 241-242
sodium bicarbonate  153-154
soft drinks  125
soluble fiber  52
soy  14, 28, 42, 45*t*, 61*t*, 190-191, 304
Soyful Smoothie  304
sport drinks  10*t*, 49, 66*t*, 118-120, 169-172
sports, power  167-168
sport supplements
    amino acids  27, 43-44, 182, 194-195, 197*t*
    androstenedione  163, 195, 197*t*
    arginine  43, 180, 197*t*
    BCAAs  27, 43-44, 182, 197*t*
    bee pollen  195, 197*t*
    beta-alanine  180-182, 197*t*
    caffeine  166-169, 197*t*, 202, 206, 268
    carbohydrate–protein sport drinks  169-172,
        197*t*, 267
    carnitine  48, 182-184, 197*t*
    chondroitin sulfate  185-186, 197*t*
    CLA  184-185, 197*t*
    confusion of  164-166
    CoQ10  134*t*, 137, 184, 197*t*
    creatine  172-176, 197*t*, 242
    DHEA  195, 197*t*
    diet and  196
    DMG  196, 197*t*
    that do not meet marketing claims  193-194
    GBL  196, 197*t*
    glucosamine sulfate  185-186, 197*t*
    glucose–electrolyte solutions  176-178, 197*t*
    glutamine  186, 197*t*
    glycerol  186-187, 197*t*
    HMB  182, 197*t*
    inosine  193, 197*t*
    MCT oil  187-188, 197*t*
    that meet marketing claims  166-179
    for muscle building  163-196, 164*t*-165*t*, 191*t*,
        197*t*
    NAC  188, 197*t*
    plant sterols  196, 197*t*
    that possibly meet marketing claims  180-
        193, 191*t*
    potentially harmful  194-196
    protein  189-191, 191*t*, 197*t*, 267
    PS  145, 189, 197*t*
    pyruvic acid  194, 197*t*
    quercetin  191, 197*t*
    rating of  197*t*
    ribose  192, 197*t*

    taurine  193, 197*t*
    tryptophan  194, 197*t*
    weight-gain powders  178-179, 197*t*
    zinc–magnesium  194, 197*t*
starch  59-60, 66*t*, 68-69, 175, 222
steroid hormone  146
steroids, anabolic  50, 96, 163, 164*t*, 195
Stout, Jeff  181
strength
    crash diets and  87
    protein and  11-12, 21-22
    training  21-22, 73-74
    water and  111-112
strength trainers
    drinking schedule for  114, 115*t*
    nutrition principles for  5-9, 10*t*
    types of  3
    vitamin and mineral supplements for  129-
        162
sugar  58-59, 67, 100, 102, 224, 237-238, 247,
    257
sugar substitutes  102
supplements. *See also* botanicals; sport supple-
    ments
    antioxidants and  130-138, 132*t*-134*t*
    calcium  154-157
    capsinoid  105, 204
    carbohydrate  49-50
    choosing  130
    fish oil  78-81
    food compared with  62, 99, 162, 196
    importance of  127-128
    iron  14-15, 39, 150*t*, 157-159
    minerals  14, 39, 129-162, 132*t*-134*t*, 149*t*-
        151*t*
    omega-3  78-81
    power and  13-14
    prudent use of  241
    vitamins  14, 129-162, 132*t*
    zinc  14-15, 39, 133*t*, 159-160, 194, 197*t*

**T**
taurine  193, 197*t*
temperature regulation  110
testosterone  163
thiamin  138, 139*t*, 141
tomatoes  62
trace minerals  150*t*-151*t*
trans fat  77, 84
tribulus terrestris  209, 215*t*
triglycerides  59, 74, 76*t*
tryptophan  28, 41, 72, 107, 194, 197*t*
tuna  31-32, 321-323
Tuna Supreme  321
turmeric  211

**U**
ubiquinone. *See* coenzyme Q10
uncoupling proteins (UCP)  104

# V

valine 43
vanadium 151*t*, 161
variation, in diet 8-9
vegan 15, 17
vegetables 45*t*, 99-100, 224
  carbohydrate and 56*t*-57*t*, 60-62, 61*t*, 65*t*
  portions 221
  recipes for 324-325
vegetarians
  creatine and 173
  Power Eating for 14-15, 17
  protein and 36-39
  weight loss for 15
very-low density lipoproteins (VLDL) 78
vitamins
  A 81, 145-146, 148*t*
  antioxidants 132*t*
  B-complex 34, 38, 129, 138-145, 139*t*-140*t*, 197*t*
  C 38, 129-130, 132*t*, 135-136, 138
  D 81, 130, 146-147, 148*t*
  DRI 131
  E 81-82, 129-130, 132*t*, 136-138
  K 81, 147, 148*t*
  multivitamins 14, 129-130, 160
  supplements 14, 129-162, 132*t*
Vitargo 68-69, 175, 239
VLDL. *See* very-low density lipoproteins

# W

water
  body weight and 121-122
  coconut 118
  fat burning and 110
  filtration 115
  glycogen and 89
  hydration and 17, 89, 109-122, 115*t*, 125
  importance of 17, 109-112
  muscle and 111-112
  requirements 112-114
  retention 241-242
  sources 115-118

weight gain
  menu plans for 264
  powders for 178-179, 197*t*
weightlifters, peak for 242-243
weight loss. *See also* diets; fat burning
  calorie needs for 226
  goal, formula for 92-93
  protein supplements and 189-191
  for vegetarians 15
whey 28, 40-41, 189-191
whole grains 60, 69-70
women
  bodybuilders 8
  calcium and 155, 157
  endurance, protein and 23
  female athlete triad and 90-91
  iron and 14, 158-159
  Kleiner's Essential Muscle-Building Formula
    for 300
  Power Eating plans for 246-249, 256-259,
    270-273, 290-293
  zinc and 8, 14, 159
workouts
  carbohydrate fueling 47-72, 53*t*-54*t*, 56*t*-57*t*,
    61*t*, 65*t*-66*t*
  hydration for 109-125

# Y

yogurt 221, 224
yohimbe 210, 215*t*

# Z

Zesty Citrus Smoothie 305
zinc
  absorption 34, 38-39
  supplements 14-15, 39, 133*t*, 159-160, 194,
    197*t*
  women and 8, 14, 159
zinc–magnesium supplementation (ZMA) 194,
    197*t*

# About the Authors

Susan M. Kleiner, PhD, RD, FACN, CNS, FISSN, is the nutrition authority on eating for strength, and her Power Eating program has reshaped the lives of thousands. She is the owner of High Performance Nutrition, LLC, a consulting firm based in Mercer Island, Washington.

Dr. Kleiner has worked as a nutrition consultant to the Seattle Seahawks (including quarterback Matt Hasselbeck), the Seattle SuperSonics, the Miami Heat, the Cleveland Browns, the Cleveland Cavaliers, and the Repertory Project Dance Company. Among her many national and international championship clients are 2008 Olympic BMX bronze medalist, three-time mountain bike 4X world champion, and two-time national downhill champion, Jill Kintner; 2006 U.S. women's ice hockey Olympian Kelly Stephens; and 2004-2006 U.S. women's masters Olympic weightlifting world champion Trish Zuccotti.

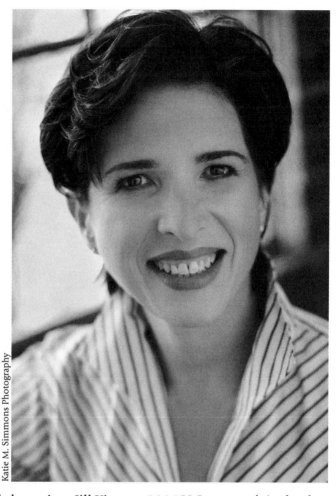

Katie M. Simmons Photography

Dr. Kleiner is an advisory board member for *Shape, FitnessRx for Women,* and *Oxygen* magazines. She is an internationally renowned author, speaker, and columnist. For her doctoral research on the cardiovascular disease risks of diet and anabolic steroid use in competitive male bodybuilders, Dr. Kleiner received a Young Investigator Award in 1987 from the American College of Nutrition. She is a fellow and cofounder of the International Society of Sports Nutrition and a fellow of the American College of Nutrition, as well as a member of the American College of Sports Medicine and the National Strength and Conditioning Association.

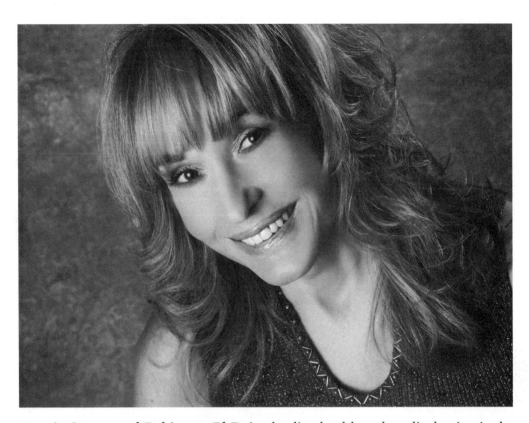

**Maggie Greenwood-Robinson, PhD,** is a leading health and medical writer in the United States. She has authored or coauthored more than 30 books on nutrition, exercise, weight loss, psychological health, and other health-related issues, among them *The Biggest Loser*, a *New York Times* best-seller that is the official diet and fitness book for NBC's hit reality show of the same name. Some of her most recent books are *20/20 Thinking*, *Good Carbs Vs. Bad Carbs*, and *Foods That Combat Cancer*. Greenwood-Robinson has appeared on numerous television and radio shows, including the *Dr. Phil Show* and NBC's *Dateline*. She has also written articles that have appeared in the magazines *Shape*, *Let's Live*, *Great Life*, *American Health*, *Physical*, *Muscle and Fitness*, and *MuscleMag International*. A frequent speaker on issues concerning health, anti-aging, nutrition, and exercise, Greenwood-Robinson is a member of the *Dr. Phil Show* advisory board and serves on the advisory board of *Physical* magazine.

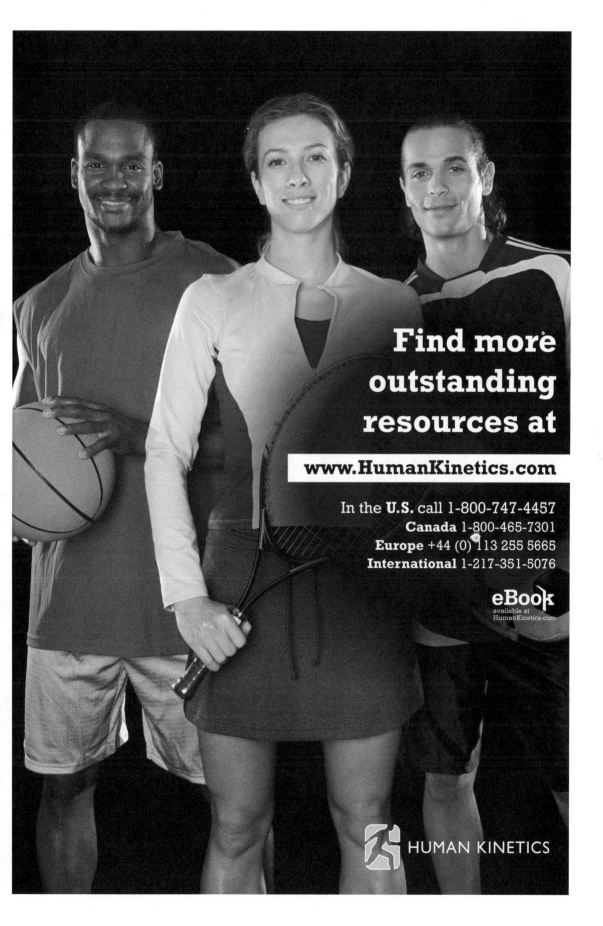